MW00680658

TABLE OF CONTENTS

About the Authors

Carol Rutenberg, RN-BC, C-TNP, MNSc, is a nationally recognized expert, speaker, and author in the field of telephone triage. She has been recognized as the foremost authority on telephone triage and scope of practice. Carol has hands-on experience, having been a telephone triage nurse in both the office and call center settings. President of Telephone Triage Consulting, Inc., she speaks and consults nationally and internationally, specializing in professional education, program design and implementation, and risk management in telephone nursing practice. Nationally certified in Telephone Nursing Practice and Ambulatory Care Nursing, she has served as an expert witness in litigation pertaining to telephone triage and ambulatory care nursing.

Carol has been published in several peer-reviewed nursing journals and is a member of the American Association of Ambulatory Care Nursing (AAACN), the Emergency Nurses Association, Sigma Theta Tau International, and the American Nurses Association. Carol is a volunteer leader in AAACN, having served that organization in numerous capacities including work groups for revision of the *Telehealth Nursing Practice Administration and Practice Standards* and development of Position Statements on the Nurse Licensure Compact and the Role of the RN in Ambulatory Care.

Carol received her BSN from Baylor University and a master's degree in nursing administration (MNSc) from the University of Arkansas for Medical Sciences College of Nursing in Little Rock. She lives in Hot Springs, Arkansas, with her husband, Howard.

M. Elizabeth Greenberg, RN-BC, C-TNP, PhD, is a nationally recognized leader in the field of telehealth nursing. A nurse for 29 years, she has extensive experience in telephone nursing practice, management, and research. For over 19 years Liz has practiced, studied, published, and presented in the field of telehealth and ambulatory care nursing. Specific practice experiences include telephone triage nursing in multi-specialty pediatric and OB/GYN ambulatory care clinics.

Liz is an Assistant Clinical Professor at Northern Arizona University School of Nursing. Liz began her career with an Associate Degree in Nursing Science. While working as a RN she progressed to a BSN and then on to a MS and in 2005 she earned her doctorate in nursing from The University of Arizona. Her thesis and dissertation research focused on telephone triage and the process of nursing care delivery over the telephone. She has numerous publications and presentations based on this research.

She is a member of the AAACN, the American Nurses Association, and Sigma Theta Tau International. Liz holds national certifications in Telephone Nursing Practice and Ambulatory Care Nursing and has served on the Editorial Board of the AAACN Newsletter, *Viewpoint,* and as a volunteer leader for the AAACN for several years. She and her husband, Jeff, currently reside in Tucson, Arizona.

ACKNOWLEDGMENTS/ DEDICATION

We understand that most people don't read acknowledgments. However, we're glad you are because we haven't gotten here by ourselves, and we have a great many people to thank and acknowledge who have helped us along the way.

We wish to dedicate this book to our parents, Cliff and Elaine, and Dick and Mitzie, who inspired us, expected us to think for ourselves, and assured us that we could do anything we set our minds to.

We owe an overwhelming debt of gratitude to our husbands, Howard and Jeff, who have been our editors, feeders, and supporters, in ways too numerous to count. A special thanks goes to Jeff for his gentle pushes, superior editing, and infinite patience.

We acknowledge the sacrifices of our children who have supported us in our careers, sometimes by being figuratively "motherless" as we each pursued our dreams and practiced our beloved nursing, a love we each share that is second only to our families. We are also grateful for their participation in the editing and design of this book.

We certainly acknowledge that we have each been blessed by unique experiences that have molded and directed us along our journeys and have brought us to this place. We are aware that the insights and passion that have made this book a reality were gifts from above, for which we are both humbly grateful.

Our reviewers, Suzi Wells, Traci Haynes, Tricia Chambers, Pete Dehnel, Anna Wahlberg, and other colleagues who looked at chapters along the way (Austin Evans, Marilyn Hudson, Margaret Verduin, Valerie Fong, Kathy Koehne, and Caroline Ellermann) were most gracious with their time and talents. Our colleagues who contributed to our Best Practices chapter were real troopers who helped bring the book to life by sharing their experience and expertise. We would especially like to thank our editor, Ken Thomas with Jannetti Publications, Inc., who has more patience than any one human should be blessed with (but we're glad he was). We want to acknowledge Jesika for holding down the fort while we concentrated on writing and editing. And last, but certainly not least, we would humbly like to thank the Board of Directors of the American Academy of Ambulatory Care Nursing for endorsing our book. We love AAACN, and you'll never know how much that recognition means to us.

We would also like to acknowledge the work done by nursing scholars and researchers in the United States and international community who have shared their knowledge, thereby validating much of the information contained in this book. Sheila Wheeler and Barton Schmitt, as pioneers and mentors, have contributed significantly to our knowledge and to the understanding of telephone triage that we have today. We also recognize our many friends and colleagues in AAACN who have accompanied us on this journey of growth and discovery.

But this book is also dedicated to the nurses and patients who have shared their unique experiences with us and have taught us about nursing over the telephone. Special recognition is offered by Liz to her nurse colleagues and mentors who participated in and supported her research to define the model of telephone nursing practice. Carol owes thanks to her seminar attendees and clients who have been the teachers and Carol the grateful student who has soaked up all they had to offer. These professionals have served as the petri dishes from which many of the concepts, stories, and insights in the book evolved. Without them, this book would certainly not have been possible. This book is truly the culmination of a dream that would have never come to fruition without each other. Finally, we would like to thank you, the reader, for picking up this book. We hope that you find it enriching and stimulating.

FOREWORD

The time has come and its time is now!

Those are the words that come to mind after reading *The Art and Science of Telephone Triage: How to Practice Nursing Over the Phone.* It has been almost 20 years since a book on the topic of telephone nursing practice has been written. This book not only supports the long-term fundamentals of telephone triage and nursing practice over the phone, but it also brings the reader up to date on current issues and trends in telephone triage. Because this book has great relevance for all ambulatory care nurses, *The Art and Science of Telephone Triage: How to Practice Nursing Over the Phone* is endorsed by the American Academy of Ambulatory Care Nursing.

The authors' collective expertise and years of experience in the field are evident chapter after chapter, as they address salient issues that impact the practice of telephone triage nursing. From the origin and evolution of telephone triage, through clinical practice and program design, the authors provide thorough discussion of the building blocks that support successful telephone triage programs, bringing the reader to the present with exemplars of best practices that exist today. The reader is also challenged to question the conventional wisdom on which a significant amount of policy and practice of telephone triage has been based over the years. As we know, examples strongly support learning. Throughout the book the authors include clinical vignettes to drive home points of discussion.

The Art and Science of Telephone Triage: How to Practice Nursing Over the Phone provides rich content to support both management and staff in telephone triage practice. The book therefore is a "must read" for each and every ambulatory care nurse leader working in clinical areas where telephone triage is performed. It is also a "must read" for each and every front-line registered nurse performing telephone triage.

One of the four key messages in the Institute of Medicine Report,[1] *The Future of Nursing*, encourages nurses to fully partner with physicians and other professionals as together we redesign health care in America. In the effort to better guide our nursing practice, there is no better opportunity to educate our colleagues, such as physicians and administrators, to the practice of telephone nursing than to have them read *The Art and Science of Telephone Triage: How to Practice Nursing Over the Phone.*

As the ending of any great book should be, the epilogue is both thought provoking and insightful. It leaves the reader to strongly consider the complex practice of telephone triage, the future of nursing in telephone triage, and nursing's professional responsibility to effect change.

The Art and Science of Telephone Triage: How to Practice Nursing Over the Phone is about our profession of nursing and the art and science of nursing practice over the phone, written *for nurses, by nurses!*

Suzanne Wells, MSN, RN
Manager, St. Louis Children's Hospital Answer Line
2012-2013 President, American Academy of Ambulatory Care Nursing

Reference

1. Institute of Medicine. (2010). *The future of nursing: Leading change, advancing health.* Washington, DC: The National Academies Press.

INTRODUCTION

This book is for anyone who plays a role in the provision of nursing care over the telephone. We will discuss how telephone triage is defined and how it evolved; we will share insights regarding critical elements necessary to support safe and effective delivery of nursing care over the telephone; and we address clinical practice, program design and implementation, risk management, and a variety of other topics.

Telephone nursing encompasses all care and services delivered using the telephone. However, in this book we will focus primarily on the practice of telephone triage, also commonly referred to as "nurse advice." This emphasis is important for four reasons.

The first is that telephone triage is a very complex, potentially ambiguous, and high-risk practice because the nurse is dealing with a patient with an unknown problem. Because this practice occurs over the telephone, the nurse is forced to make decisions with limited sensory input. In what other setting is a nurse required to perform a comprehensive assessment, make largely independent judgments, and advise patients regarding potentially life-threatening decisions without seeing or touching them? Provision of care over the telephone is like practicing nursing blindfolded with your hands tied behind your back.

Given that realization, it should not be difficult to see why telephone triage is one of the most sophisticated and potentially high-risk forms of nursing practiced today. Failure to recognize and appreciate the complexities of this practice has placed patients, nurses, and organizations at unnecessary risk.

The second reason to focus on telephone triage is that essentially all ambulatory care nurses (and many inpatient nurses) practice telephone triage, whether they recognize it as such or not. When a nurse is on the phone with a patient, regardless of the primary purpose of the call, the possibility always exists for any call to become a triage call when the patient presents the nurse with a new or unanticipated symptom. Whether a particular instance of telephone nursing is called disease management, post-op follow up, or simply reporting a test result, when the patient says, "While I have you on the phone, do you have time for one quick question?" the nurse has just stepped (or been drawn) into telephone triage. At that point, the nurse must abandon preconceived notions about the call and turn instead to a process of systematic assessment to determine the nature and urgency of the patient's problem.

In other words, every nurse/patient telephone encounter is potentially a telephone triage call. Telephone triage is simply nursing practiced over the telephone with patients for whom the diagnosis and plan of care are initially uncertain. The role of the telephone triage nurse is to assess the patient to determine the nature and urgency of his or her call and, in collaboration with the caller, develop and facilitate an appropriate plan of action.

The third reason to focus on telephone triage is that callers depend on nurses for safe and competent care. In fact, they often forsake their own instincts and defer to the advice of the nurse. Therefore, we must recognize that when we provide care over the telephone, we have an obligation to do it right. Given the lack of uniform understanding of this practice, study and discussion of this unique form of nursing are critical to providing safe and effective care over the telephone.

And finally, because of the emergence of telecommunications technologies and computerized decision support in telehealth and the limited financial and human resources of today's health care environment, the role of nursing has been called into question.[1] Therefore, we must establish what professional nurses have to offer over the phone that other, less-educated and less-expensive personnel do not.

THE PURPOSE OF THIS BOOK

In this book we explore many of the barriers and opportunities impacting the quality of patient care over the telephone. Based on current practice, nursing theory, research, and experience, we present a common-sense, reality-based approach to the practice of telephone triage and its application in a variety of clinical settings. Our goal is to provide a better, safer, and more professional approach to the practice of nursing over the telephone.

This book has been written for practicing nurses and those responsible for the development and administration of any telephone nursing services. We blend theory and practice to provide those involved in telephone triage with the knowledge and insight necessary to ensure that care is delivered in a manner that decreases organizational risk, minimizes nursing liability, and assures our patients that they will receive safe, effective care when they turn to us for advice over the telephone.

Due to the risks associated with this practice, it is essential that professional nurses providing care over the telephone be aware of the gravity of their actions. We believe there is no other form of nursing in any setting that requires more critical thinking and independent clinical judgment than telephone triage. Thus it requires RNs with experience and specialized training. We hope the information provided in this book will not only facilitate clinical and organizational knowledge and understanding but will also inspire the action necessary to support the optimal practice of telephone triage.

Throughout this book we examine and evaluate the existing, usually unwritten "rules" that currently guide the practice of telephone triage. Unfortunately, much of the conventional wisdom regarding the practice of telephone triage is not founded in fact. Many of the widely held beliefs do not facilitate care but instead interfere with our ability to provide safe, effective, patient-centered care over the telephone. We will separate the wheat from the chaff, defusing and debunking mistaken but widely held beliefs that interfere with nurses' ability to provide appropriate care. For example, we hope to put an end to the notion that, in the interest of cost savings or convenience, telephone triage can be relegated to personnel other than qualified registered nurses. By challenging many commonly held misconceptions that have molded the practice to date, we provide a blueprint for delivering safe, effective, and professional nursing care over the telephone. We ask that you shake off preconceived notions, immerse yourself in the ideas presented in this book, and be prepared to take a fresh look at telephone triage as professional nursing practice.

THE FINE PRINT

To provide a clinical perspective, patient scenarios are used to illustrate both proper and improper telephone triage. Many of these are based on actual lawsuits which illustrate the potential risk to the patient, the nurse, and the organization. Our intent is to demonstrate how telephone triage, done improperly, can result in devastating outcomes. These cases illustrate lessons learned, which we can use to improve care in the future. In the telling of these stories, we hope the overriding message is that bad things can and do happen and when they do, they happen to real people. While these stories represent actual lawsuits and are based on fact, details have been changed so that no confidential information has been disclosed.

We are not attorneys and thus do not endeavor to provide legal advice; our focus is patient care. For legal guidance, we encourage you to contact your personal or organizational attorney(s). The cases we present that represent real lawsuits have almost all been settled out of court, and thus no subsequent case law exists, nor are these cases identifiable in the general legal literature. Many of these cases didn't make it to court because the care given was indefensible due to errors in process or judgment. In other cases, good care was given, but the documentation was insufficient to defend it. We would further note, however, that often when bad outcomes occur, it is due to problems with the system rather than problems with the nurse. We will address multiple system, process, and judgment safeguards throughout the course of the book.

AUTHORS' NOTE

While we realize that many people interested in the practice of telephone triage (administrators, physicians, ancillary personnel, and even patients themselves) may read this book, it was written by nurses for nurses, and thus the "we" used throughout this book refers to those of us in the nursing profession. However, we are confident that non-nurse readers will also find the book stimulating and valuable.

Finally, as you will see in the pages of this book, telephone triage is our passion. We believe that no other area of nursing practice currently holds more potential to positively affect the lives of our patients. The time is right. Never have we been given a clearer path to follow to impact the health of our society in such a positive way. Thank you for joining us on this journey.

Reference

1. National Council of State Boards of Nursing. (1997). *Position paper on telenursing: A challenge to regulation.* Retrieved from https://www.ncsbn.org/TelenursingPaper.pdf

Chapter 1

Telephone Triage as a Vehicle for Nursing Care in the 21st Century

NURSING FOR THE NEW MILLENNIUM

In today's health care environment, strong societal, financial, and ideological forces are working, sometimes together and sometimes in conflict, to mold health care needs and delivery systems and to influence reimbursement practices.[1] These forces have provided both the impetus and the imperative for the evolution of health care in our society and for an emphasis on telephone triage in the 21st century.

Telephone triage in the United States has reached a defining moment in history. There are those who believe telephone triage is optional, or that if they ignore it, it will go away. However, the indisputable fact is that it is here to stay! Not doing triage is no longer an option. We can do it wrong, but we can't *not* do it.

Highly significant transformations have occurred simultaneously in the health care industry and in the nursing profession in general. Each has evolved separately, but they have converged in a manner that makes them inseparable. Together they underscore the value of telephone triage and assure that it will endure as an important component of health care delivery. These transformations are redefining the nature of patient care in a way that will forever change how nurses and patients interact in the future. Although in the past, telephone triage has largely been considered the domain of nurses who worked in call centers or organizations with formalized telephone triage programs, this practice can no longer be the concern of nurses in only such select settings. Telephone triage is currently taking place in primary care settings and indeed anywhere nurses talk to patients on the telephone, and the future promises even greater prevalence of this practice. The time has come that we recognize the pervasive nature and potential of telephone triage.

The average age of the population is increasing with the aging of the baby boomers. With advances in health care, a longer life span is expected but the result is that more people are living with chronic illnesses that require ongoing care.[2,3] The associated increase in health care demand is occurring at a time when resources are shrinking for both the health care industry and the health care consumer. A shortage of nurses and physicians is looming large, and the imperative has never been clearer that we must learn to do more with less.[4] More specifically, we must provide more services for more patients with less financial and human resources at our disposal.

This need, coupled with expanding technology, a multitude of sophisticated, high-risk procedures that were once performed only in the hospital, are now performed in the outpatient setting. Additionally, patients whose conditions do require hospitalization are being discharged earlier. In years past, many of today's discharged patients would have been considered too sick to go home. Home health nurses have played a significant role in providing care to these convalescing patients and a primary goal of their services is to prevent acute care rehospitalizations. Whether eligible for home health services or not, those still fragile patients, as well as many others, are looking to their primary care and specialty physicians to manage their care outside the hospital.[5] In this environment, telephone triage has been increasingly recognized and valued as an economical, efficient, and effective method of care delivery.

TELEPHONE TRIAGE IS HERE AND IT'S HERE TO STAY

In the first few years of this century, a confluence of major world events increased the visibility of telephone triage and brought it to life in a way that assures it can no longer be ignored.

First, the increasing occurrence of natural and man-made disasters potentially prevent the provision of care in the face-to-face setting. For example, incidents such as the bombing of the World Trade Center in 2001 and hurricane Katrina, which devastated the Gulf Coast in 2005, created a need for patients to receive care over distance because access to their health care providers was physically impossible.

Second was the worldwide financial crisis which began in 2007 and almost crippled the domestic and worldwide economy. The economic downturn devastated many Americans who lost their jobs and their homes and were fighting to put groceries on the table. The impact on health care spending and practices has been significant. Consumers with limited resources have stopped going to the doctor unless absolutely necessary. Elective surgeries have been cancelled, routine care has been postponed, and when patients did seek health care, it was often in the face of advanced disease. In this environment, the need for professional guidance from the telephone triage nurse is all the greater.

Finally, the global impact of new and emerging infectious diseases, such as severe acute respiratory syndrome (SARS) and the pandemic influenza, presented unique opportunities for telephone triage. The relatively unfamiliar concept of social distancing was reintroduced, and telephone triage nurses provided care to the sick and the worried well while serving an invaluable role in the health education of the public. The value of telephone triage as a public health strategy was legitimized when, in response to the H1N1 pandemic and in preparation for other emergencies, the Centers for Disease Control and Prevention (CDC) and the Department of Health and Human Services advised telephone assessment of symptomatic individuals and treatment over the telephone when indicated.[6,7] The role of telephone triage was indelibly etched on the public health landscape by development and dissemination in 2009 of a CDC publication, *Coordinating Call Centers for Pandemic Influenza and Other Public Health Emergencies,* in which medical call centers and telephone triage played a prominent role.[8] As of this writing, CDC is exploring, with its partners, the possibility of establishing a coordinated network of nurse triage lines in the event of another severe pandemic (L. Koonin, Personal Communication, January 15, 2012).

In concert with the emergence of the complex health care challenges associated with these events, the needs and expectations of health care consumers in our society have skyrocketed. Increasing the impact of these trends and forces is the rapid growth in telecommunications technology coupled with the demand for instant gratification characteristic of the information age. Thus a "perfect storm" has been created to sustain and to vastly increase the provision of patient care over the telephone.[9]

AMBULATORY CARE NURSING

Simultaneously, largely due to the same societal influences, nursing has undergone a significant transformation as well. Ambulatory care nurses compose at least a quarter of the nursing workforce and this number is likely to rise because the ambulatory care setting is where the patients (and thus the needs) will be.[10] For RNs in ambulatory care, the Bureau of Labor Statistics projects a growth rate of 48% between 2008 and 2018.[10] "Ambulatory nurse-patient encounters take place in health care facilities, in telehealth service situations…as well as in community-based settings, including outpatient office systems, private medical offices, freestanding clinics, schools, workplaces, or homes" (p. 267).[11] Nurses are increasingly assuming new responsibilities in managing complex patients in the ambulatory care setting.

Nursing has not only been physically repositioned; it has also been philosophically realigned. In the traditional inpatient setting, nurses provide and coordinate services in a relatively controlled environment. Ambulatory care nurses on the other hand are, with increasing frequency, assuming the role of patient care coordinator.[11] An integral function of the ambulatory care nurse is helping patients accurately identify their own health care needs, understand the significance of them, and determine what to do about them. Despite the recent emphasis on developing educated health care consumers, self-care management capabilities of the average patient are decreasing.[2] The role of the nurse in supporting the patient in this care is growing, and the nurse has assumed a more autonomous role in the management of ambulatory care patients. In addition to the traditional role of the nurse, new opportunities for patient coaching, collaboration, teaching, support, and various other non-technical functions have emerged. While the nurse doesn't directly provide all facets of patient care, the nurse's role in the coordination of care and patient advocacy has taken on new significance. Today's health care consumers need an advocate now more than ever to help them manage their care and to navigate the complex, convoluted, and sometimes broken health care milieu.

Telephone triage

- ***An interactive process between the nurse and client that occurs over the telephone and involves identifying the nature and urgency of client health care needs and determining the appropriate disposition.***

Telephone nursing

- ***All care and services within the scope of nursing practice that are delivered over the telephone.***

Telehealth nursing

- ***The delivery, management, and coordination of care and services provided via telecommunication technology within the domain of nursing.***

Telehealth

- ***The delivery, management, and coordination of care and services that integrate electronic information and telecommunication technologies to increase access, improve outcomes, and contain or reduce costs of health care. An umbrella term used to describe the wide range of services delivered across distances by all health-related disciplines.*** (p. 8)[12]

Nurse-patient telehealth encounters are an integral part of ambulatory care nursing.[11] Patients with increasingly complex problems are looking to the telephone triage nurse to help them make important health care decisions regarding the nature and urgency of their problem and for sound advice regarding access to care and/or appropriate self-care measures. Because of the omnipresence and convenience of telecommunications technology, the nurse is only a phone call away.

TELEPHONE TRIAGE AS A SPECIALIZED SKILL SET

The importance of telephone triage as a method to deliver nursing care and coordinate the patient's health care needs has grown by leaps and bounds. Patients have become accustomed to reaching professional nurses by telephone, often 24 hours a day, and nurse consultation and advice has become a mainstay for many American health care consumers. Due to the increasing visibility of this practice, a question has arisen regarding whether telephone triage is a specialty, a subspecialty, or a specialized skill set that nurses must acquire.

Some telephone triage nurses have specialized training and experience, and have focused specifically on this area of nursing. However, we believe that competency in telephone triage should be required by all nurses who interact with patients over the telephone. Also, because of the ubiquitous nature of telephone triage, all nurses should have some understanding of the practice of nursing over the telephone.

In years past, medical call centers dominated the telephone triage landscape, contributing to the perception of telehealth nursing as a specialty. Nurses employed in such formal settings developed an identity as "telephone triage nurses" (or other renditions thereof) and have fought to maintain that identity. Experts recognized and documented the significance of this practice area.[13,14] Professional organizations such as the American Academy of Ambulatory Care Nursing (AAACN) developed standards, continuing education programs, and a special interest group (SIG) specific to the practice of telehealth nursing.[15,16] Businesses also began to offer conferences and other continuing education opportunities specific to telephone triage. In 2001, in response to a growing cache of nurses who identified themselves as "telephone triage nurses," a national certification exam was developed and marketed to nurses engaged in Telephone Nursing Practice (TNP). Nurses who attained this certification earned the credential of RNC-TNP and were identified as experts, signifying mastery of telephone triage knowledge.[17] The addition of a certification promoted the perception of telephone triage as a specialty in nursing.

Telephone triage does require a specialized skill set which is best acquired through formalized training that is usually provided to nurses in these specialty settings. But nurses outside of the formal call center setting recognized they too were doing telephone triage, and interest began to spread. In all, over 1,200 nurses were nationally certified in TNP, not all of whom were employed in call centers (B. Grossklags, personal communication, August 16, 2011).

As this practice has garnered more attention, there has been a growing realization that telephone triage is not restricted to call centers. It is also clear that nurses from a wide variety of settings are indeed practicing telephone triage, although it is often not recognized as such. These practice settings include clinics, home health agencies, urgent care centers, correctional facilities, group homes, student health centers, emergency departments, and virtually any setting in which patients can access a nurse by telephone. In fact, it is not uncommon for patients who have recently been discharged from the hospital to get home and call their inpatient nurse for advice in the days immediately following discharge.

In 2007, the TNP certification exam was discontinued. About the same time, the AAACN began a process designed to determine the role of telehealth nursing (which includes telephone triage; see definitions earlier in this chapter) in ambulatory care. The AAACN subsequently adopted the position that telehealth nursing, instead of being a practice that is separate and apart, is an integral element of ambulatory care nursing.[18] While maintaining the Telehealth Nursing Practice SIG as a discreet entity, the AAACN decided to support efforts to incorporate telehealth nursing practice more fully into the ambulatory care nursing arena. They recognized that essentially all ambulatory care nurses may be called upon to practice various forms of telehealth nursing. Likewise, there was recognition that to be effective in the practice of telehealth nursing, a nurse must have a broad base of knowledge in ambulatory care. As a result of this position, the AAACN worked with the American Nurses Credentialing Center, an arm of the American Nurses Association, to increase the presence of telehealth nursing content in the Ambulatory Care Nursing Certification Exam (RN-BC). To date, certification in ambulatory care nursing indicates mastery of the body of knowledge related to both ambulatory care and telehealth nursing.

The Progression of Telephone Triage as Nursing Practice

To illustrate the significance of this progression, a parallel may be drawn from a more traditional patient care setting by considering for a moment the evolution of coronary care nursing. In the 1960s, EKG and basic arrhythmia recognition were not routinely included in undergraduate nursing education. Nurses who were able to perform these tasks received specialized continuing education and were regarded as an elite group.[19] Generally speaking, only nurses in coronary care units (CCUs) and intensive care units (ICUs) were able to read cardiac monitors and interpret rhythm strips.[20] In fact, it was conceivable a nurse with only a basic nursing education could fail to recognize a potentially lethal arrhythmia, such as ventricular tachycardia, or to grasp its significance. As nursing evolved, however, arrhythmia recognition was incorporated into basic nursing education and now even new graduates are able to recognize and understand the implications of potentially life-threatening arrhythmias. Instead of being limited to critical care units, cardiac monitors are now frequently found in inpatient settings and are often present in ambulatory care as well.[21] Many skills once regarded as being only within the domain of the critical care nurse are now a basic standard of nursing practice. What was once a specialty skill is now an integrated element of professional nursing.[22] In fact, yesterday's CCU patient is now often cared for on medical-surgical units or even at home. It is clear the requisite knowledge and skill required to be an RN in many settings has evolved to encompass areas of practice previously reserved for specialty nurses. As a side note of significance, in the early days of coronary care units, it was not uncommon for LPNs/LVNs to work in that setting, taking primary patient assignments. Today, due to the complexity of the practice, only RNs are employed to work in most CCUs.

A comparison of the progression of coronary care nursing and telephone triage nursing is provided in Table 1. The parallels between telephone triage and coronary care nursing are clear. And the significance of this similarity goes beyond interpretation of rhythm strips. CCUs and ICUs were the first settings in which nurses functioned autonomously in a collaborative environment under the guidance of standing orders or protocols developed for their patient population. In telephone triage, nurses are also functioning collaboratively but autonomously in the care of their patients, guided by clinical judgment and decision support tools. This analogy illustrates that historically, much of the content of what was at one time considered a specialty because of its novelty and complexity has now been integrated into the basic knowledge base and practice of nursing. And just as in the CCUs, telephone triage is being increasingly recognized as a practice that requires the skills and judgment of RNs. However, while it was once possible to maintain the discreet boundaries of coronary care nursing practice, such is not the case with telephone triage because of the ubiquitous nature of the telephone, the diversity of the patient population, and the multitude of settings in which it is performed.

SUMMARY

In summary, there is no doubt that telephone triage requires a specialized skill set not presently provided in basic nursing education. Just as a nurse would not be permitted to work in a coronary care setting

Table 1.
Comparison of the Progression of Coronary Care and Telephone Triage Nursing

	Coronary Care Nursing	Telephone Triage Nursing
Pre-Formalization		
Locus of care	Medical-Surgical unit or ICU	Multiple clinical settings
Staffing	Variable: RNs, LPNs, NAs	Variable: RNs, LPNs, clerical and medical assistants
Practice Standards	Nonexistent	Unrecognized practice, not applicable (N/A)
Special education	None or on-the-job training (OJT)	N/A
Professional organization	None	N/A
Professional identity	None	N/A
Formalization		
Locus of care	Coronary care units	Development of call centers
Staffing	RNs and LPNs	RNs
Protocols	ACLS and standing orders	Paper and computerized
Specialty Standards	Defined	Defined but variable
Special education	Continuing education only	Continuing education and OJT
Professional organization	American Association of Critical Care Nurses (AACN)	AAACN
Professional identity	Recognized specialty open to qualified RNs. Certification available (CCRN)	Recognized specialty open to qualified RNs. Certification available (RNC-TNP)
Integration		**(Predicted)**
Locus of care	CCU and other inpatient units	Primarily ambulatory care and call centers
Staffing	RNs only	RNs only
Protocols	Universally adopted	Universally adopted
Specialty Standards	Defined and integrated	Defined and integrated
Education	Basic curriculum, ACLS, and CE	Basic curriculum and CE
Professional organization	AACN and others	AAACN and others
Professional identity	Recognized specialty open to qualified RNs. Certification available	Recognized practice

without the requisite training, neither should a nurse be permitted to perform telephone triage without receiving specialized education and training. Regardless of whether the nurse practices in a formal call center or in a more informal setting such as a clinic or home health agency, it is essential that he or she be adequately prepared. Furthermore, practice must be based on sound principles of nursing because, done right, telephone triage is an effective means of patient management; but telephone triage done wrong can lead to tragic outcomes. Patients should be able to rely on the nursing advice they receive over the telephone as being of high quality and meeting the basic standards of care regardless of the nurse or the practice setting.

When a patient calls a nurse, he is depending on that nurse to provide:

- An adequate patient assessment.
- An accurate diagnosis of the nature and urgency of the patient's problem and related needs.
- Individualized goals and outcomes.
- A collaborative plan of care that considers the patient's special circumstances and preferences.
- Continuity of care to assure that the plan is implemented.
- A mechanism to evaluate the effectiveness of that care.

Anything less than these basic standards falls short of the nurse's obligation to ensure that patients receive care that is both safe and effective. Telephone triage is a sophisticated nursing practice requiring a specialized skill set. Nurses who use the telephone must have the necessary skills so that when patients turn to them for help, they will receive competent care that is individualized to their particular situation and needs. Thus all nurses, unless working in a setting that is devoid of telephones, need a thorough understanding of the practice of telephone triage – nursing for the new millennium.

References

1. Bernstein, A.B., Hing, E., Moss, A.J., Allen, K.F., Siller, A.B., & Tiggle, R.B. (2003). *Health care in America: Trends in utilization.* Hyattsville, MD: National Center for Health Statistics. Retrieved from http://www.cdc.gov/nchs/data/misc/healthcare.pdf
2. Thorpe, K.E., Ogden, L.L., & Galactionova, K. (2010). Chronic conditions account for rise in Medicare spending from 1987 to 2006. *Health Affairs, 29*(4) 718-724. doi:10.1377/hlthaff.2009.0474
3. World Health Organization (2005). *Preventing chronic diseases: A vital investment: WHO global report.* Retrieved from http://www.who.int/chp/chronic_disease_report/full_report.pdf
4. Alliance for Health Reform. (2011). *Health care workforce: Future supply vs demand.* Retreived from http://www.allhealth.org/publications/Medicare/Health_Care_Workforce_104.pdf
5. Cherry, D., Lucas, C., & Decker, S.L. (2010). Population aging and the use of office-based physician services. *NCHS Data Brief, no. 41.* Hyattsville, MD: National Center for Health Statistics. Retrieved http://www.cdc.gov/nchs/data/databriefs/db41.htm
6. Bogdan, G.M., Scherger, D.L., Brady, S., Keller, D., Seroka, A.M., ... Gabow, P.A. (2004). *Health emergency assistance line and triage hub (HEALTH) model.* Prepared by Denver Health – Rocky Mountain Poison and Drug Center under Contract No. 290-0014. AHRQ Publication No. 05-0040. Rockville, MD: Agency for Health care Research and Quality. Retrieved from http://archive.ahrq.gov/research/health/health.pdf
7. Centers for Disease Control and Prevention (CDC). (2009a). *Updated interim recommendations for the use of antiviral medications in the treatment and prevention of influenza for the 2009-2010 season.* Retrieved from http://www.cdc.gov/h1n1flu/recommendations.htm
8. Centers for Disease Control and Prevention (CDC). (2009b). *Coordinating call centers for responding to pandemic influenza and other public health emergencies: A workbook for state and local planners.* Retrieved from http://www.bt.cdc.gov/healthcare/pdf/FinalCallCenterWorkbookForWeb.pdf
9. Dolan, B. (2009, December 17). *Wireless health: State of the industry 2009 year-end report.* Retrieved from http://mobihealthnews.com/5816/wireless-health-year-end-report-2009/
10. Bureau of Labor Statistics (BLS), U.S. Department of Labor. (2010). *Occupational outlook handbook, 2010-11 Edition, registered nurses.* Retrieved from http://www.bls.gov/oco/ocos083.htm
11. Mastal, P.F. (2010). Ambulatory care nursing: Growth as a professional specialty. *Nursing Economic$, 28*(4), 267-269, 275.
12. Greenberg, M.E., Espensen, M., Becker, C., & Cartwright, J. (2003). Telehealth nursing practice special interest group adopts teleterms. *AAACN Viewpoint, 25*(1), 8-10.
13. Poole, S., Schmitt, B., Carruth, T., Peterson-Smith, A., & Slusarski, M. (1993). After-hours telephone coverage: The application of an area-wide telephone triage and advice system for pediatric practices. *Pediatrics, 92*(5), 670-679.

14. Wheeler, S.Q., & Windt, J.H. (1993). *Telephone triage: Theory, practice, & protocol development.* Albany, NY: Delmar Publishers, Inc.

15. Williams, C. (2007). Building an enriched legacy. *Viewpoint, 29*(5), 2, 11.

16. American Academy of Ambulatory Care Nursing (AAACN). (2007). *Telehealth nursing practice administration and practice standards* (4th ed.). Pitman, NJ: Author.

17. National Certification Corporation. (2011). *About NCC.* Retrieved from http://www.nccwebsite.org/about-ncc.aspx

18. American Academy of Ambulatory Care Nursing Board of Directors. (2007). AAACN holds telehealth visioning meeting. *Viewpoint, 29*(5), 4, 5.

19. American Association of Critical Care Nurses. (2011). *History of AACN.* Retrieved from http://www.aacn.org/wd/publishing/content/pressroom/historyofaacn.pcms?menu=aboutus

20. Drew, B., Califf, R., Funk, M., Kaufman, E., Krucoff, M., Laks, M., ... Van Hare, G. (2004). Practice standards for electrocardiographic monitoring in hospital settings: An American Heart Association scientific statement from the councils on cardiovascular nursing, clinical cardiology, and cardiovascular disease in the young. *Circulation, 110*(17), 2721-2746.

21. Sharman, J. (2007). Clinical skills: Cardiac rhythm recognition and monitoring. *British Journal of Nursing, 16*(5), 306-311.

22. American Association of Colleges of Nursing. (2008). *The essentials of baccalaureate education for professional nursing practice.* Washington, DC: Author.

Chapter 2

The Origin and Evolution of Telephone Triage

Health advice has been dispensed over the telephone virtually since the advent of the phone.[1] Telephone triage nursing, although not consistently recognized as a distinct practice area, has had a major presence since the 1960s in the United States,[2,3] 1970s in Canada,[4] and the 1990s in the United Kingdom.[5] Telephone triage has given rise to significant challenges in determining how to best provide care to patients over the telephone. This chapter will review factors that have influenced the evolution of telephone triage in the United States. While one might wonder what the discussion of diagnostic-related groups (DRGs) and antidumping legislation has to do with telephone triage, we believe that in order to understand how we must move forward, it will be helpful to consider where we've been.

BACKGROUND AND HISTORY

Unlike many other nations, health care in the United States has traditionally been primarily provided by private entities and not by the government. Although many states and municipalities do help fund hospitals that target primarily the uninsured or underserved in the United States, health care continues to be a free enterprise system. Many physicians are entrepreneurs and most hospitals are largely owned and operated by proprietary or commercial enterprises. Because health care is too expensive to be an out-of-pocket expense for all but the very wealthiest Americans, most funding for health care delivered in the United States is provided by insurance companies or the government, which subsidizes care for the elderly (Medicare), the poor (Medicaid), military personnel and their dependents, veterans, and Native Americans. In years past, these third-party payers (insurance companies, Medicare, and Medicaid) reimbursed hospitals and health care providers for expenses incurred.

Change from Retrospective to Prospective Reimbursement

In the mid '80s, in an effort to control health care costs, U.S. health plans went from a *retrospective* reimbursement model, or fee for service, to a closely controlled *prospective* payment scheme. This approach centered on DRGs and dictated reimbursement based on *anticipated* expenses associated with the patient's diagnosis rather than after-the-fact reimbursement for the care actually rendered. For example, if a patient was admitted to the hospital with uncomplicated congestive heart failure, the hospital received a previously contracted amount of money usually without regard for the length of the patient's hospitalization. With this strong incentive for efficiency in health care delivery, health care providers in the United States began trying to identify cost-saving measures.

Industry's Response to DRGs and Prospective Payment

One popular care delivery model that developed around this time was health maintenance organizations (HMOs). HMOs are insurance companies that contract with large groups (usually employers) to provide health services to their members, based on a fixed insurance or membership premium per person. In turn, the HMOs contract with hospitals and physicians, agreeing to pay them a flat amount, regardless of the actual health care services utilized by the population. In highly integrated systems, the HMO often employed the physicians and owned the hospitals and clinics.

For the hospitals, there were fixed fees for specific services. For example, an HMO might contract with a hospital to send all of their obstetrical patients to that hospital for delivery. However, to win this contract, the hospital often had to agree to provide the services at a greatly reduced rate.

The payment scheme was a little different for physicians. The HMOs offered doctors a certain amount per month for each insured member (per capita), and thus developed the concept of "capitation." In its purest form, capitation was intended to cover all expenses including preventative health (such as PAP smears and immunizations), management of chronic illnesses, treatment of acute illnesses, and even ancillary studies such as lab, x-ray, and other expenses associated with that care. In fact, in some cases, the provider was even held responsible for the cost of emergency department care for his or her patients who were members of the HMO. It soon became evident that it would be necessary for the physicians to find ways to significantly cut costs in order to survive economically. One way to reduce costs was to utilize nurses and other office personnel to screen patients by telephone, so those who were not thought to require an office visit could be given home care. Those patients who could not get an appointment and were not satisfied with home care advice often utilized the local emergency departments (EDs) as a primary care clinic.

Emergency Departments and Antidumping Legislation

Inability to get an appointment with their doctor, absence of a relationship with a primary care provider, lack of health care insurance, or often simple convenience, led many patients to freely utilize the emergency department as a primary care clinic. This overutilization of EDs resulted in unnecessary costs at a time that health care dollars were being tightly controlled. It was believed that if patients could be diverted from emergency departments to a more appropriate care setting, cost savings would result. To control costs and manage patient volume, EDs occasionally diverted ambulances out of their facility or sent patients out of the ED without screening and stabilization, a practice viewed as financial triage, or "dumping." In response to bad patient outcomes thought to be related to these practices, the government enacted the Emergency Medical Treatment and Labor Act (EMTALA), known as "antidumping" legislation, which ensured patient access to emergency departments regardless of their ability to pay.[6] This act imposed steep fines on hospitals that failed to provide adequate screening and stabilization to all patients who presented to their facility.

The Emergence of the Telephone Triage Nurse as a Gatekeeper

It was in this health care environment that telephone triage emerged largely as a cost-containment and demand management strategy for ED utilization in the United States. This strategy was based on the belief that if specially trained registered nurses (RNs), often referred to as *gatekeepers,* were charged with the responsibility of screening patients over the telephone, they would be able to determine which patients required care in the ED and which could be treated elsewhere. With this new practice, there was a steep learning curve for the health care industry. During this time patients were offered alternatives and even occasionally denied access to the EDs by telephone triage nurses who believed the patient's condition didn't warrant that level of care. Although the intent was to save money and manage the demand on health care resources, attempts to keep patients who were perceived to be of low acuity out of the EDs often resulted in a delay in care which eventually led to increased costs, poor outcomes, and occasionally, litigation. Additionally, this practice gave rise to a long-standing concern: the perception of telephone triage as a barrier to care.

TELEPHONE TRIAGE IN TRANSITION

The perception of nurse as gatekeeper and poor outcomes coupled with the EMTALA legislation, created an environment in which it became highly suspect for telephone triage nurses in any setting to try to divert patients from the ED. Regrettably, the term *gatekeeper* began to carry a negative connotation. Nonetheless, it was becoming apparent that telephone triage nurses provided a valuable service by redirecting patients to the appropriate level of care and otherwise facilitating good clinical outcomes and more efficient use of resources.

Although telephone triage often did result in a cost savings by offering patients lower cost options such as home care or clinic appointments, it also had the potential to legitimately result in *in-*

creased cost when the patient needed to be redirected, or "triaged," to a *higher* level of care. Although not the original goal, this higher cost was acceptable because it represented appropriate care. In evaluating telephone triage services, it became evident that the purpose of telephone triage was not to keep patients out per se, but rather to get the right patient to the right place at the right time for the right level of care, to assure safe, high-quality care, regardless of the cost.

By triaging patients over the telephone, the original goals to facilitate access to the right level of care and decrease inappropriate utilization of health care resources were met. In the process, telephone triage also facilitated effective patient education, heightened patient and physician satisfaction, improved nursing satisfaction, and provided quality patient care in a cost effective and efficient manner.[7]

TELEPHONE TRIAGE TODAY: HOW WE GOT HERE

Although telephone triage has been practiced informally in many settings for some time, due to the previously described societal and economic forces, telephone triage has come of age in the United States over the last 30 years. It has been formally recognized as a legitimate method of care delivery and is now an essential element of health care delivery in the United States.[8] Similar progress has been made in countries such as Australia and New Zealand, United Kingdom, Canada, and Sweden, where the government provides access to telephone nurses in order to manage health care access and demand.[9,10]

Telephone Triage Call Centers

Call centers are the most formal venues for the practice of telephone triage and feature nurses who field calls from patients/callers who are eligible for their services. They vary in size from less than ten to hundreds of staff and today many of them are moving to a virtual model with nurses working from home. Call centers exist either to serve specific populations or as general community resources. In these call centers, calls are managed by RNs. In some cases, clerical personnel are utilized to do the initial call intake and screening, and in other cases, the calls go directly to the triage nurses, who either take the calls live or call the patient back in a specified period of time. Virtually all of these settings use sophisticated call center software, which provides an electronic medical record, decision support, and analysis of call volume and other program metrics.

Call centers that provide telephone triage services exist in at least three types of settings.

- The first type of call center is part of an insurance company or health care plan and offers services only to patients enrolled in or eligible for their program. Examples of these programs include enrollees of a specific insurance program or those eligible for services as members of a special interest group, such as the U.S. military or veterans of the Armed Forces. Call centers serving such populations are usually owned or contracted and funded by the parent agency. These services are generally provided to patients free of charge as a benefit of the health care plan to which they are enrolled. The primary goal of these services is to facilitate access to safe and effective health care in order to contain cost and maintain and/or improve the health of that specific population.
- Call centers also exist as proprietary ventures. These call centers contract with specific entities, such as physicians or physician groups, to provide after-hours telephone triage services to their patients. The cost of the service is usually paid by the medical practice that commissioned the service. The primary goal of these programs is to relieve the physicians of the responsibility for triaging their patients after hours.
- Hospital-based call centers provide telephone triage/nurse advice as a community service. These call centers are often regarded as a marketing strategy for the community hospital in hopes of attracting patients to the services of that hospital. These services are provided free of charge to members of the community and are not offered in relationship to any particular plan or provider.

While this type of call center was common in the 1990s, many of them have lost funding and closed in the face of shrinking health care resources. Alternatively, these hospital-based call centers occasionally provide services (via contract or free of charge) to physicians on staff at the hospital.

Telephone Triage in other Ambulatory Care Settings

Telephone triage is practiced either formally or informally in virtually every ambulatory care setting. As mentioned in Chapter 1, common venues include clinics, home health and hospice agencies, urgent care centers, same-day surgery centers, college health centers, prisons, group homes for the developmentally disabled, and essentially any ambulatory care setting in which a patient can successfully access a nurse by telephone. In some of these settings, nurses have been specially trained and are dedicated to the telephone. In others, they are multitasked and provide a variety of patient care services in addition to their telephone triage duties.

If nurses in ambulatory care settings utilize decision support tools (also commonly referred to as protocols), they may be internally developed guidelines (either written or unwritten) or commercially developed manuals written by doctors and/or nurses. Sophisticated software programs which provide the opportunity for electronic documentation and decision support are also used, especially in clinics affiliated with larger institutions.

The number of medical offices and clinics utilizing RNs in this role is growing. However, even when RNs in these settings assume the responsibility for telephone triage, they are frequently multitasked and lack proper training and policy guidance. Unfortunately, due to lack of formalization and/or failure to recognize the complexity of the practice, it is not uncommon to find unlicensed personnel or licensed practical or vocational nurses (LPNs/LVNs) doing telephone triage in these settings. The boards of nursing in some states have developed language restricting the practice of telephone triage by LPNs and LVNs; and in at least one state, California, the practice of telephone triage by medical assistants is prohibited.[11] However, telephone triage by personnel other than RNs continues to be an area of concern and poses significant questions about patient safety.

Lack of Direction from Nursing

Even as telephone triage was recognized as a meaningful practice and telephone triage services began to proliferate, there continued to be an absence of clear direction from the nursing profession. This lack of nursing direction created an opportunity for businesses external to nursing to become involved in creating practices, tools, and guidelines to direct practice over the telephone. Business entities such as third-party payers, telecommunications companies, information technology companies, and developers of decision support tools (software and paper) stepped in to fill the void and mold the practice of telephone triage. While clearly focused on safe and effective patient care, these entities also had other organizational objectives which influenced their business practices and recommendations.

Telephone Triage as a Demand Management Strategy

The HMOs and other third-party payers seized an opportunity to decrease cost at a time when health care organizations had to do more with less. The role of telephone triage as a demand management strategy (as a method to direct patients to the appropriate level of care), grew rapidly with focus on cost containment and balancing risk with appropriate utilization of resources. Although the motives were more cost effective use of resources, an incidental outcome of this approach was that nurses (and others) felt actual or perceived pressure to "keep patients out," thus inadvertently representing telephone triage as a barrier to care. Poorly designed business practices in medical offices and clinics can have the same effect and thus telephone triage in any setting can be viewed as a barrier (and thus the nurse as a gatekeeper). Pressures tied to reimbursement schemes (prospective reimbursement or capitation vs. fee-for-service reimbursement) and the lack of available resources, can create situations that result in confusion among practicing nurses regarding their actual role. The following story illustrates this role confusion.

A nurse once asked a group of colleagues attending a telephone triage continuing education seminar whether they "triaged patients IN or triaged patients OUT." When asked for clarification, she replied she once worked in a practice that was not yet well established, and her physicians wanted her to triage patients "in" (to the clinic) in an effort to build the practice and generate revenue. However, she pointed out, she was now working in a practice that was basically overrun with patients and availability of appointments for acute problems was scarce. In this setting, the expectation was for her to triage patients "out" of the clinic, or to discourage appointments unless absolutely necessary.

The proper approach is to triage the patients appropriately, based on their needs and wishes, rather than on the business objectives of the organization.

Decision Support Technology

The telecommunications and information technology industries recognized potential business opportunities presented by telehealth nursing. Software companies and developers of decision support tools recognized a market niche into which they could expand their presence in the health care industry. Decision support tools were developed and promoted as tools to assure quality, standardize practice, and decrease liability. The guiding principle in their popularity was that protocol-driven triage would improve quality by standardizing advice and decision making. However, research and clinical practice have shown that the use of decision support tools do not in and of itself assure quality care delivery or standardized advice.[12,13] In fact, consistency of advice achieved by over-legislating decision making is not necessarily desirable due to the wide number of variables inherent in each specific patient encounter.[14,15] To avoid bad outcomes, nurses must base their decision making on use of sound clinical judgment.

At a national conference for telephone triage nurses, a physician developer of decision-support tools said from the podium that since physicians had developed and approved the protocols the nurses were using, if the nurses followed the guidelines precisely, were a bad outcome to occur, the physician group, not the nurse, would be held responsible.

While gallant (or patronizing, depending on your perspective), this notion flies in the face of nursing's accountability for its own practice. However, this scenario illustrates one reason nurses might tend to over-rely on decision support tools.

In an effort to control practice and reduce risk, organizations with policies promoting inflexible application of decision support tools potentially stifle critical thinking and diminish the role of clinical judgment. RNs and health care executives must realize the use of medically approved decision support tools does not relieve the RNs of accountability for their decision making. (Scope of practice for the RN is addressed in Chapter 5 and the role of decision support tools and critical thinking is more fully explored in Chapter 7.)

Meanwhile, with the proliferation of formalized telephone triage services (usually in call center settings), those responsible for organizing and managing these programs looked to the non-medical call center industry for direction. Often managers were hired who had experience and expertise in information technology, telephony, and/or customer service and efficiency in call center operations, but no experience in health care. Under their direction and leadership, telephone triage services began to be defined and evaluated primarilyin the context of customer service and efficiency. Parameters such as average speed of answer, call handling time, and other productivity measures that did not focus on the health care delivery component of these services began to assume a prominent role in practice expectations and performance evaluations of professional nurses.

One call center manager, focused on productivity measures and cost containment related to resource utilization, tracked average call length as well as the number of patients sent to the ED by each nurse. This information was shared with the nursing staff utilizing an anonymous nurse identifier known only to each nurse. During a consultation, it was later recommended that the manager discontinue this practice because of the likelihood that this information was indirectly impacting care. This would be especially true for the nurses whose practice put them at the outer edges of the bell-shaped curve. For example, the nurses who had the longest call length (considered undesirable by management) or sent the most patients to the ED (regarded as probable overutilization of the ED and thus also undesirable) might allow this information to negatively impact their practice.

The manager's response was, "No it won't. They know I don't care." However, it was obvious to the nurses that she did care, or she wouldn't have been posting that information for review. When the nurse with the highest referral rate was queried about whether this information impacted her practice, she replied, "Absolutely! Every time I think of sending a patient to the ED, I hesitate and consider what this will do to my ED referral rate." Obviously, the tracking and sharing of this information was not a good idea because the last thing a nurse should be worried about when talking to a patient who is sick enough to warrant an ED referral is how that disposition will impact his or her evaluation or workload statistics.

Thus, as illustrated, many patient care practices have been largely dictated by principles put forth by various business entities that had vested interests and varying levels of understanding of nursing practice. Efforts to standardize practice and balance safe patient care against efficiency, cost containment, and customer satisfaction had begun to emerge. This focus often resulted in program design and business imperatives that were misinterpreted by middle and first-line managers as well as by telephone triage nurses themselves. The end result was often that the policies and practices dictating patient care were not always consistent with the principles of professional nursing.

Today's Challenge

Through development of these questionable policies, apparent universal truths began to emerge. Such notions as absolute reliance on decision support tools, policies prohibiting downgrading (i.e., recommending a lower level of care than indicated by the decision support tool), call length expectations based on the belief that faster is better and the like, began to emerge and take the form of "conventional wisdom."

Conventional Wisdom

- ***"Popular notion; widespread belief" (Encarta)***
- ***"The generally accepted belief, opinion, judgment, or prediction about a particular matter" (Webster)***
- ***"May be either true or false" (Wikipedia)***
- ***May be an obstacle to introducing new explanations, theories, or approaches (Wikipedia)***

Rather than being guided by principles of professional nursing, much of what has guided our practice falls under the umbrella of conventional wisdom or widely held (presumably authoritative) beliefs. It's important to realize it takes time for conventional wisdom to become established. But often, by the time these notions are universally recognized, they're already out of date. Just as it takes ideas time to be accepted, it will likely take time for better ideas to replace them. We understand conformity is comfortable for most people. We just ask that you not be too comfortable.

For better or for worse, these are the primary forces that have molded our practice to date. Scant research has addressed the efficacy of many common beliefs and, thus far, nursing has not adequately "stepped up to the plate" to provide clear guidance about what nursing could and should look like over the telephone.

It has been said that practice often precedes policy. In other words, until a new practice emerges, there is no obvious need or incentive to develop policies directing that practice. Thus, while some boards of nursing have developed and published position statements, declaratory rulings, or FAQs addressing the practice of nursing over the telephone, many have not. The American Academy of Ambulatory Care Nursing and other professional organizations such as the Emergency Nurses Association and the Oncology Nurses Society have developed standards or other publications addressing this practice. However, many professional organizations have not yet formally recognized the practice of telephone triage and thus don't recognize the need for standards. And to date, telehealth nursing in any form has not been formally incorporated into the curriculum of schools of nursing. This is a significant oversight. The lack of ownership and direction from the nursing profession has further increased the chasm between what we're doing and what we ought to be doing. In other words, there is a disconnect between nursing theory and actual clinical practice.

SUMMARY

Lack of clear direction from nursing has helped perpetuate misconceptions about telephone triage. In Chapter 3 we will discuss many of these misconceptions because they must be put to rest before we can move forward. Based on the strength of one's conviction, some of these misconceptions will be harder to let go of than others. In fact, some of them will feel like sacred cows, and no one wants to butcher a sacred cow. However, if we are to grow, we must engage in reflection and critical analysis of these beliefs and be willing to experience a paradigm shift that might alter our view of reality.

References

1. Anonymous. (1879). Notes, Short comments, and answers to correspondents. Practice by telephone. *The Lancet, 114*(2935), 819-822.
2. Anonymous. (1996). *Telephone triage.* Retrieved from http://www.nurseone.com/essay1.htm
3. Nauright, L.P., Moneyham, L., & Williamson, J. (1999). Telephone triage and consultation: An emerging role for nurses. *Nursing Outlook, 47*(5), 219-226.
4. Canadian Institute for Health Information. (2001). *Health care in Canada.* Ottawa, Ontario: Author.
5. National Health Service. (2011). History. *NHS Direct.* Retrieved from http://www.nhsdirect.nhs.uk/About/History
6. Zibulewsky, J. (2001). The Emergency Medical and Active Labor Act (EMTALA): What it is and what it means for physicians. *Baylor University Medical Center Proceeding, 14*(4), 339-346. Retrieved from http://www.ncbi.nlm.nih.gov/pmc/articles/PMC1305897/
7. Omery, A. (2003). Advice nursing practice: On the quality of the evidence. *Journal of Nursing Administration, 33*(6), 353-360.
8. Anders, G. (1997). Telephone triage: How nurses take calls and control the care of patients from afar. *The Wall Street Journal, CCXXIX*(24), pp. A1, A2, A6.
9. Goodwin, S. (2007). Telephone nursing: An emerging practice area. *Nursing Leadership, 20*(4), 37-45.
10. St. George, I., Cullen, M, Gardiner, L., Karabatsos, G., Ng, J.Y., Patterson, A., & Wilson, A. (2008). Universal telenursing triage in Australia and New Zealand - A new primary health service. *Australian Family Physician, 37*(6), 476-479.
11. Medical Board of California. (2010). *Medical assistants - Frequently asked questions: Are medical assistants allowed to perform telephone triage?* State of California. Retrieved from http://www.mbc.ca.gov/allied/medical_assistants_questions.html#14
12. Dowding, D., Mitchell, N., Randell, R., Foster, R., Lattimer, V., & Thompson, C. (2009). Nurses' use of computerised clinical decision support systems: A case site analysis. *Journal of Clinical Nursing, 18*(8), 1159-1167. doi:10.1111/j.1365-2702.2008.02607.x

13. O'Cathain, A., Sampson, F.C., Munro, J.F., Thomas, K.J., & Nicholl, J.P. (2004). Nurses' views of using computerized decision support software in NHS Direct. *Journal of Advanced Nursing, 45*(3), 280-286.

14. Greatbatch, D., Hanlon, G., Goode, J., O'Cathain, A., Strangleman, T., & Luff, D. (2005). Telephone triage, expert systems and clinical expertise. *Sociology of Health & Illness, 27*(6), 802-830.

15. Pettinari, C.J., & Jessopp, L. (2001). 'Your ears become your eyes': Managing the absence of visibility in NHS Direct. *Journal of Advanced Nursing, 36*(5), 668-675.

Chapter 3

Misconceptions About Telephone Triage

As discussed in Chapter 2, much of what we believe we know about telephone triage is based upon widely held misconceptions and conventional wisdom which have stood in the way of progress. Before discussing the proper components and methods of telephone triage, in this chapter we will examine several misconceptions about this complex practice.

Many of the beliefs discussed in this chapter may be held by others such as your supervisor, your nursing or physician colleagues, or your patients, but they may also give rise to confusion among telephone triage nurses themselves. Unless these misconceptions are addressed, any discussion of telephone triage is likely to be fraught with misunderstanding.[1]

ANY WOMAN WORKING IN A DOCTOR'S OFFICE IS A NURSE

It is not uncommon to find a variety of personnel with different types of formal and informal education and training in various health care settings. This is particularly true in ambulatory care. For example registered nurses (RNs), licensed practical nurses (LPNs), licensed vocational nurses (LVNs), and unlicensed assistive personnel (UAP) such as medical assistants, technicians, nurse's aids, and other assistive personnel might be employed in a medical clinic. This often leads to confusion because in many health care settings, including call centers, UAP are utilized to provide patient care services, including some nursing functions. Unfortunately, in some settings it is possible to find RNs, LPNs, and UAP functioning in nearly interchangeable roles. These blurred roles contribute to the possibility that personnel with various types of education and training might be misidentified by patients and staff, especially over the telephone.

Consider the following patient's reaction to this phenomenon in her primary care provider's (PCP) office in "A Nurse's Story."[2]

A Nurse's Story

For about 7 years my husband and I (second author) had different primary care providers (PCPs) within the same ambulatory care organization. When either of us called the clinic it was not unusual to hear such phrases as, "The nurse will call you back," "I'll check with his nurse," or "This is Dr. Smith's nurse." Naturally, we thought we were speaking to the nurses who worked with our respective PCPs.

During those years, whenever I asked the "nurse" a question such as, what are my lab results?, the response was "You'll have to ask the doctor about that," or, "I'll have to check with the doctor." Although these responses gave me pause - what kind of nurse was this? - I never investigated. Imagine my surprise when after 7 years with this practice, I discovered that my health care organization did not employ registered nurses or licensed practical nurses as caregivers in the clinics. Instead, they employed UAP.

My first reaction to this revelation was one of betrayal and embarrassment. How dare you (the proverbial "you") misrepresent yourself, your staff, or your co-workers? How embarrassing to think we had been discussing our health and expecting information/advice from a medical assistant, rather than the licensed professional we had thought we were speaking to at the time. No wonder she had to check with the doctor before answering basic nursing questions. What made this more disturbing was the prob-

ability that each time I wondered why this "nurse" needed to check with the doctor, someone else in the community was equating the "I need to check with the doctor" (before I can do or say anything else) with the role of the nurse, and thus perpetuating the idea of nurse as handmaiden to the physician. Then, in processing this information further, I felt ripped off. For almost 7 years, my husband and I had taken comfort in the knowledge that a nurse was available and, in part, overseeing our care. When we felt we needed to be seen, discuss medications or lab results, or arrange a referral, we always felt reassured, believing that an RN was there to help identify and meet our needs, working with our PCPs to coordinate our care and ensure continuity and quality. Instead, the nurse in the practice was non-existent.

Although often used generically, we must shed (and help the public shed) the notion that the term *nurse* is a synonym for a woman who works in a doctor's office, and by extension, a female voice on the phone. It is no wonder that confusion exists because this misconception is perpetuated by those health care personnel who call anyone who is working with them or around them a nurse, instead of using their proper title. It is important to note the use of this term in reference to anyone other than an RN or an LPN or LVN is technically illegal in most states and subject to interpretation by the boards of nursing and others as the unlicensed practice of nursing.[3] Licensed nurses have a professional and statutory responsibility to set the record straight by informing those who misuse the title *nurse*.

Patients are most likely further confused by the variety of titles utilized by unlicensed personnel who may answer the telephone in clinics or call centers, especially those who are collecting health information. Titles such as *customer service representative, patient care representative,* and other potentially confusing terms might best be reserved for job descriptions and replaced by more descriptive and familiar terms such as *secretary, receptionist,* or *appointment clerk* when speaking with the public. Directly and clearly announcing, "This is Pat, I'm a receptionist, may I help you?" upon answering the phone will go a long way to clarify with whom the patient is speaking.

The term *nurse* specifically refers to RNs and LPNs or LVNs who are licensed by the state. A license gives the bearer permission to engage in activities that are otherwise illegal. A good analogy is the driver's license. Although it is possible for unlicensed individuals to know how to drive, unless they hold a valid driver's license conferred by the state, it is illegal for them to do so.

Medical assistants, for example, can have a wide variety of formal or informal education and training ranging from an associate degree as a Medical Office Assistant to certification as a medical assistant to individuals who have little or no formal training in health care. Of significance is the fact that, although some UAP hold degrees or certifications, most do not hold a *license.*

Moving beyond semantics, it is important to note that RNs are often reluctant to address differences in scope of practice between RNs and LPNs or LVNs and set limits on the practices of unlicensed personnel. Non-nurses often don't recognize the difference in the skill level among RNs, LPNs, LVNs, and medical assistants. Often nurses just want to get along and not ruffle feathers. Nurses may believe that discussing and trying to enforce the differences in scope of practice between RNs and LPNs or LVNs might result in hurt feelings and accusations of elitism on the part of the RN. Nurses may also lack the courage to address the problem of UAP being referred to as a nurse. However, if RNs are unwilling to address the differences in the scope and structure of nursing care in the ambulatory care setting as is consistent with educational preparation and licensure, all involved, including the patients, the organization, and the profession will suffer.

While it is obvious that an RN functioning at the level of a medical assistant is a misuse of resources, it should be just as obvious that allowing non-RNs to function at a level requiring licensure and specialized training is neither safe nor prudent. While the social, financial, and professional factors that facilitate such a situation are multiple, complex, and provide interesting fodder for analysis, only *nurses* can practice *nursing*. The bottom line is that although there is often a variety of personnel working in ambulatory care settings, the RN is not only accountable for the nursing care delivered but also responsible for the appropiate delineation of roles.

YOU'RE TAKING TOO LONG ON THAT CALL!

A frequent concern of nurses who provide telephone triage services and those who manage them is call length or call handling time. It is not unusual for programs that offer telephone triage services to attempt to establish targets for desired call length, the misconception being that faster is better. The fallacy in this thinking is the notion that call length can be controlled, and further, that it would be desirable to do so. As discussed in Chapter 2, in the early days of telephone triage, we sought guidance from the non-medical call center industry to help us identify service metrics or measurements, and consequently, we have used call length as a quality measurement. Faster has been regarded as better.

While call length is indeed a productivity measure, it does not define *quality!* Although quality has many definitions, it is clear that in the provision of health care services, quality must be associated with accurately identifying and addressing the patient's needs in order to affect a positive outcome (see Chapter 13). Regardless of how that outcome is measured, it is certain that different patients will require different call lengths in order for the nurse to complete the assessment of their needs and develop and implement a plan of care.

Individualized care has always been a basic tenet of nursing.

When assessing a patient over the telephone, the nurse must focus on more than just the patient's chief complaint. Patients are individuals, each with unique problems, symptoms, histories, and circumstances. Indeed, there are factors impacting call length that are too numerous to count, many of which are completely outside the control of the nurse. Therefore, call length may vary significantly from patient to patient, based on several factors including but not limited to:

- The complexity of the patient's problem(s)
- The caller's ability to give a clear and coherent history, respond accurately and succinctly to questions, and his or her motivation, education, and ability to understand instructions
- The patient's age, baseline health, and co-morbidities, such as elderly patients who often present challenges due to failing hearing, multiple chronic illnesses, social isolation, and other factors like polypharmacy which may significantly complicate their care
- Limited resources or family support and other social challenges such as financial concerns or lack of a relationship with a health care provider
- Types of decision support tools used, documentation required, and other organizationally dictated elements of call management such as a requirement to collaborate with a physician prior to making a disposition (often referred to as second-level triage)
- Varying responsibilities of the nurse such as performing triage, dispensing advice, coordinating services, making appointments, and placing outbound calls as necessary to complete the encounter

Even when some of the organizational variables can be predicted and/or controlled, the unique characteristics of each encounter and the resulting need for individualization of care cannot be controlled. Thus, efforts to impose arbitrary time limitations on these interactions may result in an incomplete assessment, inadequate or inappropriate instructions, and/or other process failures which may lead to disaster.

In 1995, a case was reported involving a telephone triage nurse at a large HMO call center who sent a mother with a sick infant to the "closest participating hospital," which was 42 miles away. Unfortunately, the child had meningitis and arrested enroute, losing all or part of three extremities and sustaining severe brain damage as a result of that event. There was a $47 million judgment in the lower court (later settled out of court on appeal for an undisclosed sum), because in driving to the closest network hospital, the mother bypassed four area hospitals on the way.

The HMO, which was known at the time for encouraging extremely short calls, argued that the call length was not the cause of the bad outcome because the child wasn't that sick when the nurse spoke with the mother. Assuming that's true, it begs several questions, all potentially pointing to call length. First, was the nurse on the telephone long enough to conduct an adequate assessment to accurately determine the seriousness of the problem? Second, assuming the child's situation did indeed deteriorate significantly following the call, did the nurse spend enough time with the mother to be sure she would appropriately know what to do if the child got sicker? And finally, did the nurse take the time to provide adequate teaching to assure that the mother would recognize "worse" if she saw it? If, for example, the child developed a petechial rash and became lethargic or overly fussy, would the mother have realized the potential significance of those developments without having received some direction from the nurse?

While high-acuity emergent calls can (and should) be handled quickly, a significant number of low-acuity telephone triage encounters actually take the place of an episodic visit with a provider. These calls require sufficient time to assess the patient, diagnose urgency and other needs, identify desired outcomes, collaboratively develop a plan of care, assure the plan can be carried out, and assess the effectiveness of the actions. In other words, if it takes 15-20 minutes to evaluate and manage a patient in a face-to-face setting, is it reasonable to expect a nurse to manage a call in less time over the telephone when it is not possible to see or touch the patient? Additionally, the circumstances surrounding a phone call must be addressed; for example, where is the patient calling from and is there a call-back number?

"Apart from adequate communication skills, triagists need sufficient time for telephone consultation to enable high quality performance" (p. 174).[4]

When trying to determine a reasonable length for an average call, one would do well to ask a question such as, "How long does it take to care for a patient in an emergency department?" The answer would most surely be, "It depends." That would also be the correct response in trying to predict the length of an average telephone triage call. Due to the potential risks associated with delivery of nursing care over the telephone, once nurses have received adequate training, they should be supported in spending as much time as needed to perform a thorough assessment and provide as much collaborative support as necessary for each caller.

Nurses understand the need to be efficient in their use of time. In reality, most nurses rarely have enough time to complete their assignments without having to take measures to consolidate activities or otherwise economize their use of time. When telephone triage nurses are on the phone with a patient for an extended period of time, it is more than likely it is because the patient *requires* that time!

Of course, if there are individual nurses who have difficulty staying on point or otherwise using their time wisely, a coaching opportunity would exist to help the nurse identify more time-efficient ways to conduct the encounter. However, it is a mistake to automatically assume that the nurse with the longest average call length is the one in need of remediation. In fact, it might be the nurses with the shorter calls who need to modify their approach in order to be sure they are taking ample time to perform an adequate assessment. Collaborative care planning, including sufficient patient education to ensure a successful outcome, can take time. And if the patient's needs aren't identified and addressed the first time, there will at best be additional calls, and at worst, a bad outcome.

In summary, while it is important for nurses to be as efficient as possible in their management of calls, it must be remembered that there is not a one-size-fits-all approach to patient problems. As with any other form of nursing, to be effective, care must be individualized. The unique qualities of the patient, his or her problem, the context, and the individual nurse's characteristics work in concert with organizational factors to determine the length of the call. Thus, efforts to control call length are likely to be counterproductive and potentially detrimental. Nurses who are concerned about how call length will impact their performance evaluation are likely to be distracted by concerns about their own job security. When the nurse is on the call with a patient, providing safe and effective care should be of primary concern, not the ticking clock. The bottom line on call length is that it takes as long as it takes.

Fortunately, over the course of the past several years, the pendulum has made a wide arc, with average call times gradually increasing from 3 to 7 to 12 or more minutes and, most recently, expectations in many call centers are for nurses to manage 3-4 calls per hour. The primary emphasis must be on providing quality care, resolving the caller's problem the first time (one-call resolution), and assuring customer satisfaction, rather than on enforcing an arbitrary time limit.

YOU'RE GETTING TOO INVOLVED!

Has anyone ever told you, "You're getting too involved! You should take care of their health problems and let them take care of their social problems?" Of course, the fallacy in this statement is that "getting involved" is a bad thing.

It could be argued that the practice of medicine deals with symptoms/diagnosis/treatment/cure, but the practice of nursing deals with the *human response* to those things. When dealing with the human response to illness, treatment, and wellness, we often need to get involved. So what may appear to be "too involved" is often the appropriate level of involvement, given the individual situation.

The wide variety of patient circumstances often creates a need for the nurse to get involved beyond simple symptom management. In addition to the complexity of the patient's health care needs and life situation, our current health care milieu is one in which patients, without an advocate, can get lost in the shuffle. Consider the many difficulties even we as health care professionals (who should know how to navigate the system) encounter when trying to facilitate care for ourselves or our loved ones. With that in mind, it is easy to see why our patients and their families need an advocate. The nurse's knowledge and expertise are necessary to facilitate the right care at the right time in our complex and often fragmented health care system. Additionally, patients often don't understand the significance of their symptoms or realize the potential consequences associated with failure to seek the appropriate level of care.

Take, for example, the woman of childbearing age who calls you complaining of a sudden onset of the worst abdominal pain she's ever had. It's "ripping through" her and "searing." Every time she tries to stand up straight (which she can't), she feels like she's going to faint and she's sweating profusely. She doesn't know what to do

because she's home alone. Clearly she needs an ambulance because she's too ill to drive, but your patient is reluctant to leave home because she has three small children getting off the school bus soon and if she's not there, they'll be coming home to an empty house.

Although the nurse would surely try to help the patient understand the potential seriousness of her problem, and insist that she call an ambulance, it is likely that the patient's maternal instinct would supersede her instinct for self-preservation. If unable to convince the patient to call EMS, the nurse's responsibility would then be to get involved and help the woman arrange childcare quickly. Being in severe pain and feasibly in shock, it's possible that any problem solving is beyond the patient's reach. Arranging childcare might be as simple as calling a neighbor to come to her house. The nurse might need to be a little more creative and call the school to ask them to keep the kids there until a family member could pick them up. Or, if all else fails, the nurse might need to call 911, even if over the patient's protest, advising dispatch that there is a childcare challenge in the home so they can send someone to care for the kids until more suitable arrangements can be made.

In this scenario, the nurse astutely recognized that the patient was in trouble. Maybe she was even thinking diagnostically and recognized the possibility of a ruptured ectopic pregnancy. Nevertheless, the bottom line with this scenario is that if the nurse hadn't identified what was important to the patient and developed a plan of care that was acceptable to her, the outcome was likely to be as bad as if the nurse had completely missed the significance of the clinical problem. Telephone triage is rarely straightforward. Often, getting involved is what nursing is all about.

Our goal for our patients is individualized care. Thus, the nurse must remain alert to those circumstances that offer opportunities to help the patient achieve optimum health.

TELEPHONE TRIAGE ISN'T REAL NURSING

One of the most common misconceptions about telephone triage is that it's not "real" nursing. And regrettably, that is sometimes a misconception shared by telephone triage and other nurses as well.

When I (first author) initially went into telephone triage, my son, who was in 9th grade at the time said, "Mom, don't tell anyone what you do." When I asked why, he said, "Because you used to be somebody important, and now you just sit around and talk to people over the phone all the time." Of course, as amusing as this was at the time, when I was later asked what kind of nursing I did, I am embarrassed to admit that I said, "I'm a telephone triage nurse, but I used to be an ER director." Obviously I must have felt a bit of that "I used to be a real nurse" mentality myself. I am happy to report I have gotten over that particular misconception and can now see how my entire career has prepared me to do what I am doing today.

Unfortunately, some nurses, not realizing the complexity involved in telephone triage or the risk associated with its practice, enter into telephone triage encounters somewhat lightly, failing to recognize that they are indeed practicing professional nursing. Recently, a relatively new graduate was overheard saying, "I went to school for four years and have been working as a nurse for three. I think I can manage answering the telephone."

Because talking on the telephone is a skill most people develop in childhood, the provision of nursing care over the phone is often viewed as something "anyone can do." In fact, it is not uncommon for organizations to relegate most telephone responsibilities, including taking messages on symptom-based calls, to unlicensed personnel. This is probably based on the belief that "taking messages" doesn't require an RN's level of expertise. Instead, they opt to utilize their RNs in the provision of face-to-face care.

In the hospital-based call center in which I (first author) worked, an across-the-board raise was given to the majority of the nurses in the hospital, but the telephone triage nurses were excluded. In contacting human resources to inquire why we didn't receive the raise, we were told that a deliberate decision had been made to give the increase only to the nurses who provided "direct patient care"! As an experienced nurse who has given a good deal of "direct patient care," I can say confidently that I have never given more direct patient care than when I have practiced nursing over the telephone.

Perhaps this misconception is in part due to many people regarding "nursing" as a discipline which includes "doing things," such as administering medications, taking vital signs, listening to hearts and lungs, and myriad other psychomotor tasks. Many of these skills can be delegated to others, often under the direction of a registered nurse. Although nurses *perform* psychomotor tasks, those tasks do not in and of themselves represent *nursing*. Nursing is cognitive, not psychomotor. It is the cognitive elements associated with the performance of specific psychomotor skills that places them within the domain of *nursing*.

For example, in the face-to-face setting, the professional expertise is not in giving an injection but rather in knowing when and how to administer the medication, as well as the mechanism of action, interactions, contraindications, and side effects. It is not measuring but rather interpreting the vital signs and understanding their implications in the context of each patient's condition that requires critical thinking. And it is not just listening to the heart and lungs but understanding the significance and physiology associated with the findings that constitutes *nursing*.

There are other elements of professional nursing which do not involve a psychomotor component. Nurses provide patient advocacy, health education, psycho-emotional care, care coordination, and the like; all elements of nursing that are purely cognitive. But most importantly, nurses utilize critical thinking and exercise clinical judgment in the provision of care to their patients. Many nurses find the practice of telephone triage to be especially gratifying because they practice almost exclusively in the cognitive domain without the distractions of psychomotor tasks.

Telephone triage nurses are occasionally asked, "Don't you miss the patient contact?" In reality, nurses who are on the phone 8 hours a day can conceivably spend every productive moment directly with patients or their families. And while it's not possible to *physically* touch patients during a telephone encounter, "touching patients" is still an important element of patient care over the telephone. One must recognize that *touch* isn't always *physical*. Because, patients are often more comfortable in the relative anonymity offered by the telephone, they are likely to disclose more over the telephone than in a face-to-face setting.[5] Is it possible that it is easier to disclose sensitive or personal information if one doesn't have to look into the face of another? And in the context of that level of disclosure and trust, a nurse can often make a profound difference in the life of a patient. Telephone triage is generally a pure nurse-patient interaction, largely undiluted by psychomotor tasks and other distractions. It is our belief that telephone triage is the epitome of professional nursing.

TELEPHONE TRIAGE NURSES ARE JUST GLORIFIED APPOINTMENT CLERKS

A related misconception is that telephone triage nurses are just "glorified appointment clerks." Although telephone triage can and often does involve scheduling appointments, an acute appointment is just one possible disposition the nurse might recommend for the patient. And in the process of making that appointment, critical thinking is almost always involved. For example: Is the issue urgent enough that the patient should be scheduled for the first available appointment, regardless of who it is with? Or is continuity of care so important that it would be preferable (and acceptable) for the patient to wait until later in the day to see his or her own provider? Imagine that the nurse offers a patient an 11:00 a.m. appointment but the patient states that her spouse has the car, and thus transportation won't be available until later in the day. The nurse must consider the circumstances and determine whether it's acceptable for the patient to wait for a later appointment or if instead, the problem is urgent enough that it is necessary for the nurse to help the patient find alternate transportation.

All patients requesting appointments for an acute problem (i.e., same-day appointments) should be triaged by an RN in order to determine the appropriate disposition for the patient. Although scheduling the actual appointment seems to be a task that could be relegated to others, this part of the nurse/patient interaction often requires critical thinking and negotiation and thus should be part of the triage process.

In looking at patient dispositions, it is often noted that the majority of patients requesting a same-day appointment are given a same-day appointment. In general, if a patient wants a same-day appointment, he or she should be given a same-day appointment (or sent to urgent care). This recommendation might tend to beg the question of why RNs are handling these calls. Keep in mind that the purpose of triage is not solely to determine the patient's need(s). If face-to-face evaluation is indicated or desired by the patient, the triage nurse must collaborate with the patient in determining when and where the patient should be seen and often how he or she would best be transported. Telephone triage is all about getting the right patient to the right place at the right time for the right level of care, and that requires assessment. Failure to utilize RNs in this role tempts fate in that patients might inadvertently be scheduled at the wrong time or place and/or with the wrong provider.

IT CAN'T BE SERIOUS; IT'S ONLY A PHONE CALL!

Of course, you don't have to be a health care professional to see the fallacy in the notion "it's *only* a phone call, therefore it can't be serious." However, for various reasons, it is likely that very busy, multi-tasked nurses occasionally regard patient phone calls as lower priorities than other responsibilities. For example, the nurse in a clinic might view patient calls as interfering with his or her "real" work. The nurse might believe patients who are physically present are of higher priority than those on the telephone. Or the nurse might simply be overwhelmed with the volume of work. It's not uncommon for overworked nurses to have or voice thoughts such as:

- "She's elderly and constipation is a common problem of people her age. Tell her to take her milk of magnesia and call tomorrow if she hasn't had a bowel movement." Of course, while constipation is a common problem associated with aging, the elderly also develop impactions and bowel obstructions. The conscientious nurse must rule those problems out before assuming the patient has simple constipation.

- "She's too young to be sexually active. Tell her to try a heating pad to see if that relieves her belly pain." A pregnant 10 year old, while fortunately uncommon, is not impossible. While trying to identify a pregnant child is admittedly looking for a needle in a haystack, it is a clear example of "if you don't look for it, you won't find it."

- "Oh my gosh, it's HIM again!" Our patients who call frequently are often regarded as low acuity and often don't get assessed fully with each call, especially if they have called recently with the same or similar problem. The legend goes that a tombstone in Key West sports an epitaph "See! I told you I was sick!" It is critical that patients be triaged carefully each time they call. In fact, these patients are potentially higher-risk because of their persistent complaints. Eventually even our most frequent callers are going to die of something physiologic, so we must forever remain vigilant to avoid overlooking a significant problem in someone who calls the office or call center frequently.

Telephone triage nurses must recognize that a patient who is calling with a persistent complaint is most likely sick, but perhaps we haven't made the right diagnosis or developed the proper treatment plan yet. The telephone triage nurse is in an ideal position to advocate for the patient until the underlying problem is identified and addressed. Common sense dictates that most patients have better things to do than call the doctor's office complaining of a fictitious ailment. And if the patient is indeed doing so, perhaps the underlying problem is anxiety, substance abuse, or Munchausen syndrome, all disorders that in and of themselves require treatment.

The saying goes, "If you hear hoofbeats, look for horses, not zebras." Simply put, this means that if a patient presents with a headache, it's more likely a sinus infection, migraine, or tension headache than a brain tumor or aneurysm. The usual rule of thumb in medicine is to eliminate the more common problems before looking for the needle hiding in the haystack. However, as telephone triage nurses, our job is to be zebra hunters. Is a pregnant 10 year old a zebra? Yes, thank goodness! But the prudent telephone triage nurse must keep in mind that if we're not looking for the zebras, we will never find them. No call should be taken for granted.

THERE'S A DIFFERENCE BETWEEN 'TELEPHONE TRIAGE' AND 'NURSE ADVICE'

Some organizations, either due to misunderstanding or in an effort to dodge the liability bullet, play the name game, calling telephone triage anything but. These efforts to avoid the implications of triage by disguising them are fruitless and potentially misleading. In other words, a rose by any other name is still a rose, and telephone triage by any other name is still telephone triage.

One large health care organization was deciding what to call their telephone triage program. Initial thoughts were to call it advice instead of triage in an effort to avoid the negative connotation telephone triage held for both their patients and their health care personnel. Due to previous experience, both the employees and the patients and their families regarded triage as being synonymous with "keep them out." The organizational concern was that use of the term triage would result in the program being poorly received. However, rather than spending energy trying to develop a euphemism, they would have been better served had they expended their efforts educating patients and staff about telephone triage, thereby changing the perception of triage as a barrier to care. And speaking of perception, the chief nurse executive lobbied for the title Nurse Triage because she saw telephone triage as a way to re-establish the value of nursing in her organization.

Taking this thought a step further, some organizations might claim that their nurses or other personnel aren't doing triage or nursing; instead they insist they're only collecting information for the physician, who ultimately makes the decision. There are all kinds of things wrong with this thinking! First, in order to "collect information" nurses must use critical thinking in interpreting the patient's comments, determining what to clarify, what to ask, and what to record and how. Second, nurses are nurses by virtue of their license and are thus accountable for their own actions, regardless of the decision ultimately made by the physician. For example, who is responsible if the physician makes a faulty recommendation based on incomplete or inaccurate information provided by the nurse?

It is virtually impossible for licensed nurses, especially RNs, to collect information from patients without performing some type of assessment, developing at least a preliminary conclusion about urgency, recommending some type of plan of care, and maintaining accountability for their actions. It is wrong to think that a nurse can take a message for a physician without assuming responsibility for having exercised some clinical judgment along the way. Nurses are responsible for the nursing process (see Chapter 4) regardless of whether they are cognizant that they are using it.

The extreme nature of the following example is helpful in illustrating the fundamental points necessary to understand the nurse's responsibility to the patient. Admittedly this is an absurd example, but the principles it illustrates are sound.

Imagine a patient calls with a presenting problem of "I cut my arm off with a chain saw and I'm spurting blood across the room!" The nurse will surely waste no time with history taking but will tell the patient to apply a tourniquet and call 911. In this situation, has the nurse made an assessment, diagnosed urgency, and developed a plan of care? Of course! The nurse recognized that the problem was imminently life threatening and developed a plan which included immediate life-saving intervention and rapid transport to definitive care. Although the appropriate action was almost intuitive and certainly did not represent complex decision making, the nurse did use clinical judgment in recognizing the urgency of the problem and developing a reasonable plan.

Now, conversely, consider the patient who calls complaining of a "cold." If the nurse asks only the obvious questions about fever, cough, nasal congestion, and then sends the message to the provider for action, has the nurse made an assessment? Yes. The nurse has concluded (right or wrong) that the problem is not urgent and that it can wait until the provider has a chance to review the note. But what if the patient is actually having a myocardial infarction (MI), and due to denial acknowledges only shortness of breath, which he has misinterpreted as a symptom of a "cold?" Although it appears that the nurse has only "taken a message," in reality, he or she was practicing nursing and has fallen short of the standard of care. Failure to ask about a health history or other symptoms represents an inadequate assessment, a questionable diagnosis of urgency, and a potentially unnecessary delay in care while the provider reviews the (possibly incomplete) information. Should the nurse be expected to function at a level higher than a mere "message taker?" Absolutely!

Regardless of the apparent nature of the call, one must realize that there is likely more going on than meets the eye. Message taking therefore involves assessment which requires critical thinking, specialized skills, clinical competence, and thus, a registered nurse.

ANYONE WITH A DECISION SUPPORT TOOL CAN DO TELEPHONE TRIAGE

Okay. Let's go to the next illogical idea: the belief that anyone with a decision support tool can do telephone triage. Decision support tools (marketed as triage algorithms, protocols, and guidelines) provide a recipe, if you will, for assessment of various symptoms. They also provide a standardized disposition based on preestablished criteria. If RNs are scarce in the organization or, due to perceived financial constraints the organization doesn't want to hire them, the use of protocols or guidelines by non RNs such as LPNs, LVNs, UAP, or clerks is often seen as a solution. It must be noted that when the "message taker" is a non-RN, the data becomes suspect because of the integral nature of interpretation during the process of taking a history. This is true even if efforts are made to restrict the message taker to asking and recording responses to prescribed questions. Decision support tools are often misused in this way, when non-RNs are instructed to simply ask the questions on the list. It is possible that key information might not be addressed because it is not in the protocol or on the list. Without interpretation and individualization, the history may be incomplete at best, and possibly even misleading.

As discussed previously, the process of data collection and decision making in telephone triage requires and implies assessment, independent judgment, and critical thinking. In fact, critical thinking and clinical judgment are necessary to even *choose* the right protocol. Think, for example, about the previous illustration of the patient with the MI who presented as a "cold." It is likely that a non-RN would have selected and acted upon the "cold" protocol, possibly with disastrous results. And even in the hands of the right person, many elements that must be considered in developing an individualized plan of care such as distance from care and other potentially confounding factors, are not usually addressed in decision support tools.

Data collection in the absence of these cognitive elements can indeed be done by "anyone," but at what cost? Decision support tools are just that: tools to *support* decision making. They do not qualify as artificial intelligence and thus can not stand alone in the provision of care over the telephone. Critical thinking and clinical judgment are *always* elements of appropriate telephone triage.

TELEPHONE TRIAGE EXISTS TO KEEP THE PATIENT OUT

It is not unusual for patients who are seeking appointments to be given one by an appointment clerk or secretary, unless there are no appointments available. At that point, callers are often referred to the nurse with the expectation that the RN will determine who needs to be seen and who doesn't. This approach is inappropriate and essentially sets the nurse up as the barrier to care. As previously mentioned, if a patient wants an appointment, he or she likely needs an appointment. The job of the telephone triage nurse is to help the patient determine when and where he or she should be seen.

One nurse reported a comment made to her by a patient of a practice that allowed their front office personnel to schedule same-day appointments on request. Once all the appointments were gone, the patients were directed to the nurse for triage. The patient told the nurse that when the secretary said, "Let me have the nurse call you back," his thought was, "Oh boy, I'm out of luck now!" Experience had taught him that when he was asked to speak to the nurse, it meant he would most likely be directed toward home care measures since he was never asked to speak to a nurse unless no appointments were available.

Patients such as this one obviously view the telephone triage nurse as the barrier to care and, occasionally, the perception of the nurse as patient advocate gets lost in the shuffle. It is sometimes difficult for many to remember that the role of the triage nurse is to *facilitate* care, not to *obstruct* it.

As a work-around, patients occasionally misrepresent their symptoms to get what they want. They might minimize their symptoms to avoid an appointment or they might exaggerate their symptoms to obtain an appointment. Experienced patients seem to know the "magic words" such as "chest pain," "shortness of breath," and "lethargy" that will trigger an immediate visit. Nurses often get upset when they perceive that a patient is not being honest about his or her symptoms, when in reality, this might just be an empowered patient. When a patient feels the need to fabricate or exaggerate symptoms to get an appointment, it is often indicative of a broken system and a patient who is clever enough to get his or her legitimate needs met in spite of the obstacles we pose.

If patients feel like the telephone triage nurse is the person they have to go over, under, around, or through in order to get to see their doctor, a change is needed. Here, we offer a solution.

If a patient calls asking for a same-day appointment, the prudent nurse might respond with something like, "Sure, I can get you seen. Let's figure out what is going on." It is unlikely that the patient will misrepresent his or her symptoms to the nurse then because the nurse has disarmed the patient. Lacking motivation to be anything less than candid, the patient will most likely give an accurate history. If the patient has reported a condition the nurse believes can be adequately cared for at home, and the nurse offers that alternative in an effort to facilitate appropriate care, the patient is more likely to accept the recommendation comfortably than if he or she mistrusts the motives of the nurse. The truth be told, most people, when sick, would probably prefer to be home in bed rather than fighting traffic, weather, or other obstacles to getting to the doctor's office. And besides, a doctor's office waiting room is often a breeding ground for contagious disease and isn't the healthiest place for a sick person to be, even under the best of circumstances.[6]

However, accompanying a recommendation for home care should be instructions that if the patient isn't feeling better in the appropriate time frame (this afternoon, tomorrow, in 2-3 days, etc.), he or she should call back. Employing this patient-friendly, respectful, and collaborative strategy makes obvious the nurse's interest in providing appropriate care.

Of course, some readers may be concerned that the initial response of promising the patient an appointment is risky since so many offices don't have adequate slots for same-day appointments. If this is the case, it is likely the organization isn't doing proper template (or appointment) management, a topic discussed further in Chapter 15 (Program Design and Implementation Part II). If the nurse determines that the patient needs to be seen, he or she needs to be seen whether it's convenient or not. And if the nurse determines that the patient could be cared for at home but the patient insists on a today appointment, the patient should be given that appointment.

It is likely that patients insist on a today appointment because (a) they are really sick and need to be seen, or (b) they don't trust our motives, believing that home care, when offered, represents a less desirable or ineffective plan of care. Sometimes patients are unwilling or unable to articulate their problem clearly enough to make it evident to the nurse that they really do need an appointment. Consistent, compassionate care from a nurse who has the patient's best interests at heart will go a long way in changing attitudes about triage as a barrier to care.

TELEPHONE TRIAGE EXISTS SO THE PROVIDER WON'T BE BOTHERED

Telephone triage is offered by many physician practices either through hiring their own triage nurses or contracting with a call center to provide those services. In many practices, the nurse represents not only a front-line interface with the patient but also the final barrier to the doctor. If the role of the nurse is to keep patients out, or to "protect" the doctor's schedule, eventually the actual role of the telephone triage nurse will be obscured.

On one occasion a provider commented that she "loved" telephone triage. Although this sounds like a positive, the physician went on to say, "Those triage nurses keep all that junk out of my schedule!" Although this comment devalues the role of the telephone triage nurse, if we are regarded as the schedule police, perhaps it is because we have inadvertently assumed that role.

Of course, the appropriate role of the telephone triage nurse is to determine the health care needs of the patient and then to facilitate that care.

In another instance, a more enlightened physician was approached by a telephone triage nurse who had worked a patient in for an appointment that day. The nurse apologized, saying that the patient "might not need to be seen," but she just didn't "feel right" about the patient. The physician reassured the nurse that she never had to apologize for bringing a patient in to be seen. She said, "There's a narrow line between those who need to be seen and those who don't, and if you're not leaving a wide margin on either side of that line, you're cutting it too close. I'd rather see a great many patients who don't need to be seen than miss even one who did."

Another concern is that nurses are often reluctant to call a physician after hours for fear of reprisal. Nurses may also be concerned about giving the impression that they are not doing their job adequately and are thus "bothering" the physician unnecessarily. The nurse is not there to protect the doctor from his or her patients but rather to provide professional nursing care to the patient and his or her family. Sometimes collaboration with the provider is a necessary part of care. If it is appropriate for the nurse or the patient to speak to the provider, the nurse should be willing and able to facilitate that contact.

PATIENTS DON'T KNOW WHAT IS BEST FOR THEM

Many nurses have the perception that patients don't know what's best for them. This misconception may lead the nurse to ignore the patients' priorities and worldview and to advise them in the context of the nurse's own priorities. While it's true that occasionally patients don't understand their physiologic need or don't agree with the appropriate treatment (who really *wants* an NG tube?), that assumption doesn't compute well in the outpatient setting. For example, patients who have been admitted to the hospital have essentially declared (or it has been declared for them) that today, being sick and getting well is their top priority. For these patients, health must take priority over other responsibilities such as job and family. However, in the ambulatory care setting, the patients who turn to us for advice over the telephone are still dealing with the multiple priorities of life, only one of which is their health. Our patients often must juggle work, child care, soccer games, school, choir practice, volunteer activities, car and home maintenance, and other pressures of 21st century living while trying to integrate taking care of their own health care needs and those of their family.

Many nurses naturally believe health care should be everyone's top priority, just as an auto mechanic probably thinks car maintenance is most important. Often it's all a matter of perspective. In helping patients plan their care, we must remember that once they hang up the phone, they will be free to do exactly what they want to do, with or without our blessing. Thus, we must develop a collaborative plan of care that is acceptable to and manageable for the patient. Instead of bulldozing or ignoring the patient's priorities, our job is to find a solution that allows the patient to make an informed decision that is mutually acceptable to the nurse and the patient.

OUR PATIENTS ARE UNREASONABLE AND DEMANDING

In most countries, including the United States, health care is widely regarded as a right rather than as a privilege. Patients may feel that they have earned that right by paying their insurance premium, paying their taxes, serving in the armed forces, enrolling in a particular college or university, being incarcerated, hiring a home health agency, or being a member of a particular group or community. And because patients believe they have earned that right, they are likely to become disgruntled if they aren't able to access the care they believe they need.

When a patient becomes "unreasonable and demanding," the bigger issue is *why?* Most people don't wake up in the morning looking for opportunities to be unreasonable. It is probable that patients who are behaving in an aggressive or demanding fashion have experienced something that made them that way. Perhaps they feel they have been mistreated in some way. For example, we may have failed to return their call when promised. Or worse, there may be a traumatic health history or an unmet health care need at the root of the patient's demand. Several examples illustrate this point.

- One patient called demanding a today appointment for an ingrown toenail. Efforts to persuade the patient to wait for evaluation were in vain because although the patient himself didn't have any high-risk indicators such as diabetes, his father had lost his leg and it began with an ingrown toenail.

- Another patient called complaining of an itchy patch on her face and she had just realized it was the site of the melanoma that had been removed 2 years earlier.

- A third patient demanded a same-day appointment for a Pap smear. What were the chances her abusive spouse was out of the house and this was her one chance to go to the doctor without him?

Each of these examples — an ingrown toenail, an itchy patch, and a Pap smear — appear to be low-acuity problems that could wait until tomorrow or even longer. However, each scenario represents an example of a patient in crisis — real or perceived — and the patient has turned to the nurse for help. It is interesting that the health care community has recognized physical pain as an emergency, even when it's known to be non-life-threatening, but we are reluctant to acknowledge emotional pain as an urgent need. If a patient calls complaining of a newly discovered breast lump, wouldn't the more compassionate approach be to schedule her as soon as possible for a mammogram rather than making her wait and suffer extreme, and possibly unnecessary, anxiety?

The telephone triage nurse must look through the lens of empathy, not judgment. Remember, patients likely didn't start out unpleasant or aggressive but perhaps became that way after interactions with our health care system. When patients are "demanding" or "inappropriate," keep in mind that their attitude might be more indicative of their reaction to a broken, chaotic, and dysfunctional health care system than a personal characteristic. The bottom line is that regardless of the reason for the patient's behavior, it is never appropriate for nurses to approach a patient with the attitude that he or she is being unreasonable and demanding without first trying to determine why and then taking steps to meet the patient's possibly unspoken needs.

SUMMARY

Many of these misconceptions have developed largely because of the way telephone triage has evolved. However, they remain alive and well because individuals are afraid of stepping outside the box, of being seen as different, or wrong, and do not want to accept the responsibility of working to change their organizational culture from within. This is otherwise known as "automaton conformity."[7] These issues must be pushed out in the open so they can be discussed. To provide compassionate, patient-centered care, the telephone triage nurse must realize that just as "location, location, location" is key in real estate, perhaps "attitude, attitude, attitude" should be a guiding principle in telephone triage. We all have the potential to be a positive influence in our own settings. Misconceptions impact practice. They can be changed, but many individuals must first experience a significant paradigm shift to "get in the zone" and focus on the practice of telephone triage as it should and could be.

Although access to care, efficiency, and cost containment continue to be goals of telephone triage, and information technology remains an important adjunct to practice, at the end of the day these do not assure the delivery of quality patient care. We must therefore do all we can to ensure that the basic principles of nursing provide the foundation of telephone triage training, practice, and program structure.

While knowledge, experience, clinical competence, and compliance with standards of care are essential to effective critical thinking, the role of attitude can not be underestimated in the provision of care over the telephone.[8]

References

1. Rutenberg, C. (2002). A call for understanding. *Viewpoint, 24*(4), 1, 6-10.
2. Greenberg, M.E. (2007). Nurse entitlement: Protecting what is ours. *AAACN Viewpoint, 29*(4), 4-5.
3. American Nurses Association, Inc. (2011). *Title "nurse" protection: Summary of language by state.* Retrieved from http://www.nursingworld.org/MainMenuCategories/Policy-Advocacy/State/Legislative-Agenda-Reports/State-TitleNurse/Title-Nurse-Summary-Language.html
4. Derkx, H.P., Rethans, J.J., Maiburg, B.H., Winkens, R.A., Muijtjens, A.M., van Rooij, H., & Knottnerus, J.A. (2009). Quality of communication during telephone triage at Dutch out-of-hours centres. *Patient Education & Counseling, 74*(2), 174-178.
5. Ignatius, E., & Kokkonen, M. (2007). Factors contributing to verbal self-disclosure. *Nordic Psychology, 59*(4), 362-391. doi:10.1027/1901-2276.59.4.362
6. Esposito, L., & English, T. (2008). The prepared patient: Don't let germs hitch a ride from your doctor's office. *Health Behavior News Service, 1*(6). Retrieved from http://www.cfah.org/hbns/preparedpatient/Prepared-Patient-Vol1-Issue6.cfm
7. Fromm, E. (1941). *Escape from freedom.* New York, NY: Henry Holt and Company.
8. Kayaoka-Yahiro, M., & Saylor, C. (1994). A critical thinking model for nursing judgment. *Journal of Nursing Education, 33*(8), 351-356.

Chapter 4

Telephone Triage as Professional Nursing Practice

Nursing is nursing whether practiced in the face-to-face setting or over the phone. The ability to provide care over the telephone has opened a new frontier through which nursing care can be delivered. The telephone and other forms of telecommunications technology provide access to information and advice from nurses, allow for improved communication, and enable nurses to more fully involve, support, and assist patients in making informed health care decisions. Standards exist, however, that must be incorporated into this new form of nursing care delivery. It is imperative that telephone triage nurses and other health care professionals such as physicians and administrators realize these encounters are not "just another phone call." Rather, they represent professional nursing practice.

In this chapter, we will discuss what makes nursing a professional practice in terms of four of the major characteristics of a profession.[1,2] First is the requisite education and licensure. Second is the existence of professional standards. Third is role clarity, which involves autonomy and accountability. And finally, professions must have an ethical foundation from which to practice. Each of these characteristics will be discussed in relation to the professional expectations for nursing in general and then specifically in relation to telephone triage.

EDUCATION AND LICENSURE

Nursing education from an approved school of nursing must be successfully completed as minimum preparation for entrance into nursing. Basic nursing education includes a broad liberal arts foundation followed by in-depth theoretical and practical nursing content and application. Once the degree is completed, the graduate nurse must pass the National Council Licensure Examination (NCLEX-RN) before applying for a nursing license. Upon successful completion of this exam, a nursing license may be conferred and in many states is maintained by meeting continuing education requirements. All nurses passing this exam are expected to have basic knowledge and skills which they then build upon with experience and continuing education during the course of their careers. Graduate and post-graduate degrees also exist for registered nurses (RNs). As a member of the nursing profession, the nurse is expected to engage in lifelong continuing education and professional development.

Nursing specialties require specialized education and experience and focus on specific areas of nursing. One of the newest among them is ambulatory care nursing.[3,4] Continuing education and board certification (RN-BC) are available for this specialty, and a professional organization, the American Academy of Ambulatory Care Nursing (AAACN), is devoted to the support and development of ambulatory care nurses.

Telephone triage is an integral element of ambulatory care nursing. In fact, telehealth nursing practice is one of the defining characteristics of the ambulatory care specialty.[5,6,7] Continuing education and training are available to nurses interested in developing the expertise and specialized skill set necessary for telephone triage. Despite the fact that more than 25% of the RNs in the United States practice in ambulatory care,[8] neither ambulatory care nursing nor telehealth nursing is presently included in basic nursing curricula. Although one can become certified in ambulatory care nursing and thus recognized as having specialty expertise, practice in this area requires and builds upon basic nursing education. As will become clear throughout the course of this book, skills and experience beyond basic nursing education, as it currently exists, are required for competent practice in telephone triage.

STANDARDS

Nursing standards and scope of practice define the minimum expectations for nursing practice and may be used as objective (legal and professional) guidelines for nursing performance. The American Nurses Association (ANA)[9] has written the standards and scope of practice for professional nursing. The scope of practice for all nurses is defined and regulated by state boards of nursing through nurse practice acts and related policies. For matters of common interest and concern, these state boards act and counsel collaboratively through the leadership of the National Council of State Boards of Nursing (NCSBN).[10]

In response to uncertainty as to whether telehealth nursing was professional nursing, thus requiring the expertise of an RN, the NCSBN developed a position paper in 1997. In this document, "Telenursing: A Challenge to Regulation," they clarified the issue and defined telehealth nursing as "the practice of nursing over distance using telecommunications technology" (¶ 2).[11] In this position paper, the NCSBN effectively removed two barriers to the recognition of telephone triage as professional practice. First, they affirmed that nursing does not have to occur in a face-to-face setting and thus the traditional tools of nursing, such as a stethoscope, our eyes, and our hands aren't prerequisites for nursing care. Second, they validated telecommunications technology as a legitimate tool used in the practice of professional nursing.

The NCSBN states that nursing care delivered over distance using telecommunications technology is indeed "...the practice of nursing and thus, asserts that it is regulated by the boards of nursing" (¶ 1).[11] There are three important implications of this assertion. First, as nursing care, telehealth nursing practice is subject to regulation by the boards of nursing in each state. Second, nursing's scope of practice is defined in the Nurse Practice Act and subject to the rules and regulations of the boards of nursing. In other words, any law, rule, or regulation that applies to nursing applies to telehealth nursing as well. And third, if a nurse violates those rules or otherwise fails to comply with practice guidelines, his or her license is subject to censure just as it would be if the nurse violated those regulations at the bedside. Standards specific to telehealth, and therefore telephone triage, are provided in the United States by various organizations such as the ANA[12,13] and the AAACN.[6]

Of course telephone triage, also known as telenursing, is practiced in many countries and each nation approaches the practice in its own way and/or has developed its own standards. A variety of successes and challenges have been experienced in countries such as Canada, the United Kingdom, Australia, and New Zealand, Norway, and Sweden.[14] Canada, for example, has provided stellar direction to Canadian nurses in the form of the Canadian Nurses Association Position Statement: *Telehealth, The Role of the Nurse.*[15] Other telenursing practice standards have been developed by various nursing organizations in Canada such as the *Telepractice: Practice Guideline* from the College of Nursing of Ontario[16], and the *Telenursing Practice Guidelines* from the College of Registered Nurses of Nova Scotia, which provide additional guidance.[17] It is clear from reading these documents that the Canadian Nurses Association understands that telephone triage is professional nursing practice and in fact regards it as a form of advanced practice. The International Council of Nursing[18] (ICN) developed *International Competencies for Telenursing* (2007) for the United States, Canada, and the over 130 countries in the world where telephone nursing is practiced.

Despite the widespread practice of telephone triage around the globe and the availability of standards for practice, there are still wide variations in theory and application. The nursing process, however, serves as the fundamental standard of practice for all nurses in all settings. The ANA states, "The common thread uniting different types of nurses who work in varied areas is the nursing process — the essential core of practice for the registered nurse to deliver holistic, patient-focused care" (¶ 1).[19]

Regardless of where it occurs, nursing is nursing, and use of the nursing process is necessary. It is the common denominator for every nurse-patient interaction. Whenever nursing care is delivered over the telephone, regardless of the nature of the call, the nurse must assess the patient, diagnose the actual or potential problem(s), identify desired outcomes, collaboratively develop a plan of care, facilitate implementation of that plan, and evaluate the effectiveness of their actions.

Practically speaking, if RNs are not using and documenting the nursing process for every patient encounter, they are violating the most basic standard of practice of our profession. In other words, this mandate to follow the nursing process also applies to nursing delivered over the phone. The nursing process includes assessment, diagnosis, goals and outcomes, planning, intervention, and evaluation. Each step of the nursing process is described next as they pertain to telephone nursing practice.

The Nursing Process in Telephone Triage

Many believe that telephone triage is as simple as answering the phone and following decision support tools (also commonly referred to as protocols or guidelines). Decision support tools are designed to prescribe which questions to ask and suggest associated recommendations regarding access to care and self-care interventions. While decision support tools are important to the practice of telephone triage, use of the nursing process is essential in that it not only represents the standard of care but also promotes critical thinking.

Assessment. Patient assessment is the cornerstone of the nursing process and thus a thorough patient assessment is an essential element of an effective telephone triage encounter. The nurse must perform an adequate assessment to be certain that the purpose of the call and the patient's needs have been identified accurately. Patient assessment involves collection of both subjective and objective information. The history provided by the caller constitutes the subjective information. Objective information can be gleaned by listening to the patient's breathing, clarity of speech, and appropriateness of discourse. Findings such as wheezing, tachypnea, productive (or dry) cough, slurred speech, confusion, and disorientation are examples of objective data which can be assessed over the telephone. The nurse can also gather important and sometimes unexpected information by listening for environmental cues and background noises.

Use of the nursing process represents the standard of care and promotes critical thinking.

Additional objective information can be obtained from direct observations by the patient/caller. Instrumentation is often present in the home for the caller to provide objective measurements such as temperature, blood pressure, weight, blood sugar, and peak flow volumes. In addition to information that can be measured directly, callers can also make a variety of key observations, given adequate coaching by the nurse. An example of this might involve assessment of a laceration. If asked, a caller should be able to describe the location, the size, the appearance (if the edges are well approximated), presence of any obvious foreign material, and whether or not the bleeding is controlled. Another example of self-reported objective data might be the amount, character, and odor of emesis. While these observations are unlikely to be precise (e.g., the caller probably won't be able to report emesis in milliliters), the caller can report whether it is "a lot" or "a little" (with the nurse seeking further clarification); whether the gastric contents are clear, yellow/green, bloody, like coffee grounds, etc.; and whether or not it has the odor of fecal material. A good rule of thumb to keep in mind is that anything the nurse can do with his or her eyes, hands, or nose, the caller can do with his or her eyes, hands, or nose given adequate direction from the nurse.

Diagnosis. In telephone triage, the diagnosis is a product of critical thinking and analysis of the assessment data. The diagnosis is expressed as a measure of urgency and associated patient needs. Is the problem emergent (immediately life, limb, or vision threatening), urgent (potentially life, limb, or vision threatening), or non-urgent (routine)? The determination of urgency is often based on pattern recognition and diagnostic reasoning which utilizes the nurse's education and experience (see Chapter 7). More conventional nursing diagnoses such as knowledge deficit or anxiety can be used as well. The diagnostic process also involves determination of the patient's needs and the appropriate nursing interventions, such as support, guidance, reassurance, education, and coaching. These and other nursing interventions facilitate the patient's ability to seek care and/or otherwise adequately care for him or herself or a loved one. Identification of patient needs are reflected in the desired goals and outcomes and are addressed in the plan of care.

Goal/Outcome. The nursing process has evolved over the years and the latest adaptation includes the identification of goals and outcomes.[20] These goals, when developed, are based on the diagnosis and should be reflected in the plan of care. While they may seem self-evident, occasionally there might be more than one appropriate way to meet a desired outcome. For example, it is not uncommon for decision support software to prescribe very specific dispositions such as "urgent care within 4 hours." Given the patient's specific circumstances, it is possible that there might be other referral sources that are closer or otherwise more appropriate. Using goals and outcomes to guide development of the plan of care will increase the likelihood that the plan will be effective and provide an objective basis for evaluation.

The reason conscious development of a desired outcome or goal in telephone triage is helpful is because there is usually more than one acceptable approach to managing most patients. Beginning with the preferred outcome in mind will help a nurse make the best decision for his or her patient. Three examples follow.

- For a woman of childbearing age with persistent abdominal pain, the goal (or desired outcome) might be "prompt evaluation." The disposition, given the specifics of the situation, might be office, urgent care, or emergency department, via private vehicle or ambulance.
- With someone who has a potentially life-threatening problem, such as an allergic reaction, the goal might be "definitive care prior to a catastrophic event." Again, depending on the circumstances, there might be a variety of ways to appropriately access that care.
- If your patient is a child with a non-urgent fever, your goal might be for "mother to be capable of providing home care to patient" followed by a plan to educate mother about appropriate comfort measures, use of over-the-counter (OTC) medications, and why antibiotics aren't indicated with every fever.

If the nurse has a clear idea of the desired outcome, it will give him or her a more solid basis for evaluating the appropriateness of the disposition suggested by the software. Chapter 10 elucidates the many elements that must be evaluated in determining the appropriate disposition for the patient.

Planning. Once a diagnosis is made (and desired outcomes have been identified), planning speaks to the question, "What should be done and how?" Planning must address disposition (where the patient should be seen and how quickly), transportation needs, and other elements that define the plan of care. Where does the patient need to go? How should he get there? What potential obstacles must be addressed in developing a plan? For example, if a patient needs to be seen in the emergency department, does he require EMS or is transport via private vehicle safe? And what if no transportation is available?

In telephone triage, the planning must be collaborative. It is critical that the nurse investigate the prevailing circumstances with the patient thoroughly, identify key factors important to him or her, and develop a plan of care that is acceptable to the patient. This often requires a process of negotiation and is supported by patient education. But it is the responsibility of the nurse to act in the patient's best interest and to develop a plan of care that both assures patient safety and is one that the patient is likely to follow. Collaboration is often necessary with other members of the health care team as well.

Intervention. Many nursing interventions are provided over the telephone (e.g., advice, information, support), but in the final analysis, it can be argued that telephone triage nurses can't do anything *to* or *for* patients who have needs beyond what the nurse can provide over the telephone. Someone else must do *to* or *for* these patients, and the role of the nurse is to be certain circumstances support the desired actions. For example, the nurse must assess the caller's level of understanding and may need to provide education and support to enable the caller to carry out the prescribed plan of action. If home treatments are recommended, does the caller have the resources to follow the recommendations? Or must the nurse take actions on behalf of the patient? If the patient is to be transported to a health care facility, the nurse may need to help identify, and maybe even arrange, resources to transport the patient appropriately. Sometimes an intervention can be as simple as providing information, reassurance, or advice.

Often the nurse has a key role in assuring continuity of care. If the patient is being referred for care, the nurse should advise the health care team of the referral and provide information relevant to the care the patient will require. An illustration of the importance of the nurse's role in continuity of care is reflected in the following analogy: Even an expert quarterback who has thrown the perfect touchdown pass will fail to score if he neglects to tell the receiver that he will be throwing the ball. It might be helpful for the telephone triage nurse to think of him or herself as the quarterback, the patient as the football, and the health care provider to whom the patient is being referred as the receiver. If the nurse has information critical to the care of the patient but fails to share it with the appropriate individual(s), the likelihood that the patient will receive the care he or she needs is diminished. Although telephone triage encounters are episodic, the role of the telephone triage nurse in assuring continuity of care is critical.

Evaluation. The last step in the nursing process is evaluation. There are a great many ways to evaluate telephone calls. However, in the context of the nursing process, evaluation is a measure of whether or not the actions taken were effective and answers the question, "Did this work?" Or more directly, "Did the patient get better or not?" If the patient did not get better, the nurse has a responsibility to reassess the patient, confirm the diagnosis of urgency (and be sure all elements that will impact the plan of care have been identified), revise the plan of care if necessary, implement that plan, and then re-evaluate. The encounter is not over, or closed, until the nurse has reasonable assurance that the patient will call back or seek appropriate care if his or her condition worsens or fails to improve as expected. Usually this can be accomplished by assuring that the patient understood and is comfortable with the plan of care, is willing to comply, and will call back if there are adverse outcomes. Occasionally, especially with high-risk callers or problems, it is important for the nurse to follow-up with the patient before "closing" the encounter. Table 1 illustrates the steps of the nursing process in telephone triage with a specific example.

Table 1.
Nursing Process Illustrated in a Triage Call

18-Year-Old Mother Called to Request an Appointment for Her 4-Year-Old Son Because He Has a Fever of 101 Degrees	
Assessment	4-year-old with no known allergies, in good health per mom, woke up today with fever, "he felt hot." Temp taken PO with digital thermometer, 101. Mother denies other symptoms but states son is "not eating today." States "I'm just so worried, I can't remember the last time he was sick." Child has been awake for 3 hours, has had no complaints, is sitting upright watching TV, acting "normal." Has had almost one cup of apple juice (mom measured 6 oz) and urinated once this morning "about 40 minutes ago, a usual amount." Breathing normal, denies congestion, cough, vomiting, diarrhea, or rash. Denies irritability or lethargy. Immunizations up to date per mom. Day care started 2 weeks ago. Phone call devoid of background noise except for TV.
Diagnosis	Non-urgent. Fever 101, parental anxiety and knowledge deficit (fever).
Goals/Outcomes	Mother will be less anxious, will feel confident with her ability to care for child with fever and will feel comfortable calling back if necessary.
Planning	Teach mother about fever, when to call the doctor, and home care strategies for fever management.
Intervention	Patient education and reassurance. Teaching per fever protocol. Asked mother to get pen and paper so she can write down information.
Evaluation	Mom able to identify primary S/S that indicate need to call back. States she feels "much better" and will call back if she has any questions or concerns.

The importance of using the nursing process can't be overestimated. Despite the use of decision support tools, "The nursing process provides the basis and structure for the practice of professional nursing and is used consistently with all telehealth nursing encounters" (p. 10).[20]

ROLE CLARITY: THE REGISTERED NURSE

The third characteristic of a profession is knowledge of its specific role and associated responsibilities. In addition to providing and coordinating clinical care, the role of the RN includes leadership, patient advocacy, teaching, and coaching. Utilizing the nursing process to assess, diagnose, plan, and evaluate, nurses autonomously initiate nursing interventions and provide care. The leadership role includes collaboration and communication with other members of the health care team to identify and coordinate the health care needs of their patients. Three major characteristics are inherent in the role of the professional nurse: advocacy, autonomy, and accountability.

Patient advocacy is a concept many nurses perceive as one of their primary responsibilities. RNs are patient champions, advocating and caring for patients and their families. Given the responsibilities associated with the role of the RN, there should be no one who has more knowledge of the individual patient, his or her health status, needs, fears, and desired outcomes than the nurse. The RN in all settings is in the ideal position to advocate for the patient and serve as the interface between the health care environment and the individual patient. In our health care system, particularly in the ambulatory care setting, where patients are often shifted from their primary physician to specialists to diagnostic services to treatment and then back again, it is clear that they frequently need someone to help them navigate this maze. This is especially important because patients are often provided with little or no instruction or explanation as to why they are being shuffled from place to place or how to successfully access care.

Autonomy is inherent in the nurse's role by virtue of his or her education, experience, and licensure. The RN role requires specific clinical knowledge and skills, critical thinking, decision making, and leadership. As members of the nursing profession, RNs are independent practitioners and may deliver nursing care without the direction of a physician or others. RNs function autonomously, but collaboratively, using the nursing process as the basis and structure for their practice.

The third concept inherent in the role of the professional nurse is *accountability*. This means that nurses are responsible for all of their actions. Although as nurses we do interact with other professionals, and receive and carry out orders from physicians, we are expected to use clinical judgment in carrying out those orders. If the nurse implements an order that is not in the best interest of the patient and a bad outcome ensues, the RN will likely be held responsible for that outcome. Although the physician would probably also be held accountable, this is a classic example of two wrongs not making a right.

Several years ago, a physician wrote an order for a lethal dose of potassium chloride (40 mEq of KCl) IV push and the nurse gave it! Although the physician was held responsible for the error on his part, the fact that the nurse followed the order violated the standards of nursing practice. The nurse was, of course, held accountable for her actions.

Role and Responsibilities in Telephone Triage

The increasing demand for ambulatory care and telephone triage nursing in health care today adds a special significance to the role and responsibilities of the triage nurse. The ability to provide care over the telephone has created a new venue through which nursing care can be delivered. However, although the face of nursing has changed, the vision and the cognitive elements of nursing have not. Compassionate, competent, individualized patient/family-centered care delivered in a collaborative environment is still the goal of the professional nurse even though the tools of the trade have changed.

The core elements of nursing in any setting, advocacy, autonomy, and accountability, take on much more significance in the practice of telephone triage. In the ambulatory care environment, patient *advocacy* is paramount because of the variety of sites and types of services available to patients, most of which are geographically and functionally separate. The nurse's *autonomy* is greatly enhanced in the telephone triage arena because the interactions are most often purely nurse-patient, and the oversight, input, or collaboration from other professionals is usually limited. While decision support tools and colleagues are available for backup and support, in the final analysis, decision making rests with the telephone triage nurse who is dependent upon his or her critical-thinking skills, knowledge, and experience. Decision making in nursing delivered over the telephone, even in consultation with a physician, carries undeniable *accountability* for the telephone triage nurse.

Telephone triage as professional practice requires specialized education, knowledge, skills, and licensure. Without these, patient care will suffer and the potential for liability will skyrocket.

ETHICAL FOUNDATION

The fourth and final characteristic of a profession is an imperative to follow an ethical code. To this end, the ANA has provided us with a *Code of Ethics for Professional Nurses* to which we must adhere.[21] Evidently we are succeeding because the American public has consistently responded to a Gallup poll, rating the honesty and ethical standards of nurses higher than any other profession.[22]

The ethical values of the profession serve as guiding principles. For example, a primary value is that the nurse must practice "with compassion and respect for the inherent dignity, worth, and uniqueness of every individual…"(¶ 1)[21] This principle is a reminder to all nurses that personal values and preferences are secondary to those of our patients. Awareness of our own values, beliefs, and biases can go far in assisting us to follow the ethical code of our profession and avoid ethical conflicts. In addition to respecting the values and beliefs of others, nurses have an ethical as well as a legal responsibility to safeguard patient privacy and maintain confidentiality.

In Chapter 6, we will discuss the strategy of "getting to know" our patients in an effort to respond to their individual needs. Part of this "getting to know" involves exploring values with our patients so we can help them make decisions that are right for and acceptable to them. This often requires that we subordinate our own ethics to those of our patient. Ethical dilemmas often occur because a person's underlying values are challenged.[23] Perhaps we expect some differences in values when dealing with someone from a different culture, but we also often have biases that people who are "like us" should make decisions based on values consistent with ours.[24]

Of course, when our own values are challenged, if we are not fully aware of the process at hand, it is possible that we could pressure the patient into compliance with our wishes (reflected in our plan of care for him or her). But in these cases, when we "win," the patient may lose. We must be certain, to the fullest extent possible, to inform our patients of their options and alternatives for care so that when we make a collaborative decision, it will be consistent with the patient's values rather than our own.

We must remain always aware of the disparity in the power base between nurses and patients, understanding that patients (some more than others) have the potential of deferring to our wishes, *in spite of their better judgment.* Because they respect us as professionals, coupled with our usually excellent interpersonal skills, our ability to build rapport and form a relationship is considerable. With that relationship, however, comes power — the power to persuade and the power to dissuade — and we should make every effort to get it right. Sometimes the patient's very life depends on assuring that the nurse and the patient are on the same page. Above all else, we must be certain that we protect the safety of our patients and that they have received the very best we have to offer.

Ethics Applied

The challenges and ethical dilemmas we face are often different when the decisions are made in the relative void created by an encounter over the phone. Ethical dilemmas faced by telephone triage nurses might include the following clinical, professional, and organizational examples which will be addressed in more detail in coming chapters.

Clinical. The nurse is talking with a patient who she is pretty sure is having a stroke, and although fully informed, the patient doesn't wish to seek care. In this case, the nurse must either support the patient's right to self-determination or act to assure the patient's safety, calling 911 over the patient's protest.

Professional. The nurse works in a setting in which multiple colleagues (RNs) recommend OTCs and refill prescriptions, activities which are not supported by organizational policy and are prohibited by the Nurse Practice Act in their state. The RN must either confront this practice, potentially incurring the wrath of some or all of her colleagues, or she must remain silent, passively endorsing a practice that is inconsistent with the standards, but that allows her to stay in the good graces of her colleagues.

Organizational. The nurse is expected to leave the office at 5:00 and has been requested to eliminate overtime. However, at 5:00, the nurse still has several calls to return to patients for whom the exact nature of the call is unknown. The ethical dilemma is whether to stay and return the calls, resulting in undesirable overtime and potential disciplinary action or to comply with the employer's wishes and leave, potentially putting the patients at risk.

Ethics terms have been described previously.[23] These terms and the examples provided can help individuals gain insight into the process of identifying, understanding, and resolving an ethical dilemma.

Moral Distress. The nurse feels "something is just not right here; I just don't feel good about this." Often in this situation, the nurse's underlying values are challenged. In the previous clinical, professional, and organizational examples, the moral distress first comes from the potential of letting the patient suffer a catastrophic event in an effort to respect his right to make his own decision; next allowing colleagues to violate the standards of practice in order to maintain harmony in the workplace; and finally potentially putting patients at risk in order to please the boss.

Moral Dilemma. The nurse realizes that he or she "must do either this or that" (p. 343).[23] A moral dilemma creates a forced choice situation in which the nurse is faced with two opposite and mutually exclusive choices. The moral dilemma is clear in the examples provided.

Moral Uncertainty. The nurse recognizes the moral dilemma but is uncertain which path to take.

Moral Residue. The nurse experiences a lingering feeling of concern accompanied by the feeling or knowledge that "I should have handled that situation differently" (p. 343).[23] Most nurses could, at the drop of a hat, describe one or more incidents of moral residue they have experienced, sometimes going back many, many years. It is likely that moral residue is what keeps nurses awake at night.

Moral Courage. We are "occasionally reluctant to challenge the status quo, especially when to do so would be to speak out against the majority opinion or long-established organizational cultural norms" (p. 343).[23] In the three preceding examples, moral courage requires the nurse to act on his or her beliefs and avoid the stance, "I see but I remain silent" (p. 343).[23] Does the nurse have the moral courage to dial 911 in an effort to assure the patient's safety, knowing that it will probably anger the patient and perhaps violate organizational policy? Does the nurse have the moral courage to take steps to educate his or her colleagues about the importance of practice that is consistent with the standards of nursing practice? And finally, does the nurse have the moral courage to challenge the "no overtime" policy in the interest of safe patient care?

Moral Agency. The ability to act on one's beliefs represents moral agency. However, it "may be constrained by fear, organizational policies, lack of support from colleagues, or lack of moral courage" (p. 343).[23]

Moral Sensitivity. Awareness of situations that represent moral or ethical issues is moral sensitivity. The importance of this concept is that rather than feeling disempowered and defeated by situations that don't feel right, the nurse recognizes these as ethical dilemmas and understands that they must be addressed through appropriate professional avenues.

Recognizing situations such as the ones described here as ethical, or moral, dilemmas gives the nurse a solid basis for addressing concerns, especially regarding policy or organizational norms. It is within the professional role and part of the responsibility of the RN to address the problems illustrated here: the policy barring the nurse from acting in the patient's best interest, practice inconsistent with standards, and/or an unacceptable workload. Instead of choosing to address these concerns by reacting in a passive-aggressive manner, acting out as a disgruntled employee, or complaining to others, a professional dialogue beginning with, "I have a moral dilemma..." would be a far more successful and professional approach.

SUMMARY

By this time, there should be no doubt in the mind of the reader that telephone triage is professional nursing practice. Once and for all the question of whether answering the telephone requires an RN should be put to rest. What exactly an RN brings to the table and why "someone else" can't deliver nursing care should be clear.

In the next chapter we will examine telephone nursing from a regulatory standpoint. In it, some of the information presented in this chapter will be examined in the context of the laws governing our practice.

References

1. Nursing Standards (2010, December 22). *Nursing management.* Retrieved from http://currentnursing.com/nursing_management/nursing_standards.html
2. Potter, P.A., & Perry, A.G. (2009). *Basic nursing: Essentials for practice* (7th ed.). St. Louis, MO: Mosby-Elsevier.
3. American Academy of Ambulatory Care Nursing. (2012). *Certification.* Pitman, NJ: Author. Retrieved from http://www.aaacn.org/cgi-bin/WebObjects/AAACNMain.woa/wa/viewSection?s_id=1073743906
4. Fuchs, J. (2001). The value of certification in ambulatory care nursing. *Viewpoint, 23*(3), 13.
5. American Academy of Ambulatory Care Nursing Board of Directors. (2007). AAACN holds telehealth visioning meeting. *Viewpoint, 29*(5), 4, 5.
6. American Academy of Ambulatory Care Nursing. (2011). *Scope and standards of practice for professional telehealth nurses* (5th ed.). Pitman, NJ: Author.
7. Mastal, P.F. (2010). Ambulatory care nursing: Growth as a professional specialty. *Nursing Economic$, 29*(4), 267-269, 275.
8. Bureau of Labor Statistics, U.S. Department of Labor. (2012). *Registered nurses. Occupational outlook handbook* (2010-11 ed.). Retrieved from http://www.bls.gov/oco/ocos083.htm
9. American Nurses Association (ANA). (2004) *Nursing: Scope and standards of practice.* Washington, DC: Author.
10. National Council of State Boards of Nursing. (2012). *About NCSBN.* Retrieved from https://www.ncsbn.org/about.htm
11. National Council of State Boards of Nursing (NCSBN). (1997). *Position paper on telenursing: A challenge to regulation.* Retrieved from https://www.ncsbn.org/TelenursingPaper.pdf
12. American Nurses Association (ANA). (1998). *Core principles on telehealth.* Washington, DC: Author.
13. American Nurses Association (ANA). (1999). *Competencies for telehealth technologies in nursing.* Washington, DC: Author.
14. Grady, J.L., & Schlachta-Fairchild, L. (2007). Report of the 2004-2005 international telenursing survey. *CIN: Computers, Informatics, Nursing, 25*(5), 266-272.
15. Canadian Nurses Association. (2007). *Position statement. Telehealth: The role of the nurse.* Ottowa, Canada: Author. Retrieved from http://www.cna-nurses.ca/cna/documents/pdf/publications/ps89_telehealth_e.pdf

16. College of Nurses of Ontario. (2009). *Practice guideline. Telepractice.* Toronto: Author. Retrieved from http://www.cno.org/Global/docs/prac/41041_telephone.pdf
17. College of Registered Nurses of Nova Scotia. (2008). *Telenursing practice guidelines.* Halifax, Nova Scotia: Author. Retrieved from http://www.crnns.ca/documents/TelenursingPractice2008.pdf
18. International Council of Nurses. (2007). *International competencies for telenursing.* Geneva, Switzerland: Author.
19. American Nurses Association (ANA). (2011). *The nursing process: A common thread amongst all nurses.* Washington, DC: Author. Retrieved from http://www.nursingworld.org/EspeciallyForYou/StudentNurses/Thenursingprocess.aspx
20. American Academy of Ambulatory Care Nursing (AAACN). (2007). *Telehealth nursing practice administration and practice standards* (4th ed.). Pitman, NJ: American Academy of Ambulatory Care Nursing.
21. American Nurses Association (ANA). (2001). *Provision 1. Code of ethics for nurses with interpretive statements.* Washington, DC: Author. Retrieved from http://www.nursingworld.org/mobile/code_of_ethics/provision-1.html
22. Saad, L. (2008, November). *Nurses shine, bankers slump in ethics ratings.* Gallup, Inc. Retrieved from http://www.gallup.com/poll/112264/Nurses-Shine-While-Bankers-Slump-Ethics-Ratings.aspx retrieved 6/29/11
23. Rutenberg, C., & Oberle, K. (2008). Ethics in telehealth nursing practice. *Home Healthcare Management and Practice, 20*(4), 342-348.
24. Yurak, T.J. (2007). False consensus effect. In R.F. Baumeister, & K.D. Wohs, (Eds.), *Encyclopedia of social psychology* (Vol. 1, pp. 343-344). Los Angeles, CA: Sage Publications.

Chapter 5

Nursing Regulation and Scope of Practice

The practice of nursing is regulated and licensed by the board(s) of nursing (BON). The BONs are empowered to develop rules, regulations, and policies to define and direct the practice of nursing in their state. The primary mission of the BON is to protect the public. To this end, the BON administers, interprets, and enforces the Nurse Practice Act, a law passed by the state legislature.

NURSING REGULATION AND TELEPHONE TRIAGE

Telephone triage, being a nontraditional method of nursing care delivery, raises questions about how the regulatory rules apply to nursing practiced over the telephone. Additionally, our ability to provide care over the telephone has removed the geographic barriers that have previously defined the location in which a specific nurse-patient interaction is occurring. Thus, questions exist about jurisdiction, scopes of practice, applicable policies and regulatory issues related to nursing practiced over the telephone, and therefore deserve special discussion.

The National Council of State Boards of Nursing (NCSBN) developed a position paper, "Telenursing, A Challenge to Regulation," in which they defined telenursing as "the practice of nursing over distance, using telecommunication technology" (¶ 2).[1] Further, "The National Council of State Boards of Nursing recognizes nursing practice provided by electronic means as the practice of nursing and, thus, asserts that it is regulated by boards of nursing" (¶ 1).

This declaration implies three important points:

1. The provision of care by a nurse over the telephone or via other

forms of telecommunication technology is indeed the practice of nursing and thus should be performed by duly licensed nurses.

2. Generally speaking, policies that regulate the practice of nursing apply to nursing provided via telecommunications technology as surely as they would apply to nursing in the face-to-face setting.
3. If a nurse violates these regulations, his or her license is subject to sanction, just as it would be in a traditional setting.

In other words, whether working in a virtual or face-to-face setting, nurses must be aware of and comply with the rules and regulations governing the practice of nursing in the state in which nursing care is being delivered.

THE ISSUES

In examining the practice of telephone triage from a regulatory perspective, three central issues emerge:

- Licensure and regulation of interstate practice
- RN and LPN or LVN scope of practice in telephone triage
- Scope of practice as it relates to recommendation of medications

Much of the following information has been gleaned from review of BON web sites and personal communication in the form of surveys and telephone conversations with staff of the BONs.[2,3,4] The findings reported represent formal written policy in some situations, but only the informed opinion of the executive director or his or her designee in others. It is important to realize that the question of telephone triage and scope of practice is a moving target and to date, most, if not all, of these policies or interpretations have yet to be tested.

Licensure and Regulation of Interstate Practice

The practice of nursing via telecommunications technology has raised multiple questions about nursing regulation, the most visible of which has to do with interstate practice. Because the practice of telephone triage transcends the geographic boundaries associated with face-to-face nursing care, jurisdictional questions have surfaced about the locus of responsibility in telephone triage and other forms of telehealth nursing. In other words, if a nurse is providing care over the telephone to a patient in another state, where is that nursing taking place? Is the nurse practicing in the state in which the patient is located at the time of the interaction or in the state in which the nurse is located when the encounter takes place?

Most states have taken the position that the locus of responsibility rests with the state in which the patient is physically located during his or her interaction with the nurse, rather than the state in which the nurse is located while providing care to the patient. Of course, this position has led to questions about the validity of the nurse's license in the remote state. These questions, coupled with the ever-increasing recognition of the legitimacy of nursing care delivered via telecommunications technology, led to the development in 1998 of the Nurse Licensure Compact.[5]

The Nurse Licensure Compact (NLC), patterned after the driver's license model, provides for mutual recognition of nurse licensure among the states that are members of the Compact.[6,7] According to the provisions of the NLC, the license of a nurse who resides in a member state is recognized by other states in the Compact. Specifically, nurses who are licensed in a Compact state are issued a multistate license which is valid in other Compact states. Thus, nurses in member states are able to practice in other Compact states without obtaining additional nursing licenses. An analogy would be a driver who is licensed in one state but may drive in other states on the basis of his or her driver's license in the state of residency. In 1998, Utah became the first state to sign the NLC into law, and within the next 12 years, almost one-half of the states followed suit. These measures have facilitated the delivery of care across state lines in the states that have passed the NLC. Unfortunately, since 2001, new members of the NLC have dwindled to a maximum of one to two per year as of this writing (see www.ncsbn.org for up-to-date information regarding the NLC).

In a survey of the boards of nursing,[3] the boards were queried regarding their opinions about whether nurses must have a license in their state in order to provide care to a patient physically located in their state. Ninety-eight percent of the respondents (44 of 45 states) replied that it would be necessary for nurses to be licensed in their state in order to provide care via telecommunications technology to residents of their state. Eighty percent of the respondents (36 of 45 states) replied that a nurse should be licensed in their state in order to provide care to temporary residents of their state (such as "snowbirds" or those who travel to a second home). And a startling 60% (27 of 45 states) responded that it would even be necessary for a nurse to hold a license in their state in order to provide care to vacationers or business travelers who were in their state only temporarily.

Issues associated with the interstate practice of nursing go beyond the question of licensure and have to do with the regulation of nursing practiced across state lines.[8] The states that have not passed the Compact have expressed various concerns such as loss of control over regulation of practice in their state and the subsequent limitation of the state's ability to protect the health of its citizens. In a handful of instances, state attorneys general have issued opinions that the NLC is unconstitutional in that it has the potential to limit interstate commerce.[8,9] Additional reasons for lack of adoption of the NLC include possible costs associated with disciplinary actions taken against nurses in remote states, loss of revenues related to license sales, and lack of support from their state nurses associations.[8]

Even if the NLC were to be uniformly adopted, telehealth nurses would continue to face challenges because of differing regulatory policies in each jurisdiction. Because not all BONs have yet addressed the practice of telehealth nursing, wide variability and inconsistency exist in expectations and regulations regarding this practice.

Varying opinions by the BONs, coupled with lack of uniform adoption of the Compact, have created a dilemma for nurses who provide care over the telephone. Once a nurse is on the phone with a patient, a relationship has been established, and thus the nurse owes the patient nursing services that comply with the standard of care (that, being at a minimum, the nursing process). The nurse who is obligated to assess the patient, diagnose urgency, and plan, implement, and evaluate care, if not licensed in the state from which the patient is calling, is considered by most BONs to be practicing in that state without a license. The nurse is now in a Catch-22 in which he or she must choose between providing care, potentially putting his or her license at risk, or declining to provide care to the patient, potentially putting the patient at risk (which could, of course, also jeopardize the nurse's license).

Question:

If a patient calls from another state, should I tell her I'm not licensed in that state and thus can't provide care to her?

Answer:

While this might seem like a safe approach from a regulatory perspective, it's not necessarily in the patient's best interest. In addition to the regulatory implications, each nurse must examine the moral and ethical implications of that approach. It is important to keep in mind that as soon as you pick up the phone, you've

entered into a relationship with the patient and thus owe him or her a nurse/patient interaction that meets the standard of care. In other words, once you've picked up the phone and spoken with the patient, you're already knee-deep in the provision of care. At this point, your only choice is whether you're going to provide nursing care the right way or the wrong way. Declining to provide care, or otherwise failing to perform an adequate assessment and diagnose urgency before giving advice, could result in an adverse outcome. However, in such a difficult situation, the decision is yours. It is your license and your patient!

The regulations set forth by the BONs represent state law; it is our professional responsibility and duty to know and comply with them. However, some organizations have assumed the position that if the interaction is with one of their established (or contracted) patients, provision of care is the responsibility of the organization (and therefore the nurse) regardless of the patient's location. While this could be viewed as a valid argument, it implies disregard for the prescribed policies or laws in other states.

Furthermore, many health care organizations, most notably centers of excellence, provide care to patients from all over the world. Once treatment has been initiated, and the patient has returned home, the organization has an established relationship and thus a duty to provide the patient with the standard of care.

Consider, for example, a patient who has received a bone marrow transplant at a center of excellence. Once the patient returns home (to another state), and he begins to experience graft-versus-host (GVH) problems, doesn't the organization have a responsibility to provide care to that patient even though he is no longer in their state?

An organizational attorney might advise a nurse that the organization will "cover" him or her in the event provision of care to one of his or her patients results in a disciplinary action by a BON. Because these Board policies often represent the equivalent of law, the organization can't "cover" the nurse who violates a rule any more than they can "cover" the nurse for driving 140 miles per hour down the freeway. Of course, if the nurse is ticketed and fined for reckless driving, the organization could pay his or her ticket and agree to not take disciplinary action for engaging in dangerous behavior. However, if the nurse's recklessness results in loss of his or her driver's license, the organization can't reinstate that license. And worse, if the nurse's actions result in an accident that claims the life of another, the organization can't relieve the nurse of his or her criminal, civil, or moral responsibility for the victim's death. While this example is a little far-fetched, it illustrates the principles at stake when a nurse provides care to a patient outside of his or her licensed jurisdiction. Conflicting positions of the organization and the BON creates a potential conflict for the nurse.

Organizations and individual nurses have taken a variety of approaches to resolution of this conundrum, but to date no ideal solution exists. Since it is often difficult to know the patient's physical location prior to the beginning of the call, nurses are often forced to provide care without regard for their licensure status in the state in which the patient is located. The alternative would be to purchase a license from every state (or non-Compact state, if the nurse resides in a Compact state), since it is conceivable that the nurse might receive calls from any state in the nation. To this end, a handful of organizations have decided to acquire licenses from every state not otherwise covered by the Compact for each nurse. Such a Herculean effort is difficult to sustain, however, because it is not only costly, but it poses logistical problems related to tracking of and compliance with renewal dates and continuing education requirements for each state.

Also of concern is the fact that even nurses practicing under the auspices of the NLC, or otherwise licensed in the remote state in question, are not always aware of the rules and regulations governing practice in the state in which that care is being delivered.[8] The Nurse Practice Acts and associated rules and regulations, position statements, declaratory rulings, and FAQs are state-specific. Thus, the practicing telehealth nurse potentially has 50 different sets of rules with which to be familiar and comply in order to deliver care that is within the parameters set by the responsible boards of nursing. A caveat is that due to federal supremacy and licensure portability associated with employment by the federal government, these issues are mitigated for nurses employed by such agencies as the Department of Defense, the Veterans Administration, and Indian Health Services.[9]

Uniform adoption of the NLC is strongly supported by the American Academy of Ambulatory Care Nursing (AAACN) and other professional nursing organizations such as the American Organization of Nurse Executives, the American Association of Occupational Health Nurses, and the Emergency Nurses Association as well as the American Telemedicine Association and the Center for Tele-health & e-Health Law.[6] However, until such time as the NLC is universally adopted, the importance of nurses being licensed in all states in which they provide care must be communicated clearly to both practicing nurses and their employers.

Scope of Practice: Roles of RNs, LPNs, LVNs, and UAP

Perhaps because practice often precedes policy, many BONs have not yet found it necessary to address the practice of telephone triage directly. Awareness of how interstate practice can affect care delivery over the telephone is an important first step toward change. In addition to the interstate practice issue raised, scope of practice issues regarding telephone triage have also arisen.

The first scope of practice question has to do with the roles of RNs, LPN/LVNs, and unlicensed assistive personnel (UAP). The Decision Making Model for Scope of Practice used by several BONs provides specific criteria for nurses and organizations to use in determining to what extent a practice in question (such as telephone triage) is within the scope of practice of the individual nurse. The specified criteria generally include such elements as identification of the task and determination of whether it is consistent with the standards of nursing practice; whether the task is allowed under the Nurse Practice Act and other regulatory standards; whether the nurse has the requisite education and experience, and is competent to perform the task; and finally, whether the nurse is willing to accept responsibility for his or her actions. Other BONs have addressed telephone triage and scope of practice directly through development of written policies in the form of position statements, declaratory rulings, and FAQs.

In general, nursing roles and practice parameters for telephone triage should conform to those in other settings. Registered nurses function autonomously in a collaborative practice environment, being independently responsible for assessment, diagnosis, planning, intervention, and evaluation. LPNs and LVNs, while involved in these activities, function under the supervision of RNs. They may also be supervised by physicians, dentists, podiatrists, and other licensed providers as specified by the Nurse Practice Act in the absence of RNs, but they generally may not function independently.

In a 2012 survey of BONs, approximately two-thirds of the states refute the notion that telephone triage is within the scope of practice of the LPN/LVN under any circumstances, citing the autonomous nature of the practice and the need for independent assessment and nursing judgment throughout the process.[3] A minority of states, however, still regard the practice of telephone triage as being an activity in which LPNs or LVNs may engage, provided they are supervised adequately. This calls into question the ability of one to "supervise" a telephone triage encounter without being on the phone with the LPN or LVN, resulting in unnecessary duplication. Further, a significant number of the BONs that allow supervised LPNs to perform telephone triage indicate that the supervision of LPN/LVNs must be in conjunction with the use of decision support tools. While at first glance this may seem to be a promising recommendation, it assumes that if one precisely follows decision support tools, those tools can replace or eliminate the need for the special cognitive and assessment skills the RN brings to the table. Telephone triage by LPNs or LVNs, with or without the use of decision support tools, fails to recognize the need for the critical thinking and clinical judgment inherent in the role of the RN.

The role of medical assistants (MAs) and/or other UAP in telephone triage is also an area of concern.[10] At least one state, California, has a document, written by the Department of Consumer Affairs, that expressly prohibits the practice of telephone triage by medical assistants[11] and the Board of Medicine has published an FAQ that clearly states that MAs may not perform telephone triage.[12] However, in many other states, MAs work under a Captain of the Ship Doctrine, which states that the physician, being "Captain of the Ship," is responsible for the actions of those under his or her supervision. This doctrine is adapted from the Borrowed Servant Doctrine, which applies when the MA is employed by the organization rather than directly by the physician.[13] There are important nuances associated with this relationship. Under these doctrines, the individuals supervising the unlicensed personnel are responsible for their actions. Application of this doctrine in the area of telephone triage is of concern to the public safety given the question, "How does the supervision take place?" There should be clear-cut organizational policies that establish the supervisory relationship between the physician and his or her MA (UAP).

If the RN is participating in the supervision of the UAP, he or she is at least in part responsible for any delegated acts. Because MAs and many other UAP are not regulated by the boards of nursing in most states, regulatory guidance from nursing regarding utilization of these personnel is essentially restricted to principles of delegation as outlined by the National Council of State Boards of Nursing (NCSBN)[14] and the American Nurses Association.[13] To keep the lines of authority and responsibility clear, the RN should not be involved in hiring, training, or supervising the UAP beyond those elements that comply with the Five Rights of Delegation.[14] The five rights are: the right task, the right circumstances, the right person, the right direction and communication, and the right supervision and evaluation.

One additional point of clarification is offered regarding the Captain of the Ship Doctrine as it relates to the relationship between a physician and an LPN or LVN when the physician is providing supervision in the absence of an RN. In this case, the Captain of the Ship Doctrine does not generally empower the physician to alter the LPN or LVN's scope of practice, which is prescribed by the board of nursing and standards of nursing practice. In other words, LPN/LVNs are responsible to act within their prescribed scope of practice regardless of who is supervising them.

Scope of Practice: Recommendation of Medications

The final scope of practice issue concerns the recommendation of medications by telephone triage nurses. It is understandable that patients/callers might ask questions about over-the-counter (OTC) remedies, and many calls involve symptoms that might be treated appropriately by OTC medications. It is also not uncommon for nurses (and others) in the doctor's office or clinic setting to be involved in renewal of prescriptions. In fact, in some organizations, physicians have come to rely on nurses and others in their office to initiate and renew prescriptions under certain circumstances. Unfortunately, many organizations do not have policies supporting these practices and not all of these activities are regarded by BONs as being within the scope of practice of the nurse, even if decision support tools are utilized.

Over-the-Counter Drugs. A 2012 survey of boards of nursing revealed that approximately one-third of the states believe recommendation of OTC medications is within the independent scope of practice of RNs.[3] An additional one-half believe RNs may recommend OTC medications, based on medically approved decision support tools to guide this practice.[3] It is noteworthy that a significant number of BONs (as of this writing, at least seven) regard recommendation of OTC medications, even with medically approved protocols, to be outside the scope of practice of RNs. These findings can have a huge impact on telephone triage services in general and particularly on after-hours pediatric call centers. If a nurse can't recommend an antipyretic for a febrile child in the middle of the night and must call the provider for an order, the value of that call center to both the patient and the provider is diminished dramatically.

In an effort to comply with the letter of the law but still provide care, RNs may consider a variety of approaches to the barriers imposed by those states that don't allow RNs to recommend OTCs even with a medically approved protocol.

Question:

When a mother calls asking what to give her febrile child, after I've performed an adequate assessment and determined home care is indicated, can I just advise her to give her child acetaminophen "according to package instructions" or "as her doctor has told her to do it in the past?" Since that's not a direct recommendation, wouldn't that absolve me of having "recommended" an OTC drug without an order?

Answer:

While at first this might seem like a reasonable "work-around," it could still be regarded as a recommendation. The

problem with this approach is that the nurse has, perhaps indirectly, recommended the drug without addressing associated concerns. That is to say that even if the nurse isn't explicit with his or her instructions, the mother would likely perceive the suggestion as a recommendation. However, having not received adequate associated instructions, the mother might have a knowledge deficit regarding administration of that OTC drug which could result in inappropriate dosing. Nurses have a responsibility to be sure that the patient clearly understands the recommendations made by the nurse and that the patient has no additional questions. Perhaps, after performing an adequate assessment, a better approach in this situation might be for the nurse to contact the provider for an order. Alternatively, if the call is taken after office hours, the triage nurse might advise the caller that he or she isn't licensed to recommend OTC drugs, but that the nurse would be happy to connect the caller with a local pharmacist who would be able to do so. While cumbersome, this approach would allow the nurse to function within his or her scope of practice while at the same time assuring patient safety. Conversely, obtuse efforts to avoid accountability for one's actions are less likely to be associated with sound practice, thereby increasing the likelihood of an adverse event.

One organization, perceiving that it was handicapped by its RNs' inability to recommend OTC drugs, identified one particular medication from each OTC drug class that their patients were likely to need. The selections were made from categories such as antipyretic, analgesic, anti-inflammatory, expectorant, antitussive, antacid, laxative, antidiarrheal, topical antibiotic cream, antihistamine, and antihistamine cream. After receiving education from a pharmacist on the indications, contraindications, side effects, interactions, and precautions associated with each drug, they were permitted to recommend these specific medications per an organizational protocol.

This solution worked for that particular organization because it is located in a state that allows RNs to recommend medications according to a protocol. In states that do not permit this, there is a legitimate work-around when the provider has an established relationship with the patient. If, when the patient is evaluated in the clinic, the provider places a standing order for an approved list of PRN OTCs and customizes that list for the patient, the RN would then have an order from which to work, much like orders for PRN drugs in the hospital setting. While this requires some effort, it assures compliance with the rules of the BON and, above all, protects the patient.

Legend (Prescription) Drugs. Drugs that are federally designated as requiring a prescription are referred to as *legend* drugs. According to a survey of the BONs, less than half of the states believe that RNs may renew prescription medications according to a medically approved protocol, and only about one-third permit RNs to initiate a prescription for a legend drug, also in accordance with a medically approved protocol.[3] In these cases, the protocols should include specific inclusionary and exclusionary criteria which relieve the RN of the responsibility for making an independent decision about renewing or prescribing these drugs.

Question:

My doctor has told me I can renew certain prescriptions. One such example is birth control pills. She has said I may renew the prescription for one month while scheduling the patient for an office visit within the next 30 days. Is this ok?

Answer:

While this is a common scenario, there are several problems associated with this approach. First, unless you're in a state that allows you to renew prescriptions on the basis of a medically approved protocol, or unless you are a nurse practitioner, it is not in your scope of practice to refill this prescription. Just because the doctor said you could engage in this activity does not make it within your scope of practice. Of course, if the provider's recommendation is patient-specific (i.e., you talked with that doctor about that particular patient), you are no longer renewing the medication per protocol, but rather carrying out a doctor's order. Second, even if you have a protocol and are empowered by your organization and state to use it, this still doesn't assure that renewing the medication is appropriate or safe for that particular patient. An adequate assessment must be conducted using criteria included in the protocol. For example, why is the patient requesting a refill? Has she been taking the medication consistently, or did she stop taking it 2 weeks ago and has since decided that she wants to resume it? If this is the case, has the patient had intercourse since that time? And when was her last normal PAP smear?

Question:

OK. One more question. What about benign situations such as calling in an antifungal for a patient with a vaginal yeast infection? Or eye drops for the child with conjunctivitis? Or an antibiotic for a patient with a UTI? These are familiar situations and drugs, and if I've assessed the patient for allergies, isn't it

ok for me to initiate these prescriptions based on a signed, medically approved, protocol? I've been doing that for years!

Answer:

Some states don't allow RNs to initiate prescriptions, even with a signed medically approved protocol. This position is-based on the opinion that these actions are outside the RN's scope of practice because they first require the nurse to make a presumptive medical diagnosis. However, some states do allow nurses to initiate prescriptions per protocol, based on the opinion that the nurse isn't diagnosing but rather only matching symptoms and acting according to the protocol. If you're in one of those states, and you've conducted an adequate assessment, this might be permissible provided you have an organizational policy supporting it.

Whether permitted by the BON or not, it is important that the RN involved in medication recommendation take this action seriously and utilize extreme caution when initiating or adjusting OTC or legend medications. Nurses who recommend medications must be certain they obtain an adequate history and are aware of indications and contraindications as well as the patient's current medications, current health status, co-morbid conditions, drug and food allergies, and interactions between drugs and with foods. As noted earlier, just because a drug is available OTC doesn't mean its administration is without potential consequences to the patient. For example, even if acetaminophen is appropriate and indicated for a particular patient, the prudent nurse must be aware that the patient might already be taking one or more combination drugs containing acetaminophen. This might potentially result in an overdose if the nurse were to recommend a therapeutic dose or advise the patient to take the drug "per package directions."

Discussion

Clearly, the limitations placed on nurses taking calls from patients in other states are daunting. If ever there was a no-win situation, this is it. Until further resolution is achieved, each nurse and each organization will have to decide the best course of action to take. However, it is critical for nurses to understand that just because they don't give advice doesn't mean they aren't practicing nursing. With assessment being the first step of our duty to the patient, the nurse who declines to speak further with a patient because he just has a "cold" may be violating the standard of care by not performing a more in-depth assessment to rule out other, more serious problems. Several states have provisions for nurses to accompany patients into the state for a short period of time, but few if any of those states have made the leap to recognizing that these policies might be adapted to apply to telehealth nursing. Unless significant policy change occurs in the area of interstate practice, nurses will continue to be at a loss regarding the best action to take.

Regarding telephone triage by non-RNs, of concern is the number of states that believe telephone triage can be supervised and regard the decision support tool as an acceptable substitute for critical thinking. Further, the act of "collecting data" or "taking a message" is fraught with risk because of the extent to which interpretation plays a role in deciphering the patient's concerns and recognizing the true nature of the patient's problem. In dealing with symptom-based calls, nothing less than a specially trained RN will do.

The findings of surveys of the BONs regarding scope of practice and policies directing the practice of telehealth nursing yielded interesting information that provides food for thought. For example, when asked if nurses could "recommend" OTC or prescription drugs, several Boards questioned or challenged the use of the word "recommend," recognizing it as a euphemism for "prescribe." We must define what nurses are doing when they initiate a recommendation or prescription for drugs per a medically approved decision support tool. Is that within the RN's scope of practice and, if not, is it time to re-evaluate use of decision support tools as they relate to this practice? Or is it time to take a fresh look at the capabilities and scope of practice for registered nurses?

The scope of practice issues discussed in this chapter are just the tip of the iceberg. Although RNs are providing safe and effective care over the telephone, it is sometimes questionable whether their actions are in accordance with the rules, regulations, and policies of the BON in the applicable state. Nurses and their employers need guidance from the BONs to clarify how interstate practice requirements apply in various situations such as with "snowbirds," vacationers, and those patients who have established relationships with providers. Clear and consistent language is necessary to delineate the appropriate role of LPNs and LVNs in telehealth nursing. Consistent direction by the BONs regarding nursing scope of practice in telephone triage and recommendation of medications over the telephone would be beneficial. The role of medical assistants in telehealth also needs to be formally addressed with the medical boards and/or the American Medical Association.

It is our hope that telehealth nurses and the boards of nursing will accept this information as a call to action and vigorously pursue uniform adoption of the NLC. Additionally, due to the ubiquitous practice of telephone triage across state lines, uniform language from state to state would dramatically decrease the burden on the practicing nurse and help ensure the safety of the public. In the meantime, it is the responsibility of each practicing nurse who provides patient care via telecommunications technology to be aware of and compliant with the rules and regulations of the BON in the state in which he or she is providing care, while maintaing the standards of nursing practice.

OTHER STANDARDS AND REGULATIONS

Professional practice standards for nursing have been addressed in Chapter 4. Regulatory standards are those directed by law, and the boards of nursing are significant sources of regulatory information for nursing. Additionally, nursing professionals are also required to follow the regulatory standards put forth by a variety of other municipal, state, and federal agencies. Examples of federal regulations that may impact telephone triage nurses are OSHA and HIPAA.

Occupational Safety & Health Administration (OSHA)

OSHA has regulatory requirements to help prevent workplace injuries (see www.osha.gov). Specific guidelines exist that impact call centers and other telephone triage work settings. These guidelines provide checklists for computer workstation design that address such elements as posture, seating, keyboard, monitor, work area, and accessories, as well as other general considerations.[16] Attention to OSHA standards for workplace and ergonomic safety bear careful review, especially for nurses who spend the majority of their day sitting at a computer. In fact, compliance with Professional Telehealth Nursing Standard 16 ensures that "Telehealth registered nurses perform work activities and care for patients in an internal environment that is safe, efficient, hazard-free, and ergonomically correct" (p. 37).[17]

Health Insurance Portability and Accountability Act (HIPAA)

HIPAA was enacted in 1996 to insure health care portability (or continuation of insurance) for workers who changed or lost their jobs. In 2003, HIPAA evolved to include other provisions addressing the security of health care information and protection of patient privacy. The American Telemedicine Association[18] reminds us that "Patient confidentiality and HIPAA requirements apply to telehealth nursing. Privacy policies and informed patient consent remain the same for telehealth encounters as for in-person care" (¶ 5).

HIPAA, federally mandated and regulated, is taken very seriously by health care providers and professionals. Unfortunately, misunderstandings and confusion about the application of HIPAA abound.[19] The Government Accountability Office, in a review of HIPAA implementation, found that health care providers have often been excessively cautious in the sharing of health information, even with people or entities who had a right to the information.[20]

While it is certainly not our intention to describe HIPAA in detail, we would like to make a few points based on observation and reported problems. These concerns have often involved nurses who have misunderstood HIPAA and thus have been overly guarded to the point that they negatively influenced care. We hope the following information will provide some clarity.

Simply stated, HIPAA was never intended to interfere with patient care.[21] Patient confidentiality and privacy are not new concepts for nurses. They are part of basic nursing education, and nurses have always taken them very seriously. Patient rights and nurse responsibility are also concepts addressed specifically for telephone triage nurses in the Scope and Standards of Practice for Professional Telehealth Nursing.[17] Unfortunately, there are nurses who often focus more on "complying with HIPAA" than on taking reasonable measures to protect the patient's privacy and still assure quality care. Telephone triage is designed to facilitate care, not to obstruct it. Certainly, nurses must use judgment in what, and with whom, they share and don't share. However, the bottom line is that our job is to facilitate care and advocate for our patients within the parameters outlined by not only HIPAA, but also the rules and regulations advanced by the BONs and the standards of nursing practice. A few examples highlighted on these pages might illustrate the extremes to which some nurses have taken HIPAA, based on their misunderstandings of the law.

While nurses must use judgment in what they share and don't share, the case report noted here illustrates how misinterpretation of the HIPAA rules resulted in an unfortunate outcome.

An RN's mother was admitted to the ICU in a distant state. The son called the ICU and spoke with his mother's nurse, inquiring about what was wrong with his mother. The nurse, citing HIPAA, refused to disclose the patient's diagnosis or condition. The son tried again, explaining that he needed to know whether he should come directly to the hospital or if he had time to get his affairs in order before he traveled out of state. Again, the ICU nurse declined to provide any information. The son tried a third and final time, asking, "If it was your mother, what would you do?" Once again, the ICU nurse refused to give him any information. The son took a day to make arrangements to leave town for a few days and flew to his mother's bedside the following day. When he got to the hospital, it was too late. His mother had expired just 2 hours earlier.

In this case, sharing the information with the patient's son would not have been violating patient privacy. HIPAA guidelines clearly state, "If the patient is not present or is incapacitated, a health care provider may share the patient's information with family, friends, or others as long as the health care provider determines, based on professional judgment, that it is in the best interest of the patient" (¶ 1).[22]

Another related concern deals with triage of pediatric patients who are in daycare or school and not physically with the parent who is placing the call.

A mother, who was at work, received a call from her child's day care center reporting that her child was ill. The mother called the nurse to discuss the symptoms and to see what the nurse thought she should do. The nurse advised the mother that she wouldn't be able to triage the child because the mother wasn't with her. The mother offered the information she had and provided the nurse with the number to the day care center. The nurse was reluctant to call the day care center, concerned that it would represent a HIPAA violation.

In this case, the nurse should have recognized implied consent when the mother gave her the phone number to the day care center. It is also important to note that the purpose of the call to the day care center would be for the nurse to obtain, not disclose, information about the child's condition from the day care worker. Further, it's unlikely that the opportunity to release confidential information would even present itself under such circumstances.

A wife called the triage nurse to discuss the fact that her husband had been having chest pain for several days and thus far had not sought care. She wanted to discuss her husband's symptoms with the nurse for the purpose of determining the action he should take. The nurse appropriately asked to speak with the patient but was told he was at work. The nurse asked if the wife could have the patient call her, to which the wife replied that he had been "refusing to deal with it," but had finally given her "permission" this morning to call and talk to the nurse to see if she thought there was any cause for con-

cern. Still, the nurse refused to discuss the husband's symptoms with the wife, citing HIPAA, and telling her the patient would need to make the call himself.

A more appropriate response, and fully in compliance with HIPAA, would have been for the nurse to tell the wife she would be glad to discuss her husband's symptoms with her, but she needed to be aware that the accuracy of the advice the nurse gave would depend upon the accuracy and completeness of the history the wife provided.

This is not a HIPAA violation because the nurse isn't releasing any health information but rather educating the wife and assisting her in problem solving, based on the information provided by the wife. And it's important to recognize that, because the husband was reluctant to seek care, if the nurse had refused to talk with the wife, that refusal might have deprived the couple of their only contact with a health care professional who could help them understand the potential seriousness of his condition and encourage him to seek prompt care.

In 2006, Levine stated "a major retraining of health care providers at all levels is needed to dampen the 'HIPAA scare' and clarify what HIPAA does and does not say about communication with family caregivers" (p. 51).[19] The discussion presented here is not meant as impetus to ignore patient privacy issues. However, it is a plea for nurses to use common sense and employ the Golden Rule whenever possible, making every effort to facilitate care by sharing appropriate information, within the bounds of the law, with those who need it. The bottom line is that any information shared to facilitate appropriate provision of care is generally not a HIPAA violation. Compliance with HIPAA should certainly not impede the ability of the family or other health care providers to give meaningful and responsible care to the patient.

SUMMARY

We have offered examples of how current nursing regulation falls short in relation to telephone triage practices. In this chapter, telephone triage-specific issues related to regulation and scope of practice have been highlighted. These unresolved issues create fertile breeding ground for inconsistent nursing practice and a number of patient safety concerns. Direction from boards of nursing, while present in several states, is lacking in others and is often unclear or inconsistent with the complexity of telephone triage and the subtle risks associated with the practice. Where policies do exist, they often vary significantly from state to state and create additional challenges for nurses and organizations providing telephone nursing services. Nurses need and desire direction. To ensure safe and consistent telephone nursing practice, these regulatory and scope of practice issues provide opportunities for clarity in nursing regulation and must be addressed.

Nurses in non-Compact states should consider contacting their BONs to see what they can do to help advance the Nurse Licensure Compact in their state. RNs practicing telephone triage should also remain informed of the current policies and developments in their state.[5] Telephone triage practice has preceded policy and, in the end, the nurse must decide how to best provide care to his or her patient within the bounds of reason and with consideration for moral, ethical, and legal principles.[23] OSHA and HIPAA are regulatory issues that affect all nurses but have specific implications for those who work to deliver care over the telephone.

In Chapter 6, we will continue to explore nursing principles and practice as they apply to care delivery over the telephone. We will present and apply three models to the practice of telephone triage that increase the understanding of, and provide guidance to, the practice in all its complexity. These models provide a detailed description of the complex set of processes that occur from the moment the nurse picks up the phone until the needs of the caller have been satisfied.

References

1. National Council of State Boards of Nursing (NCSBN). (1997a). *Postion paper on telenursing: A challenge to regulation.* Retrieved from https://www.ncsbn.org/TelenursingPaper.pdf
2. Rutenberg, C. (2000). Nursing licensure: States' conflicting stances pose challenges. *AAACN Viewpoint, 22*(1), 1, 5-8.
3. Rutenberg, C. (2012). [Results of the 2012 survey of the boards of nursing.] Unpublished raw data.
4. Rutenberg, C. (2008). [Results of the 2008 survey of the boards of nursing.] Unpublished raw data.
5. Hutcherson, C., & Williamson, S. (1999). Nursing regulation for the new millennium: The mutual recognition model. *Online Journal of Issues in Nursing, 4*(1). Retrieved from http://www.nursingworld.org/MainMenuCategories/ANAMarketplace/ANAPeriodicals/OJIN/TableofContents/Volume41999/No1May1999/MutualRecognitionModel.aspx
6. National Council of State Boards of Nursing (NCSBN). (2011). *Nurse licensure compact.* Retrieved from https://www.ncsbn.org/nlc.htm#
7. Ridenour, J. (2010). Nurse licensure compact 2000 to 2010: Sharing a decade of realities. *Regulatory Journal, 5*(3), 9-10, 12.
8. Stumpf, I. (2010). *The impact of the nurse licensure compact on telehealth providers.* Retrieved from from http://ctel.org/documents/The%20Impact%20of%20the%20Nurse%20Licensure%20Compact%20on%20Telehealth%20Providers.pdf
9. U.S. Department of Health and Human Services (DHHS). (2010). *Telehealth licensure report.* Retrieved from http://www.hrsa.gov/healthit/telehealth/licenserpt10.pdf
10. Otwell, D. (2008). Delegation to unlicensed personnel. *Medical Risk Management Advisor, 16*(2). Retrieved from http://www.proassurance.com/newsletter/default.aspx?f=a&k=95on
11. Bailey, L.R. (2011). *RN tele-nursing and telephone triage.* Board of Registered Nursing, State of California Department of Consumer Affairs. Retrieved from http://www.rn.ca.gov/pdfs/regulations/npr-b-35.pdf
12. The Medical Board of California. (2010). *Medical assistants – frequently asked questions.* Retrieved from http://www.mbc.ca.gov/allied/medical_assistants_questions.html#14
13. Bogart, J.B. (Ed.). (1998). *Legal nurse consulting principles & practice.* Boca Raton, FL: CRC Press.
14. National Council of State Boards of Nursing (NCSBN). (1997b). *The five rights of delegation.* Retrieved from https://www.ncsbn.org/fiverights.pdf
15. American Nurses Association. (2005). *Principles for delegation.* Silver Spring, MD: Author.
16. U.S. Department of Labor. (2003). *Computer workstations.* Retrieved from http://www.osha.gov/SLTC/etools/computerworkstations/index.html
17. American Academy of Ambulatory Care Nursing (AAACN). (2011). *Scope and standards of practice for professional telehealth nursing* (5th ed.). Pitman, NJ: Author.
18. American Telemedicine Association. (2011). *Telehealth nursing fact sheet.* Retrieved from http://www.americantelemed.org/files/public/membergroups/nursing/fact_sheet_final.pdf
19. Levine, C. (2006). HIPAA and talking with family caregivers: What does the law really say? *American Journal of Nursing, 106*(8), 51-53.
20. Wilson, J.F. (2006). Health Insurance Portability and Accountability Act privacy rule causes ongoing concerns among clinicians and researchers. *Annals of Internal Medicine, 145*(4), 313-316.

21. U.S. Department of Health and Human Services (DHHS). (2003). *Uses and disclosures for treatment, payment, and health care operations.* Retrieved from http://www.hhs.gov/ocr/privacy/hipaa/understanding/coveredentities/usesanddisclosuresfortpo.html
22. U.S. Department of Health and Human Services (DHHS). (2008). *Health information privacy.* Retrieved from http://www.hhs.gov/ocr/privacy/hipaa/faq/disclosures_to_friends_and_family/531.html
23. Kumar, S. (2011). Introduction to telenursing. In S. Kumar, & H. Snooks (Eds.), *Telenursing* (pp. 1-3). London, England: Springer.

Chapter 6

Models Directing the Practice of Telephone Triage

The practice of telephone triage is much more than "just a phone call." It has a sound theoretical basis that provides insight into why we do what we do and how we do it. In other words, there is a predictable approach to call management, and telephone triage encounters, done properly, proceed in a predictable manner.

Nursing models provide a unifying framework to guide and direct practice, an avenue for further discussion and improvement of practice, and a basis for development of clinical competencies. In this chapter, we present three models that provide structure and serve as the building blocks for the practice of telephone triage. We will first present broad supporting principles embodied in two models that underpin our practice and then conclude the chapter with a more detailed model that guides our practice, the Model of Care Delivery in Telephone Nursing Practice (referred to throughout this book as the Greenberg Model of Telephone Nursing Practice).

MODEL # 1: THE DATA TO WISDOM CONTINUUM

The Data to Wisdom Continuum,[1] shown in Figure 1, describes the relationship among data, information, knowledge, and wisdom and how these concepts inform decision making. Whether over the telephone or in person, nurses collect *data* (raw numbers or facts such as "abdominal pain" or temperature of 104). These data are combined with other relevant data to create *information.* Information is data that have been organized and interpreted (e.g., right lower quadrant, accompanied by fever and vomiting). We integrate and interpret information to develop *knowledge.* Knowledge is information that is integrated and interpreted further with previous knowledge and experience, resulting in this case in the recognition that this information might represent an acute or surgical abdomen. Wisdom is the ability to understand and apply the knowledge. In telephone nursing, wisdom is applied by making decisions appropriate for each individual patient. Nelson defines wisdom as "the appropriate use of knowledge in managing or solving human problems" (p. 13).[1] To summarize the Data to Wisdom Continuum, every telephone triage encounter involves an increasingly complex process of collecting data, organizing information, interpreting knowledge, and applying wisdom (see Schleyer & Beaudry, 2009).[2]

Figure 1.
The Data to Wisdom Continuum

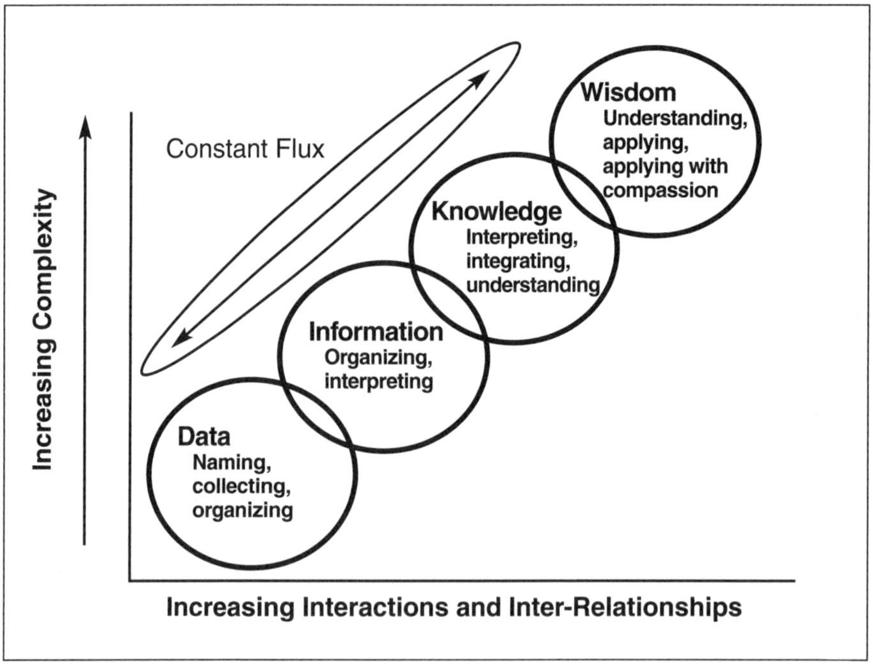

Source: Nelson (2002). Reprinted with permission.

The Data to Wisdom Continuum helps to clarify the role of decision support tools (DST) in the telephone triage process. DSTs are based on data, information, and knowledge. Important parts of data collection by the nurse include the patient context, patient preference, and other elements specific to the situation. Because DSTs are generally devoid of context, the effective use of data, knowledge, and information including decision support tools, "relies on the wisdom of the user" (p. 14).[1] "An automated decision support system uses knowledge and a set of rules for using the knowledge to interpret data and information to formulate recommendations. With a decision support system, the user decides if the recommendations will be implemented" (p. 14).[1] That is to say, while DSTs incorporate data, information, and knowledge to support clinical decision making, it is the telephone triage nurse who must apply wisdom. The Decision Making Triad, discussed below, delves further into the factors which contribute to the application of wisdom as emphasized by the Data to Wisdom Continuum.

MODEL #2: The DECISION-MAKING TRIAD

Multifaceted Aspects of Decision Making in Telephone Triage

The Decision-Making Triad featured here in Figure 2 was adapted from an original work depicting an evidence-based practice approach to nursing and clinical decision making.[3] The Decision-Making Triad illustrates the three primary sources of information used for decision making by the nurse in telephone triage: knowledge, clinical context, and patient preference. The Decision Making Triad also expands the concept of wisdom, or clinical judgment, to include consideration of the roles of clinical context, patient preferences, and established knowledge in decision making. Each component is discussed below.

Knowledge consists of scholarly works and clinical knowledge (both reflected to some degree in references such as DSTs). Clinical knowledge varies somewhat depending on the individual nurse's ed-

Figure 2.
Decision-Making Triad

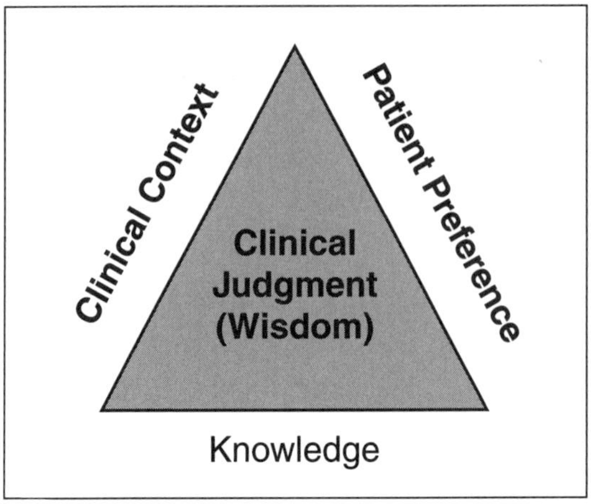

Source: Adapted from Greenberg & Pyle (2004).

ucation and experience. Scholarly works in the form of research, authoritative documents, and DSTs are based on scientific evidence and are used to guide decision making in telephone triage. It is indisputable that *clinical knowledge and experience* play a key role in decision making. Decision support tools are evidence based and provide guidance to the nurse, but their use must always be tempered with the nurse's own knowledge and experience. Professionally, the nurse who has experience in a variety of clinical settings will likely have a more diverse knowledge base from which to draw. Nurses with more general experience, more education and training, and more experience specific to the clinical specialty are more accurate with their decision making.[4,5] Personal life experience such as raising a family, caring for aging parents, and experiencing a variety of personal health care challenges also provides the nurse with invaluable information which may enhance decision making.

Clinical context provides another set of parameters which must be considered in decision making. Context consists of situational components such as relevant circumstances, available resources, and the unique characteristics of the patient.

Relevant circumstances might include (but are certainly not limited to) time of day, distance from care, and prevailing conditions. For example, the patient who calls during rush hour might be in a location that would preclude him or her from coming to the office, and thus the nurse might opt to send the patient to an urgent care center (UCC). If the weather creates potentially dangerous road conditions such as those encountered in a hurricane or ice storm, depending on the clinical condition, the more prudent course of action might be home care until the weather improves.

Available resources must be considered as well. The nurse managing a patient who calls after hours probably has fewer available resources than the nurse working during business hours. The types of diagnostic and treatment resources available in a particular facility must also be considered in many cases. For example, a DST might indicate that a patient with persistent abdominal pain should be seen in urgent care. However, based on knowledge and experience, the nurse is aware that the patient might need diagnostic procedures such as lab and x-ray which are not available at the local urgent care center. Thus, knowledge, experience, and attention to these factors might prompt the nurse to send the patient to the emergency department or bring him or her into the office, either upgrading or downgrading the disposition, based on the patient's needs and available resources. Patient resources must also be considered. For example, lack of social support and financial resources present unique challenges. Transportation or other resources such as over-the-counter medications may be lacking and thus present the need for special problem solving before making a disposition or ending the call. For example, patients who are home alone without access to an antipyretic might be encouraged to temporarily use other methods to treat a child's fever such as offering cool drinks and not overdressing the child until a suitable antipyretic can be obtained.

Context also includes *unique patient characteristics* such as age, co-morbidities, recent health status, current treatment, etc., that must also be considered. For example, a fever of 101° F is usually not a red flag unless the patient is very young, very old, or immunosuppressed. Ingrown toenails are usually of little concern except in diabetic patients or those with peripheral vascular disease. It is likely that bleeding gums will seem of little consequence unless the patient is taking an anticoagulant or suffers from a bleeding disorder. Often the emotional state of the patient is an important factor in decision making as well. An adequate investigation into the patient's current medications and past and recent medical history is often necessary to identify special circumstances.

Patient preference is the third factor which must be considered in decision making. For example, if a patient calls with symptoms consistent with an uncomplicated sinus infection of 3 days duration, the nurse might offer the patient a same-day appointment. If, however, the patient is unable to arrange transportation that day and would like to be seen the next day, it is likely the nurse would be agreeable, absent any complicating factors such as immunosuppression. If the patient says she's in critical meetings at work all week and would like to go to an UCC after work, the nurse would probably agree, given that the patient was willing to pay the associated co-pay. And finally, the patient may call just as she is boarding a plane to go on vacation and is thus unable to make an appointment. If this patient is seeking home care measures, the nurse would likely recommend those interventions outlined in the DST and insure that the patient knew the warning signs which would necessitate that she seek care while on vacation, if the situation didn't improve. Thus, as illustrated, the chief complaint associated with acute sinusitis might be treated in this case with a same-day appointment, a next-day appointment, a visit to an UCC, or home care measures, with the only variable being patient preference.

Although the diagram in Figure 2 is drawn as an equilateral triangle, it is clear that the previously described factors do not always deserve equal emphasis. This is where clinical judgment, or wisdom, comes in. Clinical judgment shapes the triangle, determining how much each of the three components of the triangle should be weighted. For example, if the nurse believes the patient might be having a myocardial infarction or a stroke, clinical knowledge takes priority. However, as illustrated previously, there will also be occasions and clinical presentations in which either context or patient preference will have the greatest influence on decision making. This is the reason DSTs, in and of themselves, are not enough. The wisdom to recognize and incorporate the patient's specific situation is what makes individualization of care possible.

THE RELATIONSHIP BETWEEN THE FIRST TWO MODELS

Having discussed the Data to Wisdom Continuum and the Decision Making Triad, let's look at an example illustrating the application and significance of these components of decision making.

The nurse receives a call from a 24-year-old female patient of childbearing age (contextual data), who has not been using birth control (contextual data) and has vaginal spotting (clinical data), abdominal pain (clinical data), and right shoulder pain (clinical data).

The nurse recognizes that this might represent an ectopic pregnancy (clinical information).

The experienced nurse knows that an ectopic pregnancy is subject to rupture and hemorrhage and is thus potentially life threatening (clinical knowledge supported by experience and decision support tools).

The nurse advises the patient to go directly to the emergency department (wisdom [application of clinical judgment]), but she would like to wait 2 hours until her husband comes home from work with the family car (preference).

The nurse learns that the patient is home alone with three small children (contextual data). The distance from her home to the hospital is several miles (contextual data) and the trip would take in excess of 30 minutes (contextual information). Given the circumstances, the nurse understands that access to care will present challenges (clinical context). The nurse knows that the UCC and doctor's offices are unable to do a vaginal ultrasound or a serum HCG (knowledge). Thus the UCC and doctor's office would be unable to perform an adequate workup (contextual knowledge) or provide definitive care if she should have a ruptured ectopic pregnancy (contextual knowledge).

The nurse concludes that the patient must be seen now in the emergency department for diagnosis and support (clinical knowledge), and she must be transported via 911 to assure her safety (clinical knowledge). The nurse recognizes she must help the patient acquire childcare or the patient will not leave home to seek care herself (clinical judgment/wisdom). Although the patient is reluctant to seek care now (patient preference), her life is potentially in danger (clinical judgment), so the nurse will work to help the patient understand the importance of being seen (clinical judgment/wisdom).

Table 1 depicts this same example using the terms of the two models in a more structured format.

Table 1.
Example of the Relationship Between Two Models

DATA

- CLINICAL
  - Abdominal pain
  - Vaginal spotting
  - Right shoulder pain

- CONTEXTUAL
  - Patient characteristics
    - Woman of childbearing age
    - Sexually active but no recent birth control measures
  - Circumstances
    - Home alone with three small children
    - 30 minutes from the hospital
  - Resources
    - No vehicle at home
    - Doctor's office and UCC don't have vaginal ultrasound or lab capabilities.

- PATIENT PREFERENCE
  - Patient would like to wait until husband gets home from work in 2 hours.

INFORMATION

- CLINICAL
  - Possible ectopic pregnancy

- CONTEXTUAL
  - Patient has childcare problem.
  - Patient is some distance from acceptable care.
  - Patient has transportation problem.

- PATIENT PREFERENCE
  - Patient is resistant to recommendation to be seen immediately.

KNOWLEDGE

- CLINICAL
  - Ectopic pregnancies are subject to rupture and life-threatening hemorrhage.

- CONTEXTUAL
  - A babysitter is needed.
  - Doctor's office and urgent care not appropriate referral sources
  - Distance to definitive care might be a problem.
  - Transportation will have to be arranged.

Table 1. (continued)

- ➤ PATIENT PREFERENCE
  - ○ Patient is unlikely to leave the house until a competent and trustworthy childcare provider has been indentified.

WISDOM

- ➤ CLINICAL
  - ○ Patient should be evaluated immediately.
- ➤ CONTEXTUAL
  - ○ A trusted neighbor can be called to watch children.
  - ○ The emergency room is the most appropriate place for evaluation and treatment.
  - ○ The patient should be transported via ambulance so that definitive care is immediately available if needed.
- ➤ PATIENT PREFERENCE
  - ○ Patient is reluctant to seek care away from home.

These examples highlight the amount of cognitive processing required to manage a telephone triage encounter and underscores points made previously in this book. A specially trained, experienced RN is the minimal level of preparation for the practice of telephone triage.

MODEL #3: THE MODEL OF CARE DELIVERY IN TELEPHONE NURSING PRACTICE

The Greenberg Model of Care Delivery in Telephone Nursing Practice provides a comprehensive description of the process used in the provision of care over the telephone (see Figure 3). The model specifically identifies and describes the essential components of telephone nursing practice. The principles described in the Data to Wisdom Continuum and the Decision Making Triad are also incorporated and elaborated upon in the Greenberg Model of Care Delivery. By presenting a clear picture of the process we are using when we manage a patient over the telephone, this model assists us in providing care that is safe, effective, and professional. Telephone triage nurses have reported that the model is valuable for:

- Articulating and validating practice
- Increasing understanding of and consistency in our practice
- Educating physicians, organizations, and the public about the telephone nursing process
- Orienting and teaching new nurses and nurses new to triage
- Developing telephone triage competencies and performance and outcome measures
- Supporting requests for organizational resources
- Providing a basis for new and ongoing research

The Greenberg Model provides insight into the structure of a call and describes the process utilized in a telephone triage encounter (see Figure 3). Analysis of the experiences of expert telephone triage nurses revealed a process that consists of three phases which are in part sequential but predominately simultaneous.[6] One of the key findings of this analysis was *interpreting,* a central activity the nurse engages in throughout each telephone encounter. Interpreting is a two-way process in which the nurse identifies and translates implicit and explicit caller information into health care information and then translates that information into language that can be understood by the caller. *Interpreting is occurrring from the beginning of the call to the end of the call and beyond.* Interpreting is a primary professional behavior that requires critical thinking, communication, listening skills, and interviewing techniques.

Interpreting involves not only listening for *explicit* information (such as "chest pain," "bleeding," "shortness of breath," or "fever of 104") but also recognition and consideration of relevant *implicit* information. Examples of implicit information include such factors as tone of voice, background noises, and contextual elements such as time of day and distance from care.

Figure 3.
The Model of Care Delivery in Telephone Nursing Practice

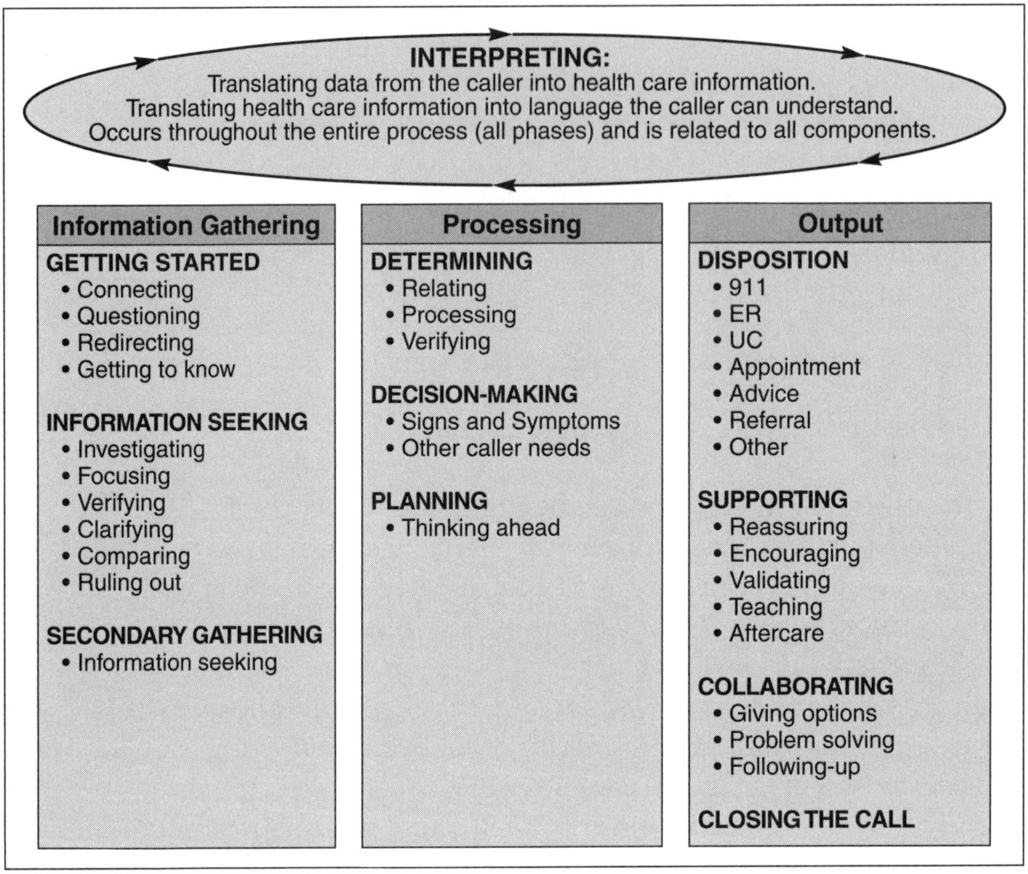
INTERPRETING:
Translating data from the caller into health care information.
Translating health care information into language the caller can understand.
Occurs throughout the entire process (all phases) and is related to all components.
Information Gathering
GETTING STARTED
• Connecting
• Questioning
• Redirecting
• Getting to know
INFORMATION SEEKING
• Investigating
• Focusing
• Verifying
• Clarifying
• Comparing
• Ruling out
SECONDARY GATHERING
• Information seeking
Processing
DETERMINING
• Relating
• Processing
• Verifying
DECISION-MAKING
• Signs and Symptoms
• Other caller needs
PLANNING
• Thinking ahead
Output
DISPOSITION
• 911
• ER
• UC
• Appointment
• Advice
• Referral
• Other
SUPPORTING
• Reassuring
• Encouraging
• Validating
• Teaching
• Aftercare
COLLABORATING
• Giving options
• Problem solving
• Following-up
CLOSING THE CALL

Source: Copyrighted © 2005 by Greenberg.

Generally speaking, calls containing a good deal of explicit information are often of high acuity but are not very complex.[7] Little interpreting is necessary to determine the significance of calls such as "I feel like there's an elephant sitting on my chest" or other obvious health care emergencies. Conversely, interpreting implicit information is more difficult, and thus these calls are generally more complex, and of lower acuity. In these cases, problem identification is often more difficult, and greater skill is required to collect and assemble all the pieces of the puzzle.[7]

Interpreting is a dynamic process which seamlessly involves the following sequence.

- In collecting the patient's history, the nurse filters and converts the data into medical information, separating the relevant from the irrelevant information.
- The nurse then processes the information, determines the nature and urgency of the patient's problem, and identifies associated needs and implications for patient management.
- Next, the nurse translates the *necessary* medical information into language the caller can understand.
- The yield, therefore, is individualized care.

In other words, what the nurse knows about the patient and the nature of his or her problem(s) has been determined in part through interpreting the information provided by the patient. The nurse will then tailor the approach to the patient, giving him or her the information necessary to ensure his or her understanding of the problem and bring about the desired action. Some patients will act simply on the recommendation of the nurse. Others will need a little more teaching and gentle coaxing, and still others will require assertive measures to assure their safety. In any event, if the nurse is not "speaking the same language" as the patient, the safety and quality of care may be compromised.

In addition to interpreting, other salient points of this model are depicted in Figure 3. The three phases include information gathering, cognitive processing, and ultimately an output phase. Each phase of the process is described below. All of the concepts in the model are addressed here and many are discussed in greater detail in Chapters 8 and 10.

Information Gathering includes data collection to assist the nurse in identifying the nature and urgency of the problem and the patient's related needs. Information gathering includes, "Getting Started," "Information Seeking," "Secondary Gathering," and associated strategies. Information Gathering is akin to the assessment phase of the nursing process.

Getting started includes multiple techniques designed to build rapport and connect with the patient. *Connecting* is an important first step in which the nurse establishes rapport. If successful, this creates a climate of trust which then facilitates communication and subsequent data collection. *Questioning* allows the nurse to determine the reason for the call, as well as what the patient perceives his or her problem to be, and what the caller wants to do about it. If the patient has an agenda, it is important for the nurse to know this at the beginning of the call. Occasionally, the nurse must *redirect* the caller from peripheral details back to more relevant information. *Getting to know* is a technique telephone triage nurses use to further establish a relationship with the patient, grasp the individual nuances of the situation, and learn important information that will be utilized in care planning, such as education level, available resources, and the patient's motivation or comfort level.

Information Seeking involves an in-depth systematic collection of information. The nurse gathers enough information to determine the nature of the caller's needs and the acuity. It is important to note that information seeking can be short (for example, if the problem is emergent) or it can be long and in-depth. Depending on the nature of the problem, the nurse may need to complete a comprehensive assessment of physical, psychosocial, historical, and resource-related factors.

Strategies used in information seeking include *investigating,* which is used to help identify the specific concerns or symptoms upon which to focus. *Focusing* involves detailed questioning about a specific element of the caller's concern. The nurse must often *verify* or *clarify* what the caller means by various terms and phrases. This is also an example of interpreting. For example, when callers use words like "lethargic," the nurse must clarify exactly what the callers mean and what they're trying to convey. *Comparing* and *ruling out* are other techniques used by experienced nurses to help identify and clarify signs and symptoms and the nature of the patient's concern. Based on their knowledge and expertise, nurses seek specific information or pertinent findings in an effort to identify or eliminate suspected illnesses or conditions.

Secondary Gathering is often necessary before the nurse is able to close the call. This is the collection of additional information that often occurs during documentation or at the end of the call but it may occur at any time after the initial information has been collected. Secondary gathering is most often based on the realization that the nurse is unable to reach a comfortable decision or plan without gathering additional information. The following are examples of secondary gathering:

- The nurse determines that the patient requires transport to the emergency department. When making the recommendation, the nurse then needs to gather information about whether or not the patient has transportation available.
- The nurse recommends an antipyretic per a decision support tool, but before instructing the mother on how to administer it, she needs to inquire whether the medication is on hand.
- The nurse or the patient deem a follow-up call necessary for reassurance or a status report. The information collected during this follow-up call represents secondary gathering. Secondary gathering often serves the purpose of confirming that it is appropriate to conclude the encounter and close the call.

Processing is the second phase of the telephone nursing process. It involves cognitive processing (discussed in-depth in Chapter 7) during which the nurse determines the nature of the problem, makes a decision about what needs to be done, and is thinking ahead to how it might be accomplished. This phase encompasses the diagnosis, goal/outcome, and planning steps of the nursing process. It is during the cognitive phase that information, knowledge, and wisdom are synthesized and applied.

Determining begins as the nurse gathers data in phase 1 and ends once the nature of the patient's problem has been identified. This process has been referred to as developing a hypothesis or determining a differential diagnosis. While determining, the nurse relates the identified problem to his or her existing knowledge and previous experience. Once determined, the nature and acuity of the problem is then verified with the patient. This cognitive processing serves as the basis for further decision making.

Decision Making is the time during which the nurse actually determines the nature and urgency of the patient's problem, based on physical *signs* and *symptoms* and psychosocial elements. Decision making includes where and when the patient should receive care. Protocols are usually available to aid decision making about the appropriate level of care. In addition to the physiologic or symptom-based concerns, the nurse also identifies other potentially important elements of care that may be needed to address the patient's problem.

Planning occurs almost from the beginning of the call. Even as the nurse is gathering information, consideration of the implications of the information and what will need to be done is taking place. This is *thinking ahead*. It is important that the nurse listens carefully, completes the assessment and diagnosis of the nature and urgency of the patient's problem, and identifies any challenges that will need to be addressed to assure that the caller will be able to carry out the plan. Knowledge of the caller, the oganization, and available community resources are usually all essential in planning interventions that will meet the patient's needs.

Output is the third and final phase of the process and includes all of the nursing interventions carried out during and at the end of the call. This phase includes explicit outputs such as recommending a *disposition* and outputs that are more implicit such as *supporting* and *collaborating*. In fact, often the primary meaningful outputs from a call come in the form of the supportive and/or collaborative strategies used to assist the patient in understanding and making good decisions regarding his or her health care problem.

Disposition includes providing a recommendation regarding the type of care to seek including when and where to be seen. For example, the disposition might be the emergency department by ambulance or private vehicle, UCC, an appointment with the doctor (now or later), home care advice, or a referral to another source.

Supporting is an implicit output which includes such actions as *reassuring, encouraging, validating, teaching,* and addressing *aftercare.* These actions occur throughout the process and are most often done automatically by the nurse in response to caller needs. It is not unusual for patients (especially the very sick ones) to presumptively know the appropriate disposition but to still call the nurse for support (perhaps in the form of "permission") to seek definitive care. For those callers who are not familiar or comfortable with the health care system, aftercare refers to advice and teaching designed specifically to increase their knowledge of and comfort with obtaining care after the call or in the future.

Collaborating is another valuable output that includes *giving options,* helping the patient with *problem solving,* and *following up* as appropriate and necessary. Similar to supporting the patient, collaboration is an implicit output that is often of greater value to the patient than the actual disposition itself. The patient, often surmising the appropriate disposition, seeks collaborative support with problem solving when care is needed but confounding factors are in the way. Consider the following example.

Susan, a nurse midwife in New England, received a call from a woman who was full term and bleeding. In response to Susan's inquiry about the amount of blood, the patient replied, "My pants are soaked, my shoes are full, and I'm standing in a 2 foot puddle of blood." While it didn't require a midwife to realize that this woman needed to go to the hospital, what was challenging about this call was that she was home alone, or essentially alone with a toddler and an infant, in the mountains of Connecticut, in the middle of a snowstorm, and the roads had not yet been cleared.

Susan marshaled her resources and stayed on the phone with the patient while her colleagues arranged childcare, called 911 for the patient, and advised the county sheriff, who got the snowplows to clear the roads. When the ambulance got the patient to the hospital, the elevator was waiting for her on the ground floor. They not only saved the patient, but they saved her baby as well. And now, every year on that baby's birthday, the mother sends Susan a card thanking her one more time for the gift of her daughter's life. Interestingly, the week before she attended a telephone triage seminar at which she related this story, Susan had received her 22nd card!

Although any call can be "just another call," the decisions we make can last a lifetime, for better or worse. This is an outstanding case of "for better." And as a post-script to this story, having been nominated by her colleagues, Susan reportedly received the New Hampshire Nurse of the Year award. Her attention to the contextual factors, not just her recognition of the patient's emergent condition, made a huge difference that day in the life of her patient and her daughter.

As discussed previously, the explicit information of "I'm bleeding" in a pregnant patient is not a difficult call in terms of identifying the nature and urgency of the patient's problem. However, as illustrated here, the challenge Susan faced was in the contextual factors, not in recognizing the significance of her signs and symptoms. This patient undoubtedly already knew the appropriate disposition. What she needed was support from and collaboration with the nurse in order to make the disposition a reality.

Closing the Call is different than hanging up the phone. Closing the call occurs after the nurse has verified the reason for the call, reviewed the recommendations, confirmed that the patient understands and is comfortable with the outcome of the call, has no further questions, and all loose ends have been addressed. For example, in closing the call, when the nurse asks the caller to "Tell me what you plan to do," the patient should be able to verbalize understanding, express the intent to comply (or not), and confirm that she has a plan and a means to carry out that plan. The nurse should also always ask the patient to confirm whether or not he or she is comfortable with the plan of care. Occasionally, in order to close the call, a follow-up call is arranged during which the nurse seeks information and confirmation (secondary gathering) that the desired outcome was met. *Note:* This follow-up call is not intended to be made in the event that the nurse or the patient is "uncomfortable" with the outcome of the call. If either party is "uncomfortable," the patient should be seen!

Influencing Factors

Several factors influence the nature of the telephone nursing process and deserve special emphasis.

Prioritization impacts the nature and length of the call. High-acuity calls will logically be shorter than low-acuity calls because of the evident nature of the complaint, the limited need for information gathering and cognitive processing, and the straightforward decision making and output.

Call complexity will likewise influence the nature of each phase of the call. Complex problems that are not readily discernable will require longer and more deliberate and comprehensive information gathering, might tax cognitive processing, and will likely require multiple output options.

Let's examine examples of low-complexity and high-complexity calls. Consider a patient complaining of extreme shortness of breath, who is wheezing and unable to speak in complete sentences. This call is not complex because of the explicit nature of the complaint and the associated objective findings (tachypnea, wheezing, and speaking in three-word phrases). In this case, the nurse would essentially limit data collection to assessment of the patient's respiratory, circulatory, and neurologic status. Cognitive processing would be occurring simultaneously with abbreviated information gathering, and the nurse would proceed directly to decision making and planning what needs to be done. The appropriate output would likely involve an emergent disposition and patient support.

On the other hand, a highly complex call, such as an elderly patient who states "I just don't feel well," replete with implicit and contextual information, would have an extended information-gathering phase. Assessment of this patient would include a significant amount of data gathering and information about the entire situation. The cognitive processing phase would likely place a significant demand on the nurse's knowledge base and clinical judgment, and the output would most likely be highly collaborative and supportive. In both of these calls, interpreting allows the nurse to "read" and relate to the patient, identify the problem and the situation, and discuss the options with the caller knowledgably.

Nurse resources also influence the telephone nursing process. Nurse resources include knowledge, past personal and professional experience and comfort level with the symptom or disease process and the telephone triage process itself. These factors can vary significantly from nurse to nurse. Since there is usually more than one "right solution" to most problems, the characteristics of the nurse influence the range of appropriate approaches to data gathering, cognitive processing, and output. Nurses with less experience, or those who are uncomfortable with the process, will be more likely to follow the decision support tool and focus on explicit information, thus providing output based on limited data. Those nurses with more experience and a higher comfort level will be more likely to listen to the caller, explore the presenting problem and situation, and adapt the output to the individual needs of the caller.

Organizational resources expand or limit intervention options and can significantly influence the telephone nursing process. Examples of relevant organizational resources include type of decision support tools and how they are used, the design of the triage encounter form, access to the patient's medical record, and the role of the physician or other provider. Additionally, the availability of resources and access to services such as provider appointments, will significantly impact the nurse's decision making. Indeed, in one study of telephone triage outcomes, 34% of the nurse errors (inappropriate dispositions) were related to lack of access to appropiate resources.[8]

Validation is an important element of successful telephone triage. Nurses need feedback to self-evaluate their practice, to address knowledge deficits, and to supplement their existing knowledge base. Formal and informal feedback make an impact, so it is important to recognize and validate positive decision making and to provide timely feedback on areas in which the nurse needs to improve. It is noteworthy that nurses frequently seek follow-up from the patient or medical record, even in cases in which the organization discourages such activity.[6] Closing the loop with feedback about the patient's outcome can be an invaluable learning activity. When it comes to the final analysis, telephone triage, with or without decision support tools, is a judgment call, and feedback about performance is critical to the professional growth of the telephone triage nurse.

Application Exercise

The concepts of interpreting, information gathering, explicit/implicit information, and influencing factors have been discussed in some depth. Let's apply those concepts to a patient scenario. As you read this example, please keep in mind that although interpreting and cognitive processing aren't mentioned at every step of the process, you can rest assured they are happening.

A patient calls with a complaint of fever and vomiting. She is requesting a suppository to stop the vomiting (information gathering). The patient history and signs and symptoms indicate the problem may be a viral gastroenteritis (determining), and the notion of an antiemetic seems appropriate to both increase the patient's comfort level and decrease the possibility of dehydration (decision making). As we think ahead, we might be wondering how we will get the suppository to her, providing the physician orders one (thinking ahead). However, let's not get ahead of ourselves...

Of course, we will need to know if the patient has any other symptoms (information gathering). We're especially concerned about pain because if the patient is vomiting, febrile, and in pain, it could represent meningitis, an acute abdomen, or pyelonephritis, depending on the location of her pain (interpreting; cognitive processing). Thus (without leading the patient), we ask for other symptoms and then more specifically, we ask "what about pain?" (information gathering).

The patient responds that she is having back pain (explicit information) but isn't concerned about it because she believes it's attributable to pulling weeds (contextual information). However, she

sounds like she's in considerable distress (interpreting, implicit information) and admits her back pain is significant, but she doesn't believe it's related to her chief complaint (information gathering: interpreting). We now have explicit information about her symptoms but implicit information that she might not be immediately compliant with a recommendation to seek care now, so our thinking ahead takes a new direction (interpreting; determining).

The decision is made that the patient needs to be seen (cognitive processing). The next questions are how, when, and where? We're no longer concerned about delivering medications to her but rather now our "thinking ahead" leads us to consider what nursing interventions will be needed to get her into the office or appropriate alternate location for an evaluation (planning). The nurse must now turn attention to what nursing support is necessary to facilitate appropriate care (output).

Looking to interpreting as an overriding element of the call, the nurse would follow the previously described process and:

- *Consider the explicit data (vomiting, fever, flank pain, pulling weeds) and implicit data (sounds to be in distress but is focused on vomiting and unconcerned about other symptoms), separating the relevant from the irrelevant, and coming up with medical information that includes flank pain accompanied by fever and vomiting.*
- *Process the information to determine the nature and urgency of the patient's problem and the implications for patient management, realizing the problem could be pyelonephritis and deciding the patient should thus be evaluated today.*
- *Translate necessary information into language the caller can understand; such as "Although it's impossible to diagnose over*

the telephone, I'm concerned you might have a kidney infection."

If the nurse recommends an immediate appointment for evaluation (disposition) and the patient says, "I'll be right there," no further information or persuasion is necessary. However, if the patient is reluctant to follow the nurse's advice, the nurse will likely continue to both gather and provide additional information (information seeking, cognitive processing, and interpreting), supporting and collaborating until the patient is convinced of the necessity of prompt evaluation. Thus, the yield is individualized care; not care that is tailored to the nurse's "style," but rather care that is individualized to the needs of the patient.

SUMMARY

The Greenberg Model provides a comprehensive look at the telephone nursing process and increases our understanding of its complexity. Consistent teaching and application of the model will reduce variations in practice and help us to provide safe care that meets the needs of our individual callers. Furthermore, the insights provided by this model should promote changes that are consistent with current evidence about telephone nursing practice. For example, current evidence shows:

- Nurses make decisions based on their knowledge, experience, judgment, and intuition.[9,10]
- Nurse decision making takes precedence over protocol advice and nurses adapt, interpret, tailor, and qualify protocol information to fit the needs of the patient.[11,12]
- The more experience and training the nurse has, the more accurate the assessment and decision making.[13,14]

- Protocols are valued by nurses as a means to augment or stimulate existing knowledge and increase their feelings of security and credibility.[15,16]

- Key aspects of telephone encounters for callers are nurse caring, listening, collaborating and communicating, and nurse ability to understand the situation and provide a solution suitable for the caller.[17,18]

Each of the three models described in this chapter highlighted the importance of nurse decision making in the practice of telephone triage. The next chapter examines an essential factor in such decision making – critical thinking.

References

1. Nelson, R. (2002). Major theories supporting health care informatics. In S.P. Englebardt & R. Nelson (Eds.), *Health care informatics: An interdisciplinary approach* (pp. 3-27). St. Louis, MO: Mosby.
2. Schleyer, R., & Beaudry, S. (2009). Data to wisdom: Informatics in telephone triage nursing practice. *AAACN Viewpoint, 31*(5), 1-5.
3. Greenberg, M.E., & Pyle, R.L. (2004). Achieving evidence-based nursing practice in ambulatory care. *AAACN Viewpoint, 26*(6), 1, 8-12.
4. Monaghan, R., Clifford, C., & McDonald, P. (2003). Seeking advice from NHS direct on common childhood complaints: Does it matter who answers the phone? *Journal of Advanced Nursing, 42*(2), 209-216.
5. O'Cathain, A., Nicholl, J., Sampson, F., Walters, S., McDonnell, A., & Munro, J. (2004). Do different types of nurses give different triage decisions in NHS direct? A mixed methods study. *Journal of Health Services Research & Policy, 9*(4), 226-233.
6. Greenberg, M.E. (2009). A comprehensive model of the process of telephone nursing. *Journal of Advanced Nursing, 65*(12), 2621-2629. doi:10.1111/j.1365-2648.2009.05132.x
7. Leprohon, J., & Patel, V. (1995). Decision-making strategies for telephone triage in emergency medical services. *Medical Decision Making, 15*(3), 240-253.
8. O'Rourke, K. M., Roddy, M., King, R., Custer, M., Sprinkle, L., & Horne, E. (2003). The impact of a nursing triage line on the use of emergency department services in a military hospital. *Military Medicine, 168*(12), 981-985.
9. Marsden, J. (1998). Decision-making in A & E by expert nurses. *Nursing Times Research, 94*(41), 62-65.
10. O'Cathain, A., Munro, J., Armstrong, I., O'Donnell, C., & Heaney, D. (2007). The effect of attitude to risk on decisions made by nurses using computerised decision support software in telephone clinical assessment: An observational study. *BMC Medical Informatics and Decision Making, 7*, 39. doi:10.1186/1472-6947-7-39.

11. Hanlon, G., Strangleman, T., Goode, J., Luff, D., O'Cathian, A., & Greatbatch, D. (2005). Knowledge, technology and nursing: The case of NHS direct. *Human Relations, 58*(2), 147-171.
12. O'Cathain, A., Sampson, F.C., Munro, J.F., Thomas, K.J., & Nicholl, J.P. (2004). Nurses' views of using computerized decision support software in NHS direct. *Journal of Advanced Nursing, 45*(3), 280-286.
13. Mayo, A.M., Chang, B.L., & Omery, A. (2002). Use of protocols and guidelines by telephone nurses. *Clinical Nursing Research, 11*(2), 204-219.
14. Valanis, B., Tanner, C., Moscato, S.R., Shapiro, S., Izumi, S., David, M., ... Mayo, A. (2003). A model for examining predictors of outcomes of telephone nursing advice. *Journal of Nursing Administration, 33*(2), 91-95.
15. Ernesäter, A., Holmström, I., & Engström, M. (2009). Telenurses' experiences of working with computerized decision support: Supporting, inhibiting and quality improving. *Journal of Advanced Nursing, 65*(5), 1074-1083. doi:10.1111/j.1365-2648.2009.04966.x
16. Purc-Stephenson, R., & Thrasher, C. (2010). Nurses' experiences with telephone triage and advice: A meta-ethnography. *Journal of Advanced Nursing, 66*(3), 482-494. doi:10.1111/j.1365-2648.2010.05275.x
17. Valanis, B.G., Gullion, C.M., Moscato, S.R., Tanner, C., Izumi, S., & Shapiro, S.E. (2007). Predicting patient follow-through on telephone nursing advice. *Clinical Nursing Research, 16*(3), 251-269.
18. Wahlberg, A.C., & Wredling, R. (2001). Telephone advice nursing – callers' experiences. *Journal of Telemedicine and Telecare, 7*(5), 272-276.

Chapter 7

Decision Making in Telephone Triage

The three models described in Chapter 6 make it abundantly clear that certain cognitive processes are essential to effective decision making in telephone triage. However, there is much more to consider about the nature of these processes. The common basis of the thought processes that lead to optimal decision making is critical thinking. This chapter therefore focuses in-depth on the nature of critical thinking, its significance for decision making, factors that facilitate and hinder the critical thinking process, and the role of critical thinking in different types of decision making.

This chapter combines research and experience to clarify critical thinking and the decision-making process in the uncertain conditions inherent in telephone triage. Although there is much more to be known, there is already a substantial body of research on the process of critical thinking in telephone triage.[1,2,3,4,5] It is clear from the existing knowledge base that the nurse's approach to critical thinking, decision making, and patient management varies, based upon the characteristics of the patient's problem and the experiences of both the nurse and the patient.[6,7,8]

In contrast to the emphasis we will be placing on critical thinking, many practice models have encouraged strict adherence to protocols for decision making in telephone triage. The conventional wisdom regarding use of decision support tools (e.g., protocols) suggests that if a nurse follows and adheres to them, (a) it will most likely prevent bad outcomes and (b) if a bad outcome does occur, compliance with the decision support tool will offer significant legal protection. We have already shown that both nursing standards and logic contradict those notions and that telephone triage is a complex process that requires critical thinking to support sound decision making. Decision support tools are valuable resources for nurses engaging in telephone triage, but they are not, and cannot be the sole basis of decision making for the telephone triage nurse.

CRITICAL THINKING

Critical thinking has been defined by the National League for Nursing Accreditation Commission as "the reasonable, reflective, responsible, and skillful thinking that is focused on deciding what to believe or do" (p. 6).[9] It is "the deliberate nonlinear process of collecting, interpreting, analyzing, drawing conclusions, presenting, and evaluating information that is both factual and belief based" (p.2).[10] Critical thinking is a complex cognitive process and much more than mere "common sense." Using critical thinking allows the nurse to identify a question (e.g., What is causing the patient's headache?), gather and analyze the relevant data (both contextual and clinical) and then determine the nature and urgency of the patient's problem and identify the necessary associated nursing interventions. Critical thinking in nursing is essential to quality nursing care.

"Being able to think critically enables the nurse to meet the needs of the patients within their context and considering their preferences; meet the needs of patients within the context of uncertainty; consider alternatives, resulting in higher quality care; and think reflectively, rather than simply accepting statements and performing tasks without significant understanding and evaluation" (p. 1).[10]

Components Supporting Critical Thinking

Good critical thinkers are confident, creative, flexible, inquisitive, intuitive, and open-minded. They understand the importance of contextual factors, and exhibit the qualities of perseverance and reflection. They have good cognitive skills and are able to analyze, adhere to standards, discriminate, seek information, think logically, predict, and apply knowledge.[10] There are five components necessary to support critical thinking: a specific knowledge base, experience, competencies, standards, and the right attitude.[11] We will discuss each of these components as they relate to telephone triage.

Specific Knowledge Base. Telephone triage nurses must have a vast clinical knowledge base. That clinical knowledge, coupled with experience and use of decision support tools, enables the nurse to consider all factors, including available patient and community resources, to individualize care. Knowledge specific to the art and science of telephone triage is also necessary to support critical thinking. Familiarity with the clinical practice perils and pearls such as the importance of erring on the side of caution, speaking directly with the patient whenever possible, and other axioms pertinent to the practice of telephone triage are elements of the specific knowledge base necessary for triage nursing. Telephone triage nurses must also have a good working knowledge of the technology they are using.

Experience. Both clinical experience and life experience are elements that enhance critical thinking abilities. Clearly the process of helping a new mother consider her options when dealing with a fussy infant is enhanced if the nurse has dealt with infants in his or her own life. Having "been there and done that" personally provides extra depth and breadth to the nurse's ability to serve as a coach and assist the patient/caller in problem solving.[12]

Although to date, no specific research has directly defined the experience necessary to support competence in telephone triage, various authors have addressed the importance of experience in the development of competence.[5,13,14] Research supports the idea that experience (both clinical and life experience) contributes to the nurse's ability to make decisions.[4,14] It is difficult to recognize a clinical entity over the telephone and understand its implications if the nurse has never encountered that particular problem in clinical practice.[5,13]

Clinical experience that is rich in both depth and breadth is also helpful because it is impossible to predict the nature of the patient's problem prior to the call. The nurse must be ready for any and all circumstances that present over the telephone. Nurses with extensive emergency department or general medical-surgical experience have often been exposed to a wide range of disease processes, providing them with experience to recognize a more diverse range of problems over the telephone. Even nurses performing triage in specialty practices would do well to be armed with varied clinical experience because of their inability to control what kinds of calls present over the telephone. For example, although a nurse might be performing telephone triage in an obstetrical/gynecological (OB/GYN) office, that does not preclude patients from calling with a variety of non-OB/GYN problems. Although it might not be the responsibility of that practice to treat a non-OB/GYN problem, it is certainly the responsibility of the RN to assess the nature and urgency of the problem and refer the patient to the appropriate level of care. Evidence suggests that nurses who are expert in a specific area make more accurate decisions on calls in that area.[4,15] Triage nurses have clearly indicated that decision making on calls/problems in which they do not consider themselves expert is enhanced by collaboration with their peers.[16,17]

In her work *From Novice to Expert,* Benner describes the continuum of Novice, Beginner, Advanced Beginner, Competent, Proficient, and Expert.[13] Characteristics of these levels of expertise are shown in Table 1. Because of the wide variety of problems that might present over the telephone and the inability to predict their complexity, it is clear that nurses who are providing telephone triage services must be able to function minimally at the level of Competent. A nurse who is only prepared to the level of Advanced Beginner might overlook the significance of seemingly obscure symptoms and thus mismanage the call.

Table 1.
Nurse Decision-Making Characteristics[13,18]

Experience	Nurse Decision-Making Characteristics
Novice to Advanced Beginner 2-3 years	Rule-governed behavior Reactive: Collects cues to determine why the problem occurred Uses smaller range of cues and a linear pattern Unable to see whole Inflexible Need support Can recognize and use recurring meaningful components Difficulty prioritizing
Competent to Expert More than 3 years	Recognizes and considers individual patient differences Proactive: Thinks ahead and collects cues to identify problem before it occurs Uses greater number, broader range, and more complex patterns of cues Perceives and understands context More holistic understanding improves decision making Learns from experiences what to expect in certain situations and how to modify plans Has intuitive grasp of clinical situations Performance is fluid, flexible, and highly proficient

An important consideration in this body of work is the realization that a nurse might be functioning as an Expert in one clinical area but able to function only at the level of Beginner in a new clinical area. Time and experience are necessary to develop full competence in a new area of clinical practice, so adequate orientation and training are also key to a successful transition from one clinical area to another, or from face-to-face nursing to nursing over the telephone.

Competency. The telephone triage nurse must possess specific competencies in order to provide appropriate care over the telephone. These competencies represent a specialized skill set and include, but are certainly not limited to, the ability to assess patients over the telephone, excellent communication and collaboration skills, the capacity to function autonomously, use of clinical judgment, appropriate utilization of decision support tools, and effective use of technology. Measurement of competency remains somewhat nebulous and difficult to pin down, but focus on performance in these areas can give good insight into how well a nurse will provide care over the telephone.

Standards. Several types of standards exist and are discussed elsewhere in this book. Both intellectual and professional standards are necessary to support critical thinking. Intellectual standards include clarity, precision, specificity, accuracy, relevancy, plausibility, consistency, logicality, depth, broadness, completeness, significance, adequacy, and fairness.[11] Professional standards for which the competent telephone triage nurse must have a good working knowledge include:

- Basic standards of professional practice, such as use of the nursing process.
- Professional standards for the practice of nursing over the telephone such as those developed by American Academy of Ambulatory Care Nursing[19] and the American Nurses Association.[20]
- Regulatory standards as promulgated by the state boards of nursing which provide the legal structure and guidance for the practice of nursing.
- Accreditation standards, promulgated by a variety of accrediting bodies, may potentially influence the practice of telephone triage. Specifically, URAC (also known as the American Accreditation Healthcare Commission) accredits call centers on a voluntary basis and has standards that can significantly impact practice.
- Organizational policies directing the practice of telephone triage.

The policies and procedures of the organization that can influence decision making are addressed in-depth in Chapters 14 and 15. However, two policies are of special significance to decision making in telephone triage. These are policies regarding call time expectations and availability of resources. It is important to note that researchers looking at time pressure, nurse experience, and decision making, concluded that time pressure negatively impacts decision performance.[21,22] Likewise, lack of organizational resources hinders decision making in telephone triage. Multiple studies have found that factors such as feedback, education, and availability of appointments will improve nurse decision making over the telephone, whereas deficits in such resources hamper it.[23,24,25]

Attitude. Having the right attitude about the practice is essential to critical thinking. Specific attitudes associated with critical thinking include confidence, perseverance, independence, creativity, fairness, curiosity, responsibility, integrity, risk taking, humility, and discipline.[11] The nurse who recognizes telephone triage as professional nursing practice and assumes the role of patient advocate in the context of the patient's own value system will likely make decisions that are in the patient's best interest. Some nurses have worked in cultures that have skewed their view of telephone triage, and occasionally a paradigm shift, as discussed in Chapter 3, is in order. It is important for the nurse to have the right idea of what his or her job is as a telephone triage nurse. For example, the nurse who believes her role is to "keep patients out" might not fully utilize critical thinking, thereby allowing organizational pressures to supersede the patient's needs.

CRITICAL THINKING AND TELEPHONE TRIAGE

The nursing process, previously discussed in Chapter 4, provides a basis for decision making that is grounded in critical thinking. With the nursing process, each step sequentially builds upon the last as the nurse makes informed decisions, makes recommendations for patient management, and works with the patient to make those recommendations a reality. Research applicable to decision making in telephone triage provides considerable insight into the process we utilize in making a decision. The models and theories presented here reflect both the capabilities and the responsibilities of the registered nurse in the practice of nursing over the telephone.

The Greenberg Model and Critical Thinking

Turner notes "critical thinking in nursing is a purposeful, self-regulatory judgment associated in some way with clinical decision making, diagnostic reasoning, the nursing process, clinical judgment, and problem solving. It is characterized by analysis, reasoning, inference, interpretation, knowledge, and open-mindedness. It requires knowledge of the area about which one is thinking and results in safe, competent practice and improved decision making, clinical judgments, and problem solving" (p. 276).[26]

Accordingly, critical thinking is inherent in the process of telephone triage as specified in the Greenberg Model of Care Delivery in Telephone Nursing Practice, dicussed at length in Chapter 6.

The *Information Gathering* phase requires active analysis, interpretation, and decision making regarding what information to collect, what information offered by the caller is relevant, and what follow-up information is necessary. During the call the nurse attends to and incorporates explicit information with the implicit information collected during the interview. Implicit information such as tone of voice, background noises, respiratory efforts, and contextual factors such as availability of resources influence the nurse's development of a hypothesis. Accurate interpretation of these cues and ultimately of the patient's needs, concerns, and situation depends on critical thinking.

The *Processing* phase is based exclusively on critical thinking and analysis of the data collected during Information Gathering. Having collected the relevant data and developed a hypothesis, the nurse utilizes processes of relating, verifying, comparing, and ruling out to identify the problem(s) and determine urgency. In planning and thinking ahead, the nurse is considering possible options, predicting outcomes, and weighing potential consequences. The ability to accurately match the individual problem, the context, and the resources with the right decision support tool and reach a decision (disposition) is dependent upon the nurse's critical thinking ability.[14,27,28]

Based on the analysis, in the *Output Phase* the nurse delivers the interventions required to meet the needs of the individual patient. The nurse recommends the appropriate disposition and provides support and collaboration as necessary to assist the patient in achieving the desired outcome.

Each step of the process requires critical thinking and interpretation. Separating relevant from irrelevant information and processing that information to determine the implications for patient management involve critical thinking. Even after the nurse has decided what needs to be done, there is a complex decision-making process required to determine how it will be done.[29,30] The fruits of that process are revealed as the nurse communicates with the caller, translating the necessary medical information into language the caller can understand. This process will vary from patient to patient, yielding in the final analysis, individualized care.

Research on nurse decision making suggests critical thinking and the resultant decision are dependent on the nurse-patient interaction, collaboration, and attention to psychosocial variables such as mood, context, and culture.[30] As previously discussed in Chapter 6, triage decision making must be based on more than clinical evidence and generalizations. Clinical context and patient preferences must be considered as well. Critical thinking is the element that determines the best balance among these three factors. All of these elements influence the experienced telephone triage nurse in making decisions that are right for each individual patient. This emphasizes the fact that telephone triage must be performed by specially trained, experienced RNs who utilize critical thinking, which then translates to the application of clinical knowledge and professional judgment.

Critical Thinking and the Use of Decision Support Tools

While critical thinking is essential for professional practice in telephone triage, the use of decision support tools presently represents the standard of care. A variety of commercially developed and home-grown decision support tools exist to help standardize practice, decrease ambiguity in decision making, and guide the nurse in performing an adequate assessment. For years there has been active debate over the meaning of the various terms used to describe decision support tools. "Guidelines," "protocols," "algorithms," and occasionally "standing orders" are terms that have been assigned differing meanings, based on their intended use. We, however, do not make a distinction among these various tools because their intent is uniformly to provide "decision support." Thus, we use the term "decision support tool" to refer to any and all of these products. References to "protocols" or "guidelines" in this book are synonyms for "decision support tools" and vice versa.

Decision support tools suggest assessment parameters and accompanying dispositions to guide the nurse in assuring collection of a relevant history and suggesting an appropriate disposition. However, although helpful, without deliberate and thoughtful use, which includes individualization of care, decision support tools can become a liability by precluding or interfering with the process of critical thinking.

To illustrate the proper use of decision support tools and the associated critical thinking, we will examine a simulated call from a mother complaining that her child has a fever.

After opening the call and establishing rapport with the mother, the nurse investigates the reason for the call. The mother states that her child has a fever and is fussy.

The first order of business is to rule out (or identify) any potentially life-threatening problems, so the nurse will interview the mother to determine the child's age and assess his airway, breathing, activity level, hydration status, temperature, and neurological status. Specifically, the nurse might ask if the child is breathing ok,

handling secretions (not drooling), if he is blue or dusky around his lips, if he has had any seizure activity, and if he is making good eye contact and behaving normally (ruling out lethargy). In assessing the child's airway, the nurse should ask the mother to hold the phone near the child so the nurse may listen to his breathing, noting stridor, tachypnea, or noisy breathing that might indicate a partial airway obstruction.

The nurse notes that the child is 2 years old and thus over 3 months of age, eliminating the need for an immediate ED evaluation to rule out sepsis in a newborn (protocol parameter). The mother reports his temperature is 102, so the nurse inquires how it was measured and learns that the mother took an axillary temperature. Many nurses might be tempted to move directly to and rely on the fever protocol at this point, but there's more assessment to do first.

Ideally, the nurse will ask the mother to tell her what's going on with her child, inviting her to share all of the information she feels is relevant, including the purpose of the call (whether she wants home care advice, an appointment, or reassurance that ED is not indicated). The nurse should listen quietly during this period, listening for relevant information and making note of comments that need additional clarification. Active listening and analysis of the information received reflects critical thinking. In most cases, it is best if the nurse doesn't interrupt the mother while she tells her story. Although the nurse already knows that the child is febrile and the mother is concerned about it, other findings or circumstances of significance might surface while the mother is providing additional history.

While the nurse is actively listening to the mother, he or she will listen for references to respiratory symptoms, signs of dehydration, and the child's general activity level. Is he making good eye contact, eating and drinking normally, playing normally, or displaying symptoms of concern? The nurse will also listen for the degree of anxiety or distress on the part of the mother.

After the mother finishes her story, with or without the use of the protocol, the nurse will seek additional information, utilizing techniques such as paraphrasing what the mother has said, restating to confirm significant findings, and exploring other information that might require clarification. The nurse will probe to explore areas of concern in order to determine the nature and extent of the child's problem. For example, if the mother states the child has a cough, the nurse will explore further to determine if it is a productive or dry cough, the color of the sputum if any, and whether the cough is interfering with the child's sleep. Additionally, based on familiarity with the protocol assessment parameters, the nurse will ask pointed questions to rule out or identify problems the mother had not previously mentioned. For example, the nurse might ask if the child has a rash. If so, the mother will be guided in describing the rash in detail, allowing the nurse to mentally visualize the child's rash. The nurse will ask if the child has been exposed to any known illnesses within the past few days, started any new drugs, traveled, been exposed to new detergents, perfumes, lotions, and other possible sources of allergy or contact dermatitis.

The telephone triage nurse will continue data collection, utilizing techniques such as connecting, questioning, redirecting, getting to know, investigating, focusing, clarifying, comparing, and ruling out. Simultaneously, using critical thinking, the nurse will be processing and verifying the information in an effort to de-

termine the nature and urgency of the problem, relating reported symptoms to known disease patterns. Having completed the bulk of data collection, based on signs and symptoms and other identified caller needs, the nurse will refer to the decision support tool to identify any information that might have been overlooked and to make a decision about what needs to be done, thinking ahead to an appropriate plan of care.

Finally, considering context and patient preference and utilizing the decision support tool, tempered by clinical judgment, the nurse will help the mother determine the appropriate disposition, providing guidance and support in the form of reassurance, encouragement, and validation. The nurse will provide necessary teaching and collaborate with the mother by providing options as outlined in the decision support tool, and/or as indicated by the patient's individual circumstances. For example, if acetaminophen is the antipyretic recommended by the protocol, but the mother only has pediatric ibuprofen in her medicine cabinet, the nurse will assist the mother in problem solving, seeking an order for ibuprofen if necessary to individualize alternative care for the patient. Once again utilizing guidance provided by the decision support tool, the nurse might explain other measures which need to be taken to help lower the child's fever. Together, the nurse and the mother will develop a plan for follow-up to assure that the child's condition is improving and that the mother is comfortable with the outcome of the call. If the mother seems uncomfortable with the recommended disposition, the nurse will explore possible reasons for this discomfort, taking steps to either adjust the disposition and/or reassure the mother in order to improve her level of comfort with the plan of care.

If, on the other hand, the disposition, and education about aftercare, recommended by the decision support tool is for the mother to seek a medical evaluation, based on contextual circumstances and the mother's preference, the nurse will exercise his or her best judgment in guiding the mother to the appropriate level of care. Time of day, distance from care, and other contextual factors will be considered in developing an individualized plan of care. Likewise, other potentially confounding circumstances such as the presence of other small children in need of childcare in the home, lack of transportation, or lack of motivation or understanding on the part of the mother will be incorporated into the nurse's planning.

Examining this scenario, it is clear that critical thinking and advanced problem solving are required throughout the encounter even though the actions of the nurse are in part guided by a well-developed decision support tool.

Factors That Influence Decision Making

In watching nurses make decisions, various themes begin to surface. Two will be discussed here: The first from personal observation and the second based on a study of how experienced nurses reach decisions.[1]

"Devloping a Hunch." Although cautioned about jumping to a conclusion, it has been observed that nurses frequently develop "first hunches" regarding the nature of their patient's problem. Although a prudent nurse would never act on a first hunch, exploration of the process at hand might provide food for thought for nurses engaged in the practice of telephone triage. An exercise frequently conducted in telephone triage seminars is to give the participants a chief complaint and then challenge them to report what immediately pops into their minds as the possible etiology of the problem. The nurses are not given an opportunity to ask questions but rather encouraged to allow their thinking to flow freely. The chief complaint most often employed is a relatively calm adult female voice announcing, "My back hurts." Participants are asked to write their first hunch and then to reflect on why they settled on that particular hunch rather than something else. Several factors have been identified that influence the nurse's decision making.

Implicit Information such as the Patient's Age, Gender, Affect, and Respirations. Although in this exercise the nurses are not given an opportunity to ask questions, they are allowed to use all of the information they are given. While many are not conscious of any information other than "my back hurts," they usually recognize and act upon the implicit information provided. For example, common hunches include urinary tract infection, labor, and gall bladder disease, all of which are gender specific for the test patient. Notably, most hunches are of relatively low acuity, with a paucity of hunches consisting of major trauma or immediately life-threatening presentations. This is probably because, whether consciously or unconsciously, the nurses take into consideration the patient's affect, tone of voice, respiratory efforts, and the like. For example, if instead of simply saying in a relatively undistressed voice, "My back hurts," the patient gasped the same words in one or two-word phrases and in obvious distress, the nurses most likely would have first hunches that were of high acuity such as a pulmonary embolism (PE) or severe trauma.

The Nurse's Past Clinical and Personal Experience. Previous clinical experience also guides nurses' first hunches. For example, oncology nurses might suggest bone metastasis. Nurses who work in pain clinics might suggest drug-seeking behavior. Labor and delivery (L&D) nurses might consider labor, while nurses from emergency departments or intensive care units might think of myocardial infarction (MI). Gastroenterology nurses often think gall bladder disease, and so forth. Personal experience also influences nurse's thinking. For example, nurses who have an initial hunch of musculoskeletal back pain, may be experiencing that problem themselves. Occasionally nurses will cite a personal history of kidney stones as the reason for that hunch. And combining clinical and personal experience, nurses often first think of clinical entities they have seen a good deal of recently. For example, during flu season, nurses are more likely to think of the aching associated with influenza than during times that flu is rare.

The Nurse's Tendency to Think Most-Common vs. Worst-Possible. It has been observed that nurses often cite "most-common" as the basis for their first hunch. For example, many nurses will suggest musculoskeletal pain because, among many populations such as the military, muscle strain is the most-common cause they see of back pain. Conversely, some nurses are "worst-possible" thinkers, immediately jumping to an abdominal aortic aneurysm (AAA) or PE when they hear the words "back pain." Based on experience, it appears that most nurses are "most-common" thinkers. This might be because we've been taught that when we hear hoof beats, we should look for horses, not zebras or because we more often see "most-common" presentations than those that would fall into the category of "worst-possible."

Nevertheless, nurses who have worked in high-acuity areas have been conditioned to think "worst-possible" because of the frequency with which they have seen it. However, regardless of whether a most-common or worst-possible thinker, nurses can discipline themselves to go against their natural instinct. An illustration of this principle would be that if you were asked to write your name, you would most likely pick up a pen and write your name with your dominant hand. In other words, you would do what came naturally to you. However, if instructed to do so, you could also write your name with your non-dominant hand, but it would take more deliberate thought. And it might be a mess. But the good news is that the more you practice writing with your non-dominant hand, the better you will likely be able to do it. The same principles apply in challenging nurses to think in ways that are contrary to their natural instincts. We can learn to think worst possible, but it might take deliberate intent. Clearly, the more that "most-common" thinkers discipline themselves to think "worst-possible," the more adept we will become at taking that approach.

Discussion. While interesting, what is the clinical application of this information, and more importantly, what is the value of this exercise? Is it designed to teach nurses to jump to a conclusion? Certainly not! Its purpose is to demonstrate that most if not all of us are capable of almost unconsciously jumping to a conclusion whether we intend to or not. While decision making in telephone triage must be based upon much more than a hunch, there is nothing wrong with developing an initial hunch. . . unless you do it and are unaware that you have done so. The value of this exercise is to help the reader reflect upon the various factors that might lead him or her to unknowingly jump to a conclusion and act preemptively without first going through a scientific thought process.

Also, it is helpful to realize that there are factors, perhaps beyond your conscious control, which influence your decision making. Each of these examples might be a double-edged sword. For example, just because a patient sounds calm doesn't mean he or she isn't experiencing a high-acuity problem. Consider past clinical experience; while it's unlikely that an L&D nurse will overlook the possibility of labor, there are a number of other unrelated problems that he or she might not consider. The same goes with past personal experience. If you had a typical case of meningitis, when talking to a patient, you might be looking for a typical presentation. However, if your meningitis was associated with atypical symptoms, your personal experience might serve to obscure your recognition of the patient's problem. And finally, knowing whether you are naturally a "most-common" or "worst-possible" thinker can serve you well in your practice of telephone triage. Because of the nature of the practice, telephone triage requires that the sound of hoof beats elicit thoughts of zebras rather than common horses. It is not prudent to spend time ruling out muscle strain or a urinary tract infection while your patient is experiencing a life-threatening emergency such as an MI or a PE. While the incidence of worst-possible presentations will be few and far between, it is likely that they will occasionally be missed unless the nurse is actively looking for them. This thought process explains the adage that "If you don't see it often, you often don't see it." Telephone triage nurses must discipline themselves to consider and look for worst-possible presentations, or it is likely that they will miss them when they do come along.

"Playing the Odds." Edwards found that in making a disposition, nurses considered what they thought was most likely going on with the patient, weighing it against the worst possible concern. They then considered the risk to the patient, and in determining the proper referral resource, weighed the risk against appropriate utilization of resources.[1] For example, the patient complaining of "indigestion" most likely has indigestion, but the potential always exists that his complaint might represent ischemic chest pain.

In an effort to conserve resources, telephone triage nurses could be tempted to "play the odds" when making decisions, opting to act on the most likely cause of the problem (in this case, indigestion). However, the nurse needs to be hypervigilant and exercise caution to rule out a myocardial etiology before recommending a lower-acuity disposition. Often, when the picture is not absolutely clear, the telephone triage nurse might "hedge his or her bets," taking a somewhat tentative approach without fully committing one way or another. In other words, instead of taking definitive action, the nurse might make a disposition that is *most likely* to be appropriate.

Let's consider a case of the 42-year-old man complaining of "indigestion" following a night of heavy beer drinking and a breakfast of cold pizza. He admits to being overweight and sedentary but states that he quit smoking 3 or 4 years ago and has been trying to improve his diet. He admits to a "touch of borderline high blood pressure" which he controls with diet and exercise. He acknowledges some slight shortness of breath and diaphoresis, but he doesn't feel that this is of significance since he has been performing manual labor outdoors in extreme heat. His family history is non-contributory.

The nurse, after careful consideration, draws the conclusion that the patient is most likely experiencing gastroesophageal reflux or gastritis, but is aware this type of ambiguous presentation might be cardiac in origin. The nurse makes the decision that the patient needs to be evaluated to rule out a cardiac event. But where? This patient is likely to be reluctant to call an ambulance for a "simple case of indigestion," and the nurse might be reluctant to force the issue because of the ambiguity of the situation. Further analysis reveals that possible dispositions in this case might be (a) home care with an antacid, (b) evaluation in the office, (c) emergency department visit via private vehicle, or (d) 911 to the nearest emergency department. Let's analyze each option.

Home treatment would be reasonable if the nurse has been able to comfortably rule out a myocardial infarction (MI). Of course, with the ambiguity of this situation as described, it would be difficult if not impossible to do so. And then there's the question of scope of practice and what over-the-counter measures might be within the purview of the RN (see Chapter 5 for more information on this topic).

If unable to rule out an MI over the phone, it is possible that the nurse's first impulse would be to refer the patient to his provider's office for a today appointment. During his office visit, it is likely that an EKG would be performed and cardiac enzymes would be drawn. However, it is known that EKG changes and enzyme elevations associated with an MI may be delayed, and therefore even a normal EKG and enzymes wouldn't definitively rule-out a cardiac etiology. So the nurse, in spite of his or her best intentions, might have unwittingly sent the patient with an acute MI to an office, certainly a less-than-ideal setting to treat such an emergency.

A third option would be to recommend evaluation in the emergency department (ED). To avoid excessive cost, the nurse might be tempted (with encouragement from the patient) to recommend that the patient have another adult drive him to the hospital. Of course, a risk associated with this mode of transport would be that if the patient is having an MI, he might suffer a cardiac arrest en route, with predictably disastrous consequences.

A final option might be to refer the patient to the ED via EMS, a safe but potentially costly disposition, particularly if the diagnosis turns out to be indigestion. This is where the nurse must be clear about the desired outcome. If the goal is to *rule out* an MI, there's only one appropriate place to send him and only one appropriate mode of transportation: that is via 911 to the ED.

With the clarity this thought sequence offers, one might wonder why nurses would even consider an office visit or to permit the patient to be transported to the hospital by private vehicle. Some insight might be gained by reviewing the work of Edwards[1] in which he studied the decision making processes of telephone triage nurses. He found that in determining a disposition, the nurses in his study identified the most likely cause of the patient's problem, weighed the worst possible against the most probable etiology, assessed the risk to the patient, and balanced that risk against appropriate utilization of resources. He also identified the fact that in making triage decisions in this category, the nurses often considered their own vulnerability, perhaps being afraid of being "wrong."

So given that referring the patient to the clinic or to the hospital by private vehicle might both predictably result in an unfavorable outcome, it is worthwhile to examine why nurses might select those options. Giving these thought processes careful consideration, it is possible that the nurse might be afraid of being "wrong" by over or under-referring the patient. Obviously, if the nurse sends the patient to the hospital via 911, everyone knows what she is thinking and if she's wrong, she's *really* wrong. And if the nurse leaves the patient at home to take an antacid, her thinking is obvious, and again, if she's wrong, she's *really* wrong. But if she sends the patient to the clinic or to the hospital via private vehicle, her conclusion about the nature of the patient's problem isn't so obvious. And she might justify that if she's wrong, she's just a *little* wrong. However, if the patient suffers an adverse outcome because the nurse hedged her bets, dead is dead whether it occurs at home, in the office, or in the car.

Understanding the nurse's potential concern about "getting it wrong," it's easier to see why the nurse might take a more "middle of the road" approach. However, the telephone triage nurse must at all times keep in mind that the safety of his or her patient must always supersede the nurse's fear of being wrong. This concept, being of great potential significance, will be discussed further later in this chapter.

In looking at the previously discussed dispositions, it becomes clear that if the nurse is unable to comfortably rule out an MI, there's only one appropriate place to send the patient and only one appropriate mode of transport that will assure the patient the best possible outcome. That would be via EMS to the closest ED. Taken to an extreme, this notion could potentially result in a knee-jerk response to send every patient with indigestion or a similarly ambiguous chief complaint to the emergency department via ambulance. This, of course, would not be an appropriate approach to triage (in fact, it would be no triage at all).

This is where critical thinking comes in! Herein lies another reason telephone triage must be performed by experienced RNs with specialized training. While it is not the responsibility of the RN to diagnose the etiology of the patient's symptoms, the nurse must act prudently by ruling out life-threatening emergencies before assigning a disposition consistent with a lower-acuity problem. In addition to critical thinking, telephone triage nurses utilize decision support tools that are designed to guide the nurse in consideration of the worst-case scenario before settling on a problem of lesser concern. This approach, coupled with erring on the side of caution, dramatically increases the likelihood that a patient will be given a disposition that will protect him from a bad outcome. The primary point of this exercise is that the nurse must make a decision about what he or she thinks is (or isn't) the patient's problem, and then take the appropriate action.

The problem with the alternative approach is that it results in "playing the odds" with a patient's life. Although the "odds" of the patient depicted here having an MI are slim, if he is indeed having an MI, then he is 100% having an MI. The following story illustrates the risk in "playing the odds."

On one particular occasion of a cardiologist referring his patient for bypass surgery, the patient asked, "So, Doc, what are my odds?" to which the cardiologist replied "100%." The patient said, "No, I mean, what are the odds that I will live or die in surgery?" and the cardiologist again replied "100%." The frustrated patient then asked, "So do you think I'm going to live or die?" and the cardiologist succinctly replied "Yes."

As a patient advocate, the RN in the office approached the cardiologist and indignantly inquired, "For heaven's sake, why are you playing these word games? Why don't you just answer the man's question? You know what he wants to know!"

The wise physician replied, "You're right. He wants to know what is going to happen to him. ***He doesn't really care about the 'odds.' I believe he will likely survive the surgery and wouldn't be recommending it if I didn't, but only God knows which way that***

pendulum will swing. There are very few things in medicine where we don't get a second chance. But once I've given a patient false reassurance in the form of an inflated percentage, if he dies on the table, it's too late to explain that even with a 99% survival rate, 1 person out of 100 will die, and that one might be him. Simply put, I'm not going to play the odds with a patient's life! He's either going to survive or he isn't. Thus his odds are 100%."

The moral to this story is that triage is a practice of *exclusion*. The RN must utilize the process of elimination in identifying what is *not* going on with the patient before deciding to follow a course of action based on a lower acuity. In conjunction with the patient's story, decision support tools are excellent adjuncts to the application of clinical judgment. The RN, using all available resources including education, experience, critical thinking, intuition, and decision support tools, will evaluate the situation, ruling out possibilities by starting with the worst possible problems and then take action at the point that it is no longer possible to rule out the next most significant potential problems. The prudent nurse must keep in mind that statistics don't apply to *individuals*. They apply to *populations!* Regardless of how remote the possibility, if the possibility does exist, it is impossible to predict which patient will be the exception and which will be the rule. Because telephone triage nurses are not equipped with crystal balls, perhaps the most important guiding principle would be the Golden Rule. Each nurse should triage every patient as if he or she were the nurse's parent, spouse, sibling, child, or very best friend. Often there are no second chances to "get it right."

Types of Decision Making

A study examined decision making by RNs who were doing EMS dispatch in Ontario, Canada.[5] While these circumstances are not specifically telephone triage, the study did involve RNs making triage decisions over the telephone in conditions of uncertainty, and multiple parallels may be drawn. Although critical thinking, appropriate use of decision support tools, and caution are common elements to all telephone triage decision making, an important finding of this study was that the specific decision-making approach used by the nurse will vary, based on the nature of the patient's problem.

In looking at how expert nurses make decisions in uncertain conditions, Leprohon and Patel identified three types of decision making based on three types of problems.[5] Nurses utilize different approaches and decision making processes for patients with each problem type, and thus to provide clarity, each type of problem is illustrated in Table 2.

Table 2.
Decision Making in Conditions of Uncertainty[5]

Characteristic	EMERGENT *Life Threatening* Pattern Recognition Immediate Response (e.g., Airway Compromise/Severe Dyspnea)	URGENT *Potentially Life Threatening* Focused Limited Problem Solving (e.g., Abdominal Pain/Headache)	NON-URGENT *Not Life Threatening* Deliberative Deliberate Problem Solving (e.g., Minor/Vague/ Chronic)
Acuity/Urgency	High	Moderate	Low
Accuracy	Perfect	Highest % of error	Middle
Timing	Shortest (<2 min 93% of time)	Longer	Longest
Trigger	Symptoms only	Hypothesis (R/O diagnosis)	Whole situation
Process	Little deliberation or problem solving	Information seeking Clarifying	Options/Alternatives Negotiation
Comment	Rules of thumb Intuition/Gut	Most complex Greatest demand on knowledge base	Much reasoning Holistic

Adapted from Leprohon and Patel (1995).

Pattern Recognition Decision Making. Patients in this category are experiencing life-threatening emergencies. These calls are short, accuracy in decision making is excellent, and there is little deliberation or problem solving regarding the nature of the call because the disposition is made on the basis of symptoms alone.[5] This category is called "pattern recognition" because the primary decision-making process used here is almost intuitive and requires little conscious thought for the experienced nurse. The pattern recognized for patients in this category would be problems with airway, breathing, circulation, or neurological deficit (ABCD) such as airway obstruction, hemorrhage, or shock. Severe pain and psychiatric emergencies would also fall into this category.

An example of this type of patient would be someone gasping in two-word phrases, "I can't catch my breath!" The "pattern" recognized in this case would be one of respiratory distress. Because these patients are experiencing immediate life-threatening problems, they will often be triaged directly to the ED via emergency ambulance. The triage category assigned to these patients will be Emergent/Immediate. Much of the information collected from this category of patient will be explicit in nature[2] and, generally speaking, documentation for these calls will be limited to the information necessary to support the emergent disposition.

Focused Decision Making. Focused decision making is utilized for patients with problems that are *potentially* life threatening. Therefore, patients in this category have specific problems which must be targeted and evaluated closely by the telephone triage nurse. These calls focus on the problem at hand, with the primary goal of determining where the patient should be seen and how quickly. The assessment will be longer than that seen with Pattern Recognition because the nurse must develop a hypothesis regarding the nature of the patient's problem before arriving at a disposition.[5,31] It was noted that this is the category in which the most errors are made, an unfortunate observation discussed further below.

An example of this patient type would be a woman who calls with persistent abdominal pain of several hours. The information collected from patients in this category will be both explicit and implicit. While most of these patients will receive a same-day appointment, or will certainly be seen within 24 hours, documentation should justify why the patient was not triaged as emergent or non-urgent and include other relevant information to facilitate collaboration and communication.

Deliberative Decision Making. Patients requiring deliberative decision making have problems that are often either obscure or otherwise very complicated. An example of this patient type might be the patient who calls complaining of an uncomplicated rash of 3 days duration. This is the category of patients with problems considered to be non-life threatening.[5]

Home care is often recommended for patients in this category, and if given an appointment, they are likely seen routinely. The urgency and acuity of these problems is the lowest of the three types: non-urgent. However, this is the category for which the nurse must collect the greatest amount of information, much of it being implicit. Paradoxically this is the patient with whom the nurse will often spend the longest time on the phone and will consequently do the greatest amount of documentation.[5]

Comparison of Different Call Types

Acuity/Urgency. As discussed previously, callers in the *emergent* (pattern recognition) category are of high acuity and urgency, presenting with life, limb, and vision-threatening problems. Those in the *urgent* (focused) category will generally represent patients who need to be seen within 24 hours, and callers in the *non-urgent* (deliberative) category will often benefit from routine or home care.

Accuracy in Decision Making and Thought Processes Utilized. Decision making in the *emergent* (pattern recognition) category was observed to be accurate 100% of the time.[5] The nurses relied heavily on experience and rules of thumb, or heuristics, in making these decisions, doing little sophisticated problem solving, due to the explicit nature of these problems. Previous studies have had similar findings.[32,33]

As mentioned previously, an important observation about *urgent* (focused) decision making is that this is the category in which the most errors are made,[5] a worrisome finding since these patients have potentially life-threatening problems. Previous studies have shown similar findings; for example, there are more frequent errors in decision making with increased number of cues, information complexity, or information non-relevance.[30] Several explanations can be hypothesized.

- *Failure to consider all calls life-threatening until proven otherwise.* This approach could cause the nurse to overlook the potentially life-threatening nature of the patient's call.
- *Failure to err on the side of caution.* The trigger for action with these calls is development of a hypothesis, a hunch, or a differential diagnosis.[5] Nurses who act on their hunches, but fail to err on the side of caution, risk delay in treatment for patients with potentially life-threatening problems.
- *Fear of being wrong.* As mentioned previously, Edwards identified fear of their own vulnerability as being a factor that impacts nurses' decision making.[1] The nurse, fearing retribution or ridicule for "overreacting," might be hesitant to send patients to the hospital unless the indications are clear-cut. Telephone triage nurses must have sufficient self-confidence and ego-strength to withstand criticism associated with erring on the side of caution.

- *Knowledge deficit.* This is the category which requires the most complex decision making, placing the greatest demand on the nurse's knowledge base.[5] For this reason, it is imperative that telephone triage nurses possess knowledge and experience that is extensive in both depth and breadth. With this category of patients, knowledge deficits could result in disastrous outcomes. Conscientious and consistent use of decision support tools will help supplement knowledge deficits and guide the nurse in making decisions when they are less than clear-cut.

Considering every call life-threatening until proven otherwise, erring on the side of caution, and judicious use of decision support tools will help prevent undesirable outcomes in patients who fall into the urgent category. It should be noted, however, that when nurses do appropriately err on the side of caution, it will occasionally result in referral of patients who *in retrospect* did not require urgent treatment. Those who do not understand the role of the triage nurse might regard these referrals as "inappropriate," when in fact, this is not the case. Telephone triage nurses, and those who work with them, must become comfortable with the notion that "crying wolf" in this context is often a patient safety measure and not a sign of "overreacting."

Accuracy in decision making for *non-urgent* (deliberative) problem solving is mid-range,[5] probably because the amount of information that must be collected and analyzed to make an accurate decision is significant. The nurse also relies heavily on implicit information in assessment of these patients,[2] so excellent listening and communication skills are essential.

Trigger for Action. The trigger for action is significantly different among the three types of decision making. In the *emergent* (pattern recognition) category, the trigger is symptoms alone. The ABCD problems are frequently so severe that the underlying cause of the symptoms is largely irrelevant and the nurse relies heavily on explicit information indicating respiratory, circulatory, neurological, or psychiatric emergencies.

Another more controversial characteristic specific to *urgent* (focused) decision making is the finding that nurses do base their decisions on development of a hypothesis[5] or a "working diagnosis" (p. 90).[31] Even though it is clearly impossible (and outside of the nurse's scope of practice) to *diagnose* the cause of the patient's pain over the telephone, nurses often do *think diagnostically.* While decision support tools are very helpful in decision making for these patients, it is unlikely that the nurse will act prior to forming that hypothesis or working diagnosis. For this reason among others (including the fact that this is a category in which the nurse is most likely to err), it is imperative that the nurse always err on the side of caution, regardless of the formulated hypothesis.

The trigger in *non-urgent* (deliberative) decision making is the entire situation.[5] This is often the category of patient for whom the statement, "If they don't need an appointment, they need *something*" will apply.

Timing/Anticipated Call Length. In today's health care environment, concern for cost effectiveness and efficiency is essential, often resulting in monitoring of call length. However, it was observed that emergent calls were managed in less than 2 minutes 93% of the time, urgent calls took longer, and non-urgent calls resulted in the longest call lengths.[5] This information clearly illustrates that the length of time a nurse is on the telephone is usually far more dependent upon the nature of the patient's problem and his or her ability to articulate that problem than any particular skill on the part of the nurse. While call length is a parameter frequently tracked for overall program evaluation and is important information used to predict staffing needs, it is essential that the primary focus be on quality of care rather than on call length. Since telephone triage is a high-risk practice, undue emphasis on call length can be counterproductive and even dangerous.

Likewise, it is interesting to note that the greatest amount of time is spent on deliberative decision making, and thus on the lowest-acuity patients. It may seem paradoxical that our greatest resources would be spent on our least "sick" patients. However, while Pattern Recognition patients are often seen in the ED and Focused decisions result in urgent appointments, the patients in the non-urgent or the deliberative decision making categories will often receive the majority of their care directly from the triage nurse. Thus, the nurse must spend adequate time to assess, plan, facilitate continuity of care, and develop a plan for evaluation of the effectiveness of the care delivered.

Approach to Collaborative Planning. The approach to collaborative planning can vary somewhat with patients in each of these categories. With patients who have life-threatening problems, there is often little, if any, room for negotiation. With patients in this *emergent* category, nurses occasionally involve EMS over the protests of the patient, especially when the nurse believes that the patient isn't competent to refuse care or doesn't fully understand the probable consequences of failure to act.[7]

If a patient with an *urgent* problem is reluctant to act in his or her own best interest, the nurse might exercise his or her "duty to terrify" (p. 34)[31] in order to persuade the patient to take appropriate action. Informing the patient directly of the possible or likely consequences of failure to act might provide the patient with adequate motivation to act according to the nurse's recommendation. Occasionally, this requires advising the patient of the worst-case scenario, an action that many nurses tend to shy away from because it might require mention of a particular diagnosis. Nurses are often concerned that naming a particular disease or condition might appear to constitute "diagnosing." On the contrary; advising a patient that he or she might be experiencing a heart attack (for example) is simply providing the patient with sufficient information to make a more informed decision. Education about possible causes of their problem and likely outcomes will often provide the patient with adequate motivation to act in his or her own best interest.

With patients in the *non-urgent* category, a variety of options frequently exist for their care, and therefore the possibility exists for a fair amount of negotiation if necessary. Context and patient preference are key factors in making decisions with patients who have non-urgent problems.

Holistic or Limited Approach. Often the telephone triage nurse must deal with multiple health and social issues in addressing patient needs, and a holistic approach is desirable. This is especially true for the patient with the *non-urgent* problem. It is also probable that these patients, many of whom will receive home care recommendations, will require more teaching and counseling than the other two groups. In contrast, however, the nurse might find it necessary to take a very limited approach to patients with life-threatening problems. *Emergent* patients require immediate decision making,[5] in which even factors such as gender and age are not always relevant considerations.

Implications for Clinical Practice

To understand the implications of the previously described types of decision making, let's look at examples of each and try to understand how the underlying process is impacted by each patient type.

***"I Can't Catch My Breath..."* (Pattern Recognition/Emergent).** The patient who calls complaining of shortness of breath and is gasping in one or two-word phrases, requires immediate action. While the cause of the patient's problem is unclear, what is clear is that the patient is experiencing a life-threatening emergency as evidenced by the symptom of *extreme dyspnea*. While this symptom could represent airway obstruction, respiratory compromise, circulatory impairment, or even a neurological deficit, the exact cause of the problem is essentially irrelevant. As predicted by the research findings,[5] it is likely that the nurse will quickly and accurately identify that this patient requires an *emergent* disposition. The appropriate course of action for this patient would be for the nurse to activate EMS in order to facilitate immediate transport to definitive care.

These calls are usually very short in duration because, after identifying a symptom such as severe dyspnea, little information is needed beyond confirming the location of the patient and that their front door is unlocked. Information such as additional symptoms, the history of the present illness, past medical history, and other routine information is not only usually unnecessary, but collecting this type of information is usually contraindicated because it could result in a delay in care. Thus, the documentation with these patients is often minimal.[34] Appropriate documentation for this patient might include a comment such as "Patient gasping in two-word phrases. Interview was interrupted to activate EMS." (Note: In some cases, the nurse will call the ambulance, and in others, the patient will be instructed to do so. This policy will vary from community to community, based upon the preferences of EMS personnel but the decision should also be influenced by the nurse's perception of whether it is advisable to allow the patient to hang up and place the call himself.)

***"I Have Pain in My Belly. I've Tried Everything But It Still Hurts. What Should I Do?"* (Focused/Urgent).** This is an example of a call that will require limited problem solving and focused decision making. This patient will be assigned an urgent disposition based on her need to be seen for evaluation within the next 24 hours. Questioning of this patient will be directed toward determining where she needs to be seen and how quickly; thus history taking will be limited to questions that facilitate this decision making. For example, after determining that the patient doesn't have signs and symptoms of shock (related to a life-threatening intra-abdominal event), the nurse will want to know characteristics of the pain (e.g., severity, location, quality, duration, and radiation), whether the onset was sudden or gradual, associated symptoms (specifically including GI and GU or other generalized symptoms relevant to abdominal pain such as fever), and pertinent history (relevant to abdominal pain or associated problems). While the nurse will want to know what factors precipitate the problem, make it better or worse, and if time of day, week, month, or year is a factor, again these questions will be specific to the abdomen (such as whether or not antacids, bowel movements, micturation, etc., impact the problem).[35] Since information is collected for the primary purpose of determining where and when the patient needs to be seen,[5] documentation will be limited to information included in decision making for the appropriate disposition.

***"I Have a Rash."* (Deliberative/Non-Urgent).** The patient with a rash provides a good example of a call in which the nurse must engage in deliberative problem solving. Assuming the nurse determines that the patient isn't experiencing signs and symptoms of anaphylaxis, meningococcemia, or another emergent or urgent cause of rash, the nurse will usually be on the phone longer with this category of patient than with any other because a significant amount of information is necessary to determine a disposition.[5] Not only does the nurse need to determine what the patient means by "rash" (Is it localized or generalized? What does it looks like? Does it itch or hurt? Is it scaling, sloughing, or does it represent new onset petechiae or purpura?), but it is also necessary to take a very precise history regarding a variety of other topics. Examples of necessary information would include chronic illnesses, recent acute illnesses, current medications (prescription and over-the-counter), allergies, exposures to infectious diseases, new substances ingested or contacted, recent travel, exposure to animals, and other historical questions.

While it is not necessary (or possible) to diagnose the cause of the rash (or other vague and non-specific complaints) over the phone, it is frequently impossible to assign a disposition until the nurse has a clear picture of the entire situation. Clearly, this line of questioning could be carried too far, but in most cases, history taking for these patients is more comprehensive and will take longer than with the other two categories. Another factor adding to the length of time required to manage these patients is that the plan of care must often be negotiated.[5] In other words, there are frequently a variety of appropriate dispositions for this patient, and factors such as time of day, distance from care, availability of transportation, and patient preference will impact the plan of care. And remember, this is the patient with whom the nurse will most often take a holistic approach, another factor that adds to call length.[5]

Decision Making as a Dynamic Process

We would like to make one final comment before we end our discussion of different types of decision making. While we have provided neat and tidy examples of Pattern Recognition, Focused, and Deliberative decision making, telephone calls do not clearly or automatically fit into one category or another. It is best to think of these three types of decision making as being on a continuum. The nurse should first address any obvious high-risk patterns, and then conduct a focused assessment to determine the nature and urgency of the patient's problem. Once satisfied that the patient's problem is neither emergent nor urgent, the nurse would take a more deliberative approach to decision making.

Intuition

Nothing can replace experience. Earlier in this chapter, we discussed the many factors involved when nurses are making decisions in uncertain conditions. However, there is one element of decision making, intuition, which is a highly valued component of nursing, but is difficult to explain. Nonetheless, nurses know that when they have "a feeling," they better pay attention.

Intuition represents recognition on a less than fully conscious basis.[13,36] That is, the nurse, sometimes without realizing what he or she is seeing, recognizes a pattern or a red flag that leads him or her to a high-acuity disposition even without hard evidence to explain the decision. Because most nurses reading this book have probably worked in an inpatient setting, we will start with an inpatient example of intuition and then provide an example specific to telephone triage.

In the hospital, it is not uncommon for a nurse to call a doctor in the middle of the night reporting, "I can't put my finger on it, but there's something wrong here." In this situation, it is possible that the patient is experiencing subtle signs and symptoms that in and of themselves don't trigger a concern. However, when taken together, perhaps subconsciously, the nurse realizes that the patient's condition is deteriorating. Take, for example, the cardiac patient in a coronary care unit who has been stable, but now the nurse has an uneasy feeling about him. Perhaps the nurse is observing subtle signs such as a decreasing urine output, decreasing blood pressure, or an increasing heart rate. Additionally, although the patient's color isn't exactly abnormal, it's not exactly good either and his skin, while usually dry, is just slightly moist. And finally, this usually jovial and outgoing patient is now behaving in a more reserved manner. If the nurse were able to say he was oliguric, hypotensive, tachycardic, pale, diaphoretic, and obtunded, it would be clear that the patient might be experiencing pump failure. However, since the findings are still subtle and generally "unnamable," the nurse might merely be noticing a slight change in the wrong direction, but experience leads the nurse to realize that these subtle signs are potentially ominous.

A classic telephone triage example of intuition is a situation in which a nurse carefully assesses a child, double checks against the decision support tools, and concludes that the child's condition doesn't require evaluation today. However, the mother is concerned and feels like her child needs to be seen. Although the nurse isn't able to say exactly why, she feels uneasy about the child as well, recognizing the mother's concern, and thus brings the child in for a same-day appointment. This is not only an example of nursing intuition, but it also illustrates that mothers (in fact, patients and callers of all varieties) also have intuition. It could be that they are unwilling or unable to articulate the specific source of their concern, but experienced telephone triage nurses know to trust the mother (or patient's) instincts, nonetheless.

One such example of nursing intuition involves a woman who called an after-hours call center complaining of a headache, GI upset, and a feeling that things just weren't "quite right." She wasn't exactly dizzy, but her "equilibrium felt a little off." The nurse, for reasons she couldn't explain, asked the patient if she had any children at home. Getting an affirmative response, she advised the mother to awaken her children to check on them. Fortunately, the mother complied. At that point, two of her five children were already unconscious secondary to carbon monoxide poisoning.

Although the nurse involved can't specify what made her think of carbon monoxide, it is possible that the symptoms, coupled with other factors such as the time of year and/or part of the country, contributed to the nurse's intuitive need for the mother to check on her children. Had the nurse not provided that instruction, by morning, the two youngest, and possibly all five of the children might have succumbed.

Occasionally, feelings attributed to intuition occur when nurses can't explain what they heard, thought, or said, but they follow their instincts nonetheless, often with a surprisingly favorable outcome. While we make no effort to explain those experiences, we do encourage nurses to listen to their inner voice when something "pops into their head" that they just can't otherwise explain.

Although nurses don't generally need to be convinced of the value of intuition in clinical practice, one distinct difference exists between the significance of intuition in the face-to-face setting versus over the telephone. In the hospital setting, for example, the nurse with a bad "gut" feeling has opportunities to watch the patient more closely, reviewing labs, vital signs, and otherwise remaining hypervigilant for signs of deterioration. However, the nurse with an intuitive feeling over the telephone has no such opportunities. Given the hypothesis that intuition represents a recognition that the nurse is unable to specify, intuition probably represents clinical judgment that can't be articulated. It wouldn't be prudent to delay care for an unknown problem. Thus, because the nurse is aware that "something is wrong" but not able to specify the problem, it is important for the nurse with an intuitive thought or feeling to facilitate evaluation of the patient immediately.

SUMMARY

While information about types of decision making does not provide a consistent blueprint for patient management, it does illuminate factors integral to the critical thought process in conditions of uncertainty. More research is needed to determine the cognitive processes that the expert telephone triage nurse uses to determine urgency, with or without the benefit of decision support tools, and to identify factors critical to success. In the meantime, it is essential that telephone triage nurses and nursing leaders alike recognize that, due to the complex nature of the practice of nursing by telephone, a "cookie cutter" approach to patient management is not appropriate. Decision support tools, while important to the practice of telephone triage, should be used judiciously, and nurses must realize that critical thinking and professional judgment must be the basis of their decision making and thus their provision of care over the telephone.

References

1. Edwards, B. (1994). Telephone triage: How experienced nurses reach decisions. *Journal of Advanced Nursing, 19*(4), 717-724.
2. Greenberg, M.E. (2009). A comprehensive model of the process of telephone nursing. *Journal of Advanced Nursing, 65*(12), 2621-2629. doi:10.1111/j.1365-2648.2009.05132.x
3. Mayo, A., Chang, B., & Omery, A. (2002). Use of protocols and guidelines by telephone nurses. *Clinical Nursing Research, 11*(2), 204-219.
4. Valanis, B., Tanner, C., Moscato, S., Shapiro, S., Izumi, S., David, M., Keyes, C., & Mayo, A. (2003). A model for examining predictors of outcomes of telephone nursing advice. *Journal of Nursing Administration, 33*(2), 91-95.

5. Leprohon, J., & Patel, V. (1995). Decision-making strategies for telephone triage in emergency medical services. *Medical Decision Making, 15*(3), 240-253.
6. Greatbatch, D., Hanlon, G., Goode, J., O'Cathain, A., Strangleman, T., & Luff, D. (2005). Telephone triage, expert systems and clinical expertise. *Sociology of Health & Illness, 27*(6), 802-830.
7. Rutenberg, C., & Oberle, K. (2008) Ethics in telehealth nursing practice. *Home Healthcare Management and Practice, 20*(4), 342-348.
8. Smith, C. (2008). Knowledge and the discourse of labour process transformation: Nurses and the case of NHS direct for England. *Work, Employment & Society, 22*(4), 581-599.
9. Ennis, R.H. (1991). Critical thinking: A streamlined conception. *Teaching Philosophy, 14*(1), 5-25. Retrieved from http://faculty.ed.uiuc.edu/rhennis/documents/Ennis StreamlinedConception_000.pdf
10. Benner, P., Hughes, R.G., & Sutphen, M. (2008). Clinical reasoning, decision making, and action: Thinking critically and clinically. In R.G. Hughes (Ed.), *Patient safety and quality: An evidence-based handbook for nurses.* (Prepared with support from the Robert Wood Johnson Foundation). AHRQ Publication No. 08-0043. Rockville, MD: Agency for Healthcare Research and Quality.
11. Kataoka-Yahiro, J., & Saylor, C. (1994). A critical thinking model for nursing judgment. *Journal of Nursing Education, 33*(8), 351-356.
12. Ström, M., Marklund, B., & Hildingh, C. (2009). Callers' perceptions of receiving advice via a medical care help line. *Scandinavian Journal of Caring Sciences, 23*(4), 682-690. doi:10.1111/j.1471-6712.2008.00661.x
13. Benner, P. (1984). *From novice to expert: Excellence and power in clinical nursing practice.* Menlo Park, CA: Addison-Wesley.
14. Dowding, D., Mitchell, N., Randell, R., Foster, R., Lattimer, V., & Thompson, C. (2009). Nurses' use of computerised clinical decision support systems: A case site analysis. *Journal of Clinical Nursing, 18*(8), 1159-1167. doi:10.1111/j.1365-2702.2008.02607.x
15. Giesen, P., Ferwerda, R., Tijssen, R., Mokkink, H., Drijver, R.W., & Grol, R. (2007). Safety of telephone triage in general practitioner cooperatives: Do triage nurses correctly estimate urgency? *Quality & Safety in Health Care, 16*(3), 181-184.
16. Hanlon, G., Strangleman, T., Goode, J., Luff, D., O'Cathian, A., & Greatbatch, D. (2005). Knowledge, technology and nursing: The case of NHS direct. *Human Relations, 58*(2), 147-171.
17. Knowles, E., O'Cathain, A., Morrell, J., Munro, J.F., & Nicholl, J.P. (2002). NHS direct and nurses – opportunity or monotony? *International Journal of Nursing Studies, 39*(8), 857-866.
18. Hoffman, K.A. Aitken, L.M., & Duffield, C. (2009). A comparison of novice and expert nurses' cue collection during clinical decision-making: Verbal protocol analysis. *International Journal of Nursing Studies, 46,* 1335-1344. doi.10.1016/j.ijnurstu.2009.04001
19. American Academy of Ambulatory Care Nursing. (2011). *Scope and standards of practice for professional telehealth nurses* (5th ed.). Pitman, NJ: American Academy of Ambulatory Care Nursing.

20. American Nurses Association. (1999). *Competencies for telehealth technologies in nursing.* Washington, DC: Author.
21. Thompson, C., Bucknall, T., Estabrooks, C.A., Hutchinson, A., Fraser, K., de Vos, R., Binnecade, J., Barrat, G., & Saunders, J. (2007). Nurses' critical event risk assessments: A judgement analysis. *Journal of Clinical Nursing, 18*, 601-612. doi: 10.1111/j.1365-2702.2007.02191.x
22. Thompson, C., Dalgleish, L., Bucknall, T., Estabrooks, C.A., Hutchinson, A., Fraser, K., ... Saunders, J. (2008). The effects of time pressure and experience on nurses' risk assessment decisions. *Nursing Research, 57*(5), 302-311.
23. Hagbaghery, M.A., Salsali, M., & Ahmadi, F. (2004). The factors facilitating and inhibiting effective clinical decision-making in nursing: A qualitative study. *BioMed Central Nursing, 3*(1), 2.
24. Valanis, B., Moscato, S., Tanner, C., Shapiro, S., Izumi, S., David, M., & Mayo, A. (2003). Making it work: Organization and processes of telephone nursing advice services. *Journal of Nursing Administration, 33*(4), 216-223.
25. Wahlberg, A.C., Cedersund, E., & Wredling, R. (2003). Telephone nurses' experience of problems with telephone advice in Sweden. *Journal of Clinical Nursing, 12*(1), 37-45.
26. Turner, P. (2005). Critical thinking in nursing education and practice as defined in the literature. *Nursing Education Perspectives, 26*(5), 272-277.
27. Collin-Jacques, C., & Smith, C. (2005). Nursing on the line: Experiences from England and Quebec (Canada). *Human Relations, 58*(1), 5-32.
28. Wilson, R., & Hubert, J. (2002). Resurfacing the care in nursing by telephone: Lessons from ambulatory oncology. *Nursing Outlook, 50*(4), 160-164.
29. Boblin-Cummings, S., Baumann, A., & Deber, R. (1999). Critical elements in the process of decision making: A nursing perspective. *Canadian Journal of Nursing Leadership, 12*(1), 6-13.
30. Lee, J., Chan, A.C.M., & Phillips, D.R. (2006). Diagnostic practice in nursing: A critical review of the literature. *Nursing and Health Sciences, 8*, 57-65. doi:10.1111/j.1442-2018.2006.00267.x
31. Wheeler, S.Q., & Windt, J.H. (1993). *Telephone triage: Therapy, practice, & protocol development.* Albany, NY: Delmar Publishers, Inc.
32. Benner, P., & Tanner, C. (1987). Clinical judgment: How expert nurses use intuition. *American Journal of Nursing, 87*(1), 23-34.
33. Corcoran-Perry, S., & Narayan, S. (1991). Lines of reasoning used by triage nurses in cases of varying complexity: A pilot study. In W.H. Lake (Ed.), *Perspectives on judgment and decision-making* (pp. 104-110). Metuchen, NJ: Scarecrow Press.
34. Schmitt, B.D., & Thompson, D.A. (2005), Triage documentation: Setting a best practice. *Answerstat.* Retrieved from http://www.answerstat.com/articles/5/42.html
35. Rutenberg, C. (2000). Telephone triage: When the only thing connecting you to your patient is the telephone. *American Journal of Nursing, 100*(3), 77-78, 80-81.
36. Kahneman, D., & Klein, G. (2009). Conditions for intuitive expertise. *American Psychologist, 64*(6), 515-526.

Chapter 8

Clinical Practice Part I: The Patient Interview

Patients using telephone triage services expect the nurse to understand their concerns and provide solutions that are tailored to the individual and his or her particular situation.[1,2,3] Consistent with these expectations, patients are more satisfied with the services when the interaction is seen as collaborative and personalized.[2,4,5]

Providing such individualized care without benefit of sight, touch, or smell can be tricky and requires superior communication skills. Along with clinical competency and a robust knowledge base, communication skills can make or break a telephone triage nurse. The ability to connect with the caller at the outset of the call and then to listen and hear the caller's concerns provide the basis for a meaningful telephone triage encounter. The telephone triage nurse must also be proficient at teaching, supporting, collaborating, and other nursing skills that are dependent upon the ability to communicate successfully.

We know that most nurses pride themselves at being effective communicators. Nurses learn basic communication skills in nursing school and incorporate them into practice throughout their careers. However, a fair amount of effective and meaningful communication in the face-to-face setting is nonverbal. Nurses have learned the importance of touch, eye contact, and occasionally the value of merely being a silent presence to meet our patients' unspoken needs. But the practice of telephone triage compels us to learn how to communicate with our patients entirely over the telephone and thus without nonverbal communication tools as basic as touch or eye contact. As telephone triage nurses, our verbal skills will be tested to the hilt, and our nonverbal communication is limited to such subtleties as tone of voice and background sounds.

Because of these challenges, telephone triage services sometime fall short of optimal communication. One study of the quality of communication found that triage nurses often do not "elicit the concerns of the patient and [they] obtained little information about patients' perception of the problem or about the physical, emotional, or social impact of the problem" (p. 177).[6]

The significance of these findings is twofold. First, highly developed communication skills are required to engage the caller and to build an accurate picture of the patient, the context, and the patient's problem. And second, rushing through a call will decrease both the quality of the interaction and the patient's satisfaction with the care delivered. Researchers have found that the longer the call, the more satisfied the patient was with the telephone encounter. Further analysis suggested that this longer call length improved satisfaction because it enhanced the nurse's ability to understand and address the patient's individual concerns. Researchers concluded that "Apart from adequate communication skills, triagists need sufficient time for telephone consultation to enable high quality performance" (p. 177).[6]

"Patients' dissatisfaction with telephone consultation is often due to the lack of acknowledgement of physical or emotional needs or not to meet patients' expectations" (p. 174).[6]

In some settings, efforts are made to limit the length of nurses' calls, although as previously discussed, rushing through a call will usually decrease both the quality of the interaction and the patient's satisfaction with the care delivered. Thus, the telephone triage nurse should allow enough time to open the call properly, let the patient tell his or her story, conduct an adequate assessment, provide necessary teaching, and close the call properly with attention to patient understanding of and comfort with the plan of care.[7]

According to national standards for the United Kingdom's NHS Direct, a telephone consultation ought to last 8-10 minutes.[8] Call center management in Sweden recommends 6-8 calls per hour.[8] It is important to note that for many national call centers, these average time expectations include non-triage calls about health care information such as phone numbers, as well as nurse triage and advice calls (A.C. Wahlberg, personal communication, January 27, 2012). However, prescribing call times is not in the best interest of the patient. Experienced telephone triage nurses indicate that prescribed call times limit their professional practice and decrease their morale.[9,10] Pressure to do calls within a predetermined time frame is counterproductive, and evidence suggests that time pressure negatively affects decision making.[11,12] Patients require adequate time to tell their story, receive the necessary education, and make informed decisions. Although it is important for a telephone triage manager to know average call length as a parameter upon which to base staffing, the trend in call center management is to move away from set time expectations and to allow the nurses to focus on meeting the patients' needs, regardless of the resulting call length. It is not unusual for call centers to "budget" 15-20 minutes per call, depending on the population being served.

A flexible approach to call length is helpful but what matters most is the quality of the nurse-patient interaction. In this chapter, we will discuss strategies for patient-centered care, how to open a call, close a call, and everything in between, focusing on the communication techniques necessary to facilitate a meaningful telephone triage encounter. To accomplish this, we will discuss techniques nurses use to compensate for the absence of visual cues.[13] In the process, we will move beyond the basics and look at how these strategies are used to develop the competencies that must be included in the specialized skill set of a telephone triage nurse.

PATIENT-CENTERED CARE

Common Courtesy

When talking on the telephone, it is important to remember that without eye contact or body language, the patient has no idea what you're doing or if you're even listening. Here are a few tips that might enhance the quality of your interaction.

- ***Explain Long Silences and Typing Noises.*** If you are making notes, consulting a decision support tool, or just thinking, it is perfectly appropriate to tell patients what you're doing. Otherwise, they're liable to think you're not listening or perhaps even typing an email to a friend. Comments such as, "You've given me a lot of good information. Just give me a minute to get it all documented" and/or "Just give me a minute to think to see if we've overlooked anything" will help the caller understand that you are still an active participant on the call. And patients will appreciate your attention to detail.

- ***Thank the Caller for Holding.*** If you have a display on your phone that indicates how long the patient has been on hold, it can help defuse the potentially angry patient if you open the call by apologizing and thanking her for holding "for over 6 minutes." That type of announcement lets patients know you're aware they had to hold and you're really sorry about it. It also keeps them from overestimating and inflating the amount of time they had to wait. And if you have to put the caller on hold to, for example, consult with a colleague, ask their permission, tell them what you're doing, and let them know approximately how long the hold time will be.

- ***Handle Transfers Appropriately.*** If you have to transfer a call, tell the patient where you're transferring him or her and why. Then, instead of just transferring the call and leaving the patient alone to start from scratch, do it as a "warm transfer" (or conference call). It's helpful to explain the situation to the person on the other end of the phone, ideally with the patient listening, so he or she will know where to begin with this new person.

- ***Don't Chew Gum or Eat While on the Phone.*** This seems self-evident, but when we don't feel like we can get away from our desks for a meal or a break and decide to work through lunch, everything and everybody suffers, including our professional appearance.

- ***Call Patients by Name (The One They Prefer).*** It is likely that most people prefer to be called by their first name rather than their last name. It's more personal, and thus often makes it easier to connect with the patient. However, if you make that assumption, and it's wrong, your patient might be highly offended. And there are some populations, such as the military, where retirees might like to be called by their previous rank. Instead of guessing, the best policy is to ask, "How would you like for me to address you?" Patients will be grateful for the personal touch.

- ***Be Real! We're All People.*** Speaking of the personal touch, please try to produce it. No one wants to speak to an automaton. One nurse had so mastered the skill of answering the phone warmly, one caller actually commented that she felt like she had been "hugged." Selected as one of the 100 most effective advertising campaigns of the 20th century, Tom Bodett, with his folksy voice, invited the listener to stay at Motel 6, closing with the tagline, "We'll leave the light on for you."[14] This created a wonderful warm feeling for many travelers. In fact, larger and more expensive hotel chains followed suit, not with their advertising campaigns but by actually leaving the light on for their guests. Walking into a hotel room away from home doesn't feel so empty and cold when the light is on, the TV or music is playing softly, and the bed is turned down, even before the patron checks in. We need to do the best we can to replicate the feeling left with us by Tom Bodett. We need to convey the message that we are figuratively "leaving the light on" for our patients.

So when you are listening to somebody, completely, attentively, then you are listening not only to the words, but also to the feeling of what is being conveyed, to the whole of it, not part of it.
~Jiddu Krishnamurti

- ***Listen as if You Were in Their Shoes.*** Although we try to empathize, it's worth reflecting on the fact that we usually can't really feel what it's like to be in the patient's shoes because we're nurses and have a unique understanding of matters related to health and the human condition. This is one example of the importance of interpreting. Because of our nursing knowledge, when we're sick ourselves, our understanding of the situation will feel different (for better or for worse) than that of our patients. Equate this situation to a person who doesn't speak German in a room full of Germans. He probably wouldn't understand a word except Gesundheit! But once he learned German, it would be impossible to be in the room and not comprehend at least some of what was being said. Apply that analogy to our patients and their lack of knowledge about health and their bodies. Listen, interpret what you hear, be gentle, and try to imagine (or remember) what it was like before you became a nurse (and figuratively "learned to speak German").

In a study comparing physicians who had never been sued to those who had been sued two or more times (excluding surgeons), the behaviors cited in Table 1 were observed in each group.[15] While admittedly, this was a study of physicians in the face-to-face setting, the applicability to telephone triage is clear. Notice how the "never sued" group demonstrated behaviors that would serve a nurse well over the telephone.

Table 1.
Physician-Observed Behaviors

Never Sued	Sued
Average 18 minutes with patient	Average 15 minutes with patient
Showed concern	Ignored patients
Accessible	Rushed exam
Good listeners who invited questions	Unwilling to listen or answer questions
"Go on"… "Tell me more"	Interrupted after 18 seconds
First exam, then we'll talk	
Used humor	
Involved the family	
Explained and checked for understanding	
Negotiated	
Expressed interest	
Encouraged conversation ("Anything else?"). Talked an average of 90 seconds but not more than 150 seconds.	Failed to respond when patients, at or near the end of their visit said, "Oh, by the way."

GETTING STARTED

Our discussion about interviewing will begin at the beginning — opening the call. It is well known that you only get one chance to make a first impression, and for better or worse, it is lasting. Several of the techniques discussed have been identified in the Greenberg Model of Telephone Nursing Practice (see Chapter 6), but in this chapter we address their practical application.

Opening the Call and Connecting

Answering the phone or beginning your call with a caring, concerned, unhurried tone of voice is essential in establishing rapport, conveying interest and empathy, and thus facilitating a more complete and accurate assessment. Although circumstances such as heavy call volume or callers who have difficulty expressing themselves can lead to frustration for the nurse, this should never be conveyed in the nurse's tone of voice. Any indication of impatience or lack of concern might sharply curtail the caller's interest in telling his or her story and expressing the details that will bring the situation to life. If the nurse is rushed, the patient is likely to mirror the nurse's approach and try to rush through his or her history, which is not a good thing. One organization, in an effort to make a good first impression, recorded a pleasant greeting from each nurse and initiated each inbound call with the recording, so that regardless of the nurse's state of mind, the patient would first hear an inviting greeting. Whether or not this is an option for you, be certain to give adequate attention to how you answer the call. And be sure to let them hear you smile.

Greeting. The actual verbiage used in opening the call also sets the tone. In addition to giving attention to tone of voice and cadence, the words you choose convey a powerful message and begin the direction of the call on the right or wrong foot. Although this seems very elementary, let's review the basics. It is surprising how many organizations, or nurses, don't give ample thought to this very important part of the call.

When answering a cold call (the phone rings and you don't know who is calling or the nature of the call), it is always appropriate to begin with the name of your organization and your name. Use of your first name sets the tone for a more intimate interaction, and at this point, your last name probably falls into the category of too much information. If you prefer to be called Mr., Ms., or Mrs., then introduce yourself slowly to be sure the caller catches your last name.

Because of confusion about the professional identity of the various types of personnel employed in health care settings, especially over the telephone, it is important for the RN to be clear about his or her level of licensure. Following your name, say "I'm a registered nurse" or "I'm an RN" to be sure the caller realizes he is talking to an RN rather than a customer service representative. Here, we would like to make a special comment to active duty military personnel. Although you are an officer and, of course, must use your rank, it is also appropriate and desirable to follow your name with your license. Remember, in the military setting, callers probably have no idea what level of preparation or licensure the person answering the phone has unless they are told. You might answer, "Family Practice Clinic. This is Captain Johnson, RN."

In the past, some call centers have allowed nurses to use pseudonyms and discouraged or forbid them to disclose their real name. The rationale was to protect the nurse's privacy. However, the call center environment already provides functional anonymity and physical isolation from the patient, so what can by gained by further obscuring the identity of the nurse? And it is a common requirement of the Nurse Practice Act in most states that licensed nurses identify themselves to their patients by name and title.

An executive director of one of the boards of nursing (let's call her Janice) placed a call to the 800 number on the back of her insurance card in an effort to "see who these people are and how this thing works." When the phone was answered, the greeting was, "This is a nurse. How can I help you today?" Janice inquired as to the name and location of the nurse, to which the nurse responded that she was "not allowed" to release that information. Imagine her surprise when her caller responded, "Listen, young woman. You're talking to the executive director of the board of nursing in (state), and thus you're practicing in my state, possibly without a license. Now, once again, may I please have your name and location?"

Although Janice had no interest in taking any type of disciplinary action, it hit her the wrong way when the nurse refused to disclose her name and location. Just because we practice in an untraditional setting doesn't permit us to disregard professional standards or legislated requirements. Individually we are accountable for our practice, and should be willing to provide our name and credentials. How would you feel about conferring with a professional (e.g., doctor or lawyer) who refused to provide his or her real name?

Like the introduction, it is important to give some specific thought to the last part of your greeting. If you finish with "How may I help you?" you are inviting a barrage of information for which you might not yet be ready. Depending on how you locate your patient's record in your database (or how you initiate a new record), you might want to ask directly for that identifying information. Several software programs allow the nurse to search for a name phonetically, so asking for a name and date of birth might give you enough information to find the patient's medical record promptly. Once the patient's identifying information appears, all the nurse has to do is confirm it.

So, for example, you might answer the phone, "Community Nurse Line. This is Carol. I'm a registered nurse. May I please have your last name and date of birth?" This greeting, spoken warmly, slowly, and distinctly, gives the caller the impression that you care, that you're qualified to help her, and that you have time to listen to her concerns. *Note:* Because many software programs require the nurse to identify the patient before accessing the record, the nurse must try to identify the patient so that the documentation can be initiated promptly. The caveat is that it is clearly not acceptable to focus on demographic or other clinically irrelevant information when a nurse is dealing with a patient with an obvious life-threatening emergency.

If you return calls in your setting rather than answering them live, a suggestion would be to identify yourself by organization, first (or last) name, title, and then let the patient know that you and the initial message taker have communicated without leading the patient into his history. For example, if the note says "nausea and vomiting," instead of saying "I understand you have been vomiting," you might say something to the effect of "I understand you're not feeling well. Can you tell me what's going on?" Occasionally, what the message taker chooses to record might not be the most meaningful symptom or problem. If you start with the wrong question, you might misdirect the patient from the very beginning of the call, making it more difficult for him or her to get back on track.

Attending to the Caller. Throughout the conversation, it is important for the caller to feel that the nurse is listening and really hearing his or her concerns. There's nothing like speaking to a "real" human being, especially when in distress. Sometimes efforts to locate the caller's record in the database, document patient information, and/or access and reference the decision support tool will divert the nurse's attention. The result can be overlooking key comments or phrases that would provide insight into the patient's problem and request. It is ideal to have a template (discussed in Chapter 11) that will allow the nurse to do real-time documentation while listening carefully to everything the patient says. Difficulty typing or using the software proficiently will distract the nurse from the patient, potentially altering the quality of the nurse/patient interaction in multiple ways.

Establishing rapport quickly is an important element of a successful call and must be given ample attention. One important strategy identified by nurses that is used to develop rapport is to allow the caller to present his or her problem uninterrupted.[13] Policies and practices that interfere with the nurse's ability to establish rapport should be identified and addressed. For example, some organizations require nurses to follow scripts to a greater or lesser degree. Some even require the nurse to read the script and then ask every protocol question verbatim, even if unsuitable. This approach creates the potential for a variety of problems. Nurses who are obliged by organizational policy to read scripts may have a difficult time maintaining a sense of humanity and compassion in their voice. This approach may also deprive the nurse of the ability to individualize the interaction. Strict adherence to the script may also force the nurse to ask unsuitable or unnecessary questions, utilize verbiage that is inappropriate for the specific patient, and thus impair the quality of the interpersonal interaction.

Caring. In addition to using a warm, caring, unrushed tone of voice, nurses are accustomed to using other techniques to connect with their patients such as introducing themselves, calling the patients by name (the one they prefer), using eye contact and touch, sitting at their level, using open body language, and other verbal and non-verbal strategies. Other, more intimate strategies such as holding a patient's hand, providing a gentle presence, or even occasionally embracing or crying with a patient or family member who is grieving or otherwise distraught are powerful ways to connect and say "I care." However, many of these techniques cannot be used in a telephone encounter. Telephone triage nurses must be able to verbally express warmth, sympathy, concern, and confidence, and to compensate for the inability to use meaningful eye contact and touch.

Confidence. The self-confidence that the nurse exudes in his or her telephone demeanor can be extremely comforting to the caller. Comments such as, "I'm glad you called. I can help you with that," or "Yes, we have talked to quite a few people experiencing what you are experiencing," or (if true) "I have 20 years of pediatric experience; let's see how we can get your little guy feeling better," will get the call off to the right start and boost the caller's confidence. Of course, if you don't know the answer to a patient's question, one advantage of being in a call center or centralized telephone triage setting is that the nurse can say, "I don't know the answer to that, but my colleague sitting right beside me is an expert in that area. Let me consult with her."

The most important thing in communication is to hear what isn't being said.
~Peter F. Drucker

Self-Disclosure. A strategy that can be as powerful as some of those we use when we are physically with the patient is the technique of self-disclosure. There are times when a gentle comment indicating "I understand because I have been in that situation too" can be both appropriate and effective.

A patient called because her child had been sent home from school with head lice. She was so upset she could hardly get the words out of her mouth. In an effort to decrease her obvious embarrassment, the nurse said, "Oh I can relate to what you're going through. The first time my kids brought home head lice, I was horrified!" That simple bit of self-disclosure (a) validated the mother's feelings and (b) reassured her that head lice were equal opportunity pests, infesting the families of health care professionals as well as others. And the nurse not only admitted to her children having had head lice, but she intimated that they had contracted them more than once. In a discussion of how lice spread, the nurse explained that her son had a special baseball cap he wore to school every day, and it was frequently passed around the class for every other boy in his class to try on. And her daughter had been at the age that little girls liked to play "beauty shop," sharing hairbrushes and barrettes regularly. Subsequently during the conversation when the nurse was advising the mother about the seemingly extreme measures necessary to rid her child and their house of the lice, the nurse was able to reassure the mother that although seemingly overwhelming, she had firsthand experience that the process was manageable.

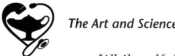

While self-disclosure wasn't absolutely necessary on this occasion, the nurse in this particular situation felt it was an acceptable way to both reduce the mother's emotional discomfort and provide information.

In another case, a nurse reported receiving a call from a woman whose husband was recently diagnosed with Lou Gehrig's Disease, or amyotrophic lateral sclerosis (ALS). Coincidentally, that nurse's husband and father-in-law also had ALS. What a blessing it must have been for that caller to speak to a nurse who had been through the experience herself! Although every nurse should be empathetic and able to manage the call properly, there's nothing like having "been there." And one might wonder whether it was only a coincidence that particular nurse had received that particular call.

These examples are offered to illustrate the potential value of self-disclosure; however, we acknowledge that it is not always appropriate to utilize that strategy. One nurse reported having made a comment to a patient, "Oh, my kids had that too," and her comment was met with dead silence. Apparently, the patient was telling the nurse, "I don't care. This is about my kids, not yours." The patient may have also felt that the nurse was minimizing the seriousness of her situation.

The point of this discussion isn't necessary to advise you to use self-disclosure (nor to discourage you from doing so), but rather to give you *permission* to do so if you believe it's indicated. Most of us were taught in nursing school that we should not share personal information with our patients. However, most of our instructors never dreamed that we would be trying to develop therapeutic relationships with our patients entirely over the telephone. An old African proverb says it all: "When the music changes, so does the dance"

In self-disclosing, it's helpful to keep in mind that the litmus test to determine whether self-disclosure is appropriate or not is to reflect on *whose needs you are meeting*. If you are disclosing information about yourself to comfort or connect with your patient, it may be appropriate to do so. If not, stifle the urge, keep it focused on the patient, and find another way to connect.

Questioning

Questioning is thought by many to be the crux of the interview, but we believe that as far as the nurse talking, less is more. In reality, history taking in telephone triage requires a subtle balance of listening and talking, with heavy emphasis on the listening. For example, some callers will feel a need to share a good deal of background and circumstantial information, occasionally being slow at "getting to the point" of the call. These callers require patience in allowing them to share the information that they believe is important. For example, with your patients who are storytellers (you'll recognize them when you hear them), just let them talk. If you interrupt them in an effort to move them along, you might succeed in shifting their focus off of the important information they are willingly ready and able to give you. Nurses are often so anxious to help the caller that they intervene too soon.[8] If the nurse fails to allow callers the opportunity to share information in a way that is meaningful to them and consistent with the way they organize their thoughts, critical pieces of information might be overlooked or omitted.

In contrast to patients who have a lot to say, some patients offer only the bare minimum in hopes of gaining direction from the nurse and perhaps getting off the phone more quickly. In so doing, they might understate the nature of the problem and inadvertently or deliberately withhold key information. These patients often need a little coaxing to come forth with all of the relevant information. In such cases the nurse will have to employ other interviewing techniques such as direct questioning to determine the nature of the call. Patients don't always know what's relevant and what isn't relevant, and you won't either, until you hear their story, told in their own words. Remember, the interview is about the patient, and since he or she is essentially your only source of information, you need to take full advantage of the caller's willingness and ability to share information he or she believes is germane to his or her particular situation. Questioning, therefore, should be used with discretion until the nurse has heard the concerns of the caller or unless there is a clinical reason to interrupt the caller's story.

Redirecting

Of course, with some patients, there will come a time when they need to be redirected. This is occasionally necessary if the caller is off-track and providing seemingly irrelevant information. However, the nurse must use extreme caution and exercise patience in first allowing the caller to tell his story in his own way. Aggressive or premature attempts to redirect the patient might prevent the nurse from learning key pieces of information that would be relevant to the patient's care. There will also be occasions such as when a patient mentions "swelling," that you might need to interrupt him or her and inquire further about the swelling (questioning), redirecting him or her to the relevant information you need to rule out a potentially life-threatening emergency. The risk with redirecting lies in doing it too early or redirecting the patient to information that isn't as relevant as you might think. So, early in the encounter, it is probably best to restrict efforts at redirecting to those necessary to rule out problems requiring immediate lifesaving intervention.

Getting to Know

Getting to know the patient is another listening exercise. While the patient tells his or her story, the telephone triage nurse should listen for cues that help the nurse "get to know" the patient. For example, the nurse can get to know the patient's age, level of education, ethnicity, socioeconomic status, and often even his or her values and beliefs. Listen for the patient's chief complaint and try to identify what he or she wants to do about it. Note the patient's concerns. If he or she is worried about a medical condition or that of a loved one, take him or her seriously. Other factors such as being home alone, having seen the doctor yesterday, or concerns about missing work will help the astute nurse build context that is important to collaborative care planning with the patient.

INFORMATION SEEKING

Information seeking is a critical part of the "Information Gathering" phase of the interview. Unfortunately, this is also often one of the most mistreated portions of the call. Many of us have probably heard that "good telephone triage nurses" will "take control" of the call, directing the interview. As discussed previously, this is often an unworkable strategy, derailing the patient before he gets to the bottom line in telling his history. Respect for the patient and his individual style of communication will serve a telephone triage nurse well and increase the quality of the information obtained from the patient.

Active listening is essential to reassure the caller that the nurse is interested and engaged. It is helpful for the nurse to use terms of encouragement or "listening noises" such as "Go on," "What happened then?" "Tell me more about that" and so forth. These forms of active listening serve to "prime the pump," encouraging the patient to continue to talk, exhausting all of the information he or she believes is important.

Always Speak to the Patient

To assure complete and accurate assessment, it is important for the nurse to speak directly to the patient whenever possible. This permits direct assessment of certain objective information such as the patient's respiratory efforts, cognition, quality of speech, and other parameters amenable to direct observation. Although not all patients will be good historians, a great deal can be gleaned from even a casual conversation with the patient. This rule of thumb also applies to patients such as the very young, those with dementia, and those who are generally non-verbal, such as infants or the developmentally disabled. Even to patients who are comatose, the ability to assess the patient's audible respiratory efforts is invaluable.

"Training in active listening for telephone nurses should be compulsory, including regular listening to authentic calls by the individual nurse, but also discussing calls in a group" (p. 407).[16]

Speak with the Family when Offered or Indicated

It is also important for the nurse to speak with the patient's family or friend when indicated in order to ascertain their concerns or obtain additional information. In many cases, the caller represents a family member who has information that the patient might not be able or willing to share. For example, in some households, especially those of previous generations, an unspoken social contract exists between husband and wife that lends itself to the husband being the bread winner and the wife being, among other things, the family's health care manager. In other cases, a family member may be the primary caregiver for a chronically ill patient. If that caregiver is deprived of the opportunity to share his or her observations and concerns with the nurse, the caller might experience unnecessary frustration, and a less than optimal outcome might result. In other words, although it's important to speak to the patient whenever possible, do not exclude speaking with a concerned friend or family member, providing that the patient has no objection. Although patient confidentiality is always a concern, attentively listening to the caller and responding appropriately to information provided by the family is not in and of itself a violation of patient confidentiality (see also Third-Party and/or Surrogate Callers in Chapter 9).

Investigating

Of course, we must determine why the patient called. However, once again, letting the patient talk is probably your best strategy for figuring out what is going on. As soon as is feasible in the conversation, the nurse should try to determine why the patient is calling. This answer, properly investigated, will have two parts. First, the nurse needs to identify the patient's concern, but second (and this is often overlooked), the nurse needs to know what action the caller is seeking (i.e., what he or she wants to do about it). Patients usually have an agenda when they call the nurse. Does the caller want an appointment with his or her primary care provider or is he or she seeking a referral to a specialist? Would the caller prefer home care? Is he or she seeking health information or reassurance or does he or she just need someone to talk to?

Erma Bombeck once said that human gestation is "as long as you can stand it, plus 10 days." A pregnant woman, well into her "10 days," had already been seen in labor and delivery twice and sent home, both demoralizing experiences. She was once again calling labor and delivery to see if the nurse thought she might be in labor. After listening to the patient a while, the nurse said, "Julie, do you want to come in again to be checked?" to which Julie wailed, "No! I just want someone to promise me I'm not going to be pregnant for the rest of my life!" The nurse reassured her they wouldn't allow her to go more than 14 days past due before they induced her, giving the patient the peace of mind that there was a guaranteed end in sight, allowing her to relax and enjoy, as best she could, the remaining few days of her pregnancy.

Thus it is helpful to know the caller's expectations and keep his or her wishes in mind. This will help avoid misunderstandings and increase the likelihood that the caller will feel that his or her needs have been met at the end of the call. To this end, early in the encounter and after identifying the patient's main concern, the nurse might pose the question, "What can I help you decide today?" Without knowing what the patient's problem is and what he or she wants to do about it, the well-intentioned nurse might provide misguided advice, overlooking the patient's actual need or the caller's wishes. Admittedly, while the caller's wishes might not ultimately be in his or her best interest (such as an antibiotic for a cold or an office visit for chest pain), in many cases, there is more than one acceptable approach to problem solving. Knowing the patient's expectations is an important element of care planning and may avert a misunderstanding or development of a plan of care that the patient won't carry out.

A mother whose child had a cough called the triage nurse for advice about getting him seen that day. The nurse performed a thorough assessment and concluded that the patient was a candidate for home treatment. The nurse took quite a bit of time reassuring the mother and teaching her about the care of her son and the warning signs to watch for, should his condition worsen or not improve as expected. Although the nurse had done an excellent job, providing every bit of information she thought necessary to support home care of the child, the mother seemed reluctant to end the call.

After approximately 20 minutes on the phone with the nurse, the mother finally mustered the courage to ask the nurse if she thought her son needed an antibiotic. It was only then that the nurse realized the mother's real agenda had been to get an antibiotic for her son, whether she was advised to get an appoint-

ment or not. The nurse recognized this as a teachable moment and explained why antibiotics would not only be unnecessary but also probably contraindicated in this clinical situation. The extra time spent by the nurse in teaching the mother about appropriate use of antibiotics gave the mother more confidence in caring for her son on this occasion and likely averted unnecessary calls in the future. Of course, had the nurse recognized the mother's true agenda earlier in the call, perhaps the call would have been shorter. However, it is fortunate that although she initially didn't know why, the nurse was sensitive to the hesitancy of the mother to conclude the call, and the proper information was eventually shared.

This example illustrates why the nurse should try to establish the patient's agenda early in the call and listen for the "message behind the message" (p. 50).[17] The nurse who is really engaged in the call will seize those "teachable moments" when they present themselves. This speaks to the fact that long calls can be extremely good calls. There is often more than one path to a favorable outcome, but the nurse needs to remain vigilant to not allow golden opportunities to pass unnoticed. This also illustrates that tending to the strategies available to us such as verifying, clarifying, and investigating can make the difference between a 10-minute and a 20-minute call or between an effective encounter and one that leaves much to be desired.

Open-ended questions such as "What do you hope is the outcome of today's call?" are important in the telephone triage interview. It is important to avoid jumping to a conclusion about the patient's needs or desires and approaching the call in a way that might lead the patient down an unnecessary or inappropriate path.

Use of terms such as "Can you tell me more about that?" "What happened then?" and "Is there anything else going on?" are other examples of open-ended questions and techniques used to investigate the clinical problem and the patient's agenda.

General, open-ended questions are best used at the beginning of the call. Conversely, leading questions should be avoided unless they are used late in the call to rule out important problems not previously addressed, and then only with caution. Direct questioning is best conducted after the patient has told his or her story in his or her own words. The more specific questions should be used to narrow the inquiry once a clear picture begins to emerge.

Prior to guideline selection, the nurse must do a sufficient assessment (enough investigating) to accurately ascertain the nature of the patient's problem(s). This topic is addressed in-depth in Chapters 10 and 11. Patients often initially express their "most worrisome associated symptom" instead of their actual primary problem. For example, a patient with pyelonephritis might first complain of fever and vomiting, but only after careful assessment will the nurse be able to identify other symptoms such as flank pain, hematuria, or a recent history of cystitis. It should be noted that prematurely choosing the protocol (e.g., vomiting or fever) may extend the length of the call and decrease the effectiveness of the telephone triage process.

Callers will often couch their request in the form of a health information question when, in reality, they have a deeper health care concern. An example of this might be the mother who asks about the symptoms of chickenpox or the "right dose of acetaminophen" for her baby. Indeed, these might be straightforward health information calls but the possibility always exists that the mother may be worried about a sick child. For example, if she is inquiring about the symptoms of chickenpox because her child has been exposed and not vaccinated, and she doesn't know what to watch for, that is probably indeed a health information call. But on the other hand, if the child is covered with blisters, the nurse had better assess the child.

Perhaps it *is* chickenpox, but it could also be poison ivy, impetigo, Stevens-Johnson syndrome, anthrax, smallpox, or varous other pustular rashes. The nurse won't know until he or she assesses the child.

The other example is the mother who calls asking for dosing information for acetaminophen for her child. If the reason for the call is that she wants to leave an over-the-counter (OTC) medication list for the babysitter, it is appropriate for the nurse to inquire about the weight of the child and the medication the mother has on hand. However, if her call is because her child has a fever, the nurse must assess the child to be sure that nothing serious is going on. The bottom line is assess, assess, assess. Remember, every call is a triage call until proven otherwise.

One nurse received a call from a patient who had "one quick question." Her question was "Is nitroglycerine still good after 10 years?" Being conscientious, the nurse asked, "Is someone having chest pain?" The caller's response was, "Oh no, honey! I'm just cleaning out my medicine cabinet and want to know if this stuff is still any good or not." This might launch a response directed at a teachable moment which would include information about brown bottles, cotton, refrigerators, and the like, along with confirmation from the nurse that the medication probably had no potency and should be discarded and replaced. However, the reality of the situation was that the caller had thrown the expired medication in the trash. Subsequently her 18-month-old grandson was found sitting on the floor playing with an empty nitroglycerine bottle with the lid and the cotton on the floor next to him. As a result, this nurse's new response to anyone with "one quick question" is that she'd be happy to answer their one quick question, but they would have to answer several long questions for her first!

Focusing

As the patient provides information and the nurse investigates, a pattern will likely begin to emerge or key symptoms will surface that require additional investigation. At this point, the nurse "focuses" on the symptom or pattern in question, first listening for, and then asking about other findings that could be ruled out or would be consistent with the suspected problem.

Verifying

Verifying requires active listening and paraphrasing to confirm that the nurse understands what the patient is trying to convey. This is also known as reflective listening, and is an example of one way to use interpreting. An example would be, "So what I'm hearing you say is…" This is an especially important technique not only because of the opportunity to assure accuracy of the data collected, but also to be sure nothing important to the patient has been overlooked.

Clarifying

Clarifying is necessary when the information the patient has provided is unclear or the nurse needs more specificity from the patient. It is also necessary to watch for and clarify ambiguous terms that might have a specific meaning to a health care professional but have a somewhat different meaning for your caller (interpreting). Examples of potentially ambiguous or misunderstood words might include "lethargic," "indigestion," and "stomach." One patient, experiencing dysuria, urgency, and frequency, complained that her "kidneys" were bothering her. Likewise, it is important to avoid medical jargon and realize that there are seemingly simple terms we use that patients might not understand such as "abdomen."

A nurse reported having assessed her patient, asking about abdominal pain on more than one occasion during the call, with a negative response from the patient each time. Then, later in the interview, the word "abdomen" came up again and the patient asked, "What's an abdomen?" This illustrates the necessity of interpreting, asking key questions in more than one way, and adapting the terms as necessary.

The example provided about the patient not knowing what an abdomen is illustrates the value of "getting to know" the patient, listening to the spoken and the unspoken, and using terminology consistent with what you know about the patient. The example also illustrates the importance of developing rapport, thus allowing the patient to feel comfortable enough to ask, "What is an abdomen?"

Comparing

The process of comparing is a technique used to expand upon information that has been elicited. This process gives patients a point of reference to which they may compare their current sign or symptom in an effort to paint a clearer picture for the nurse. For example, if the patient is complaining of pain in an extremity and the nurse is interested in the presence of swelling or discoloration, the patient may be instructed to compare the affected to the non-affected extremity. It is also important to establish how today's complaint compares to the patient's baseline. Patients with chronic pain might be asked to use a pain scale to compare today's pain to their usual pain. And for patients with acute illnesses, whether it's better or worse today than yesterday can provide key information about the course of the illness.

Ruling Out

Ruling out is a process the nurse uses to eliminate key symptoms that might be consistent with a specific problem or disease entity. This is an example of nurses' use of differential diagnoses, and thinking in terms of medical diagnoses to help determine the nature and urgency of the patient's problem. The process of ruling out results in a list of pertinent negatives that must be documented in order to paint a clear clinical picture and demonstrate the critical thinking process of the nurse.

CLOSING THE CALL

Closing the call properly is essential to a successful telephone encounter and is different than just hanging up the phone. Closing the call requires the nurse to review the plan with the patient, confirming his or her understanding and intent to comply. Of the three primary outputs in a telephone nursing encounter, two of them, supporting and collaborating, are strongly dependent upon good communication skills.[18] The following is a description of some of the techniques to use before closing a call.

Supporting

Often patients, especially the really sick ones, already know what their appropriate disposition should be but they call the nurse for support, or permission, to seek that care. Sometimes callers just need "someone who can confirm that one's thinking is correct" (p. 686).[3] An example of this phenomenon is the patient who has been to the emergency department (ED), diagnosed, and sent home but is still sick and feels the evaluation or treatment was inadequate. Because evaluation in the ED is based upon a snapshot of a moment in time, if the patient's problem has evolved, or if the ED provider missed a diagnosis, repeat visits might be necessary to achieve satisfactory resolution for the patient. If the patient is still concerned (and the assessment indicates a return to the ED is appropriate), the fact that the patient has already been to the ED should not dissuade the nurse from sending him or her back for re-evaluation. It is critical to keep in mind that patients may not be able or willing to articulate what is going on with them, but they *know* when something is amiss with their own body or with that of their child. A good telephone triage nurse will recognize this and provide apropriate patient support.

Along with a thorough assessment, reassuring, encouraging, and validating are supportive techniques nurses utilize when helping a patient through a new or challenging experience. In fact, Wheeler (2009) reports that "one study showed that reassurance was more important than the relief of symptoms" (¶ 6).[19] The following example illustrates supporting, reassuring, encouraging, and validating.

A mother of a 1 year old called at the end of the day worried about her daughter who had come home from daycare with a fever of 102.4. As it turned out, today was the first day ever in daycare for this child, who had never been sick before. The nurse carefully assessed the child who was breathing, eating, and playing, normally, making good eye contact, voiding regularly, and whose color was normal. The nurse recommended the appropriate dose of an antipyretic, instructing the mother on other fever interventions. The mother seemed reluctant to hang up the phone, so the nurse offered to stay on the phone with the mother while she gave the acetaminophen, took excess clothing off the child, and offered her a popsicle to eat. The call lasted approximately 25 minutes, about 12 minutes longer than the nurse's average call length, but the support and encouragement provided by the nurse reassured the mother and prepared her to manage her daughter's next illness with confidence, knowing that the telephone triage nurse was only a call away.

Teaching

Teaching is also an important element of the call and must be individualized for each patient. Although decision support tools include a variety of home care instructions, some of them will not be appropriate in certain situations, for a number of reasons. Perhaps the family doesn't have the recommended resources (such as a humidifier) and the nurse needs to consider alternatives for the family such as placing pans of water around the house or creating steam with boiling water or a shower. If the family doesn't have the protocol-recommended antibiotic cream in the house but has a different one, perhaps the nurse could work with a provider to get an order for the alternative ointment. And if the patient is being referred for care today, she should not be given homecare instructions beyond the time of the recommended evaluation. The provider who manages the patient at her appointment will provide appropriate aftercare instructions, based on the diagnosis and treatment plan at the time the patient is seen.

A patient called the nurse with a complaint of an "infected bug bite." Upon assessment, it appeared that the patient might have cellulitis. Based on her judgment and the decision support tool, the nurse referred the patient for same-day evaluation by her primary care provider. The nurse then moved into the home care section of the protocol and proceeded to read all of the instructions to the patient, including how to care for the bite the next day. The nurse, realizing the folly in this line of reasoning, back-pedaled saying, "This is what you would do if you weren't going to see the doctor, or what you should do the next time this happens." Nope! Giving the patient instructions, "If you don't see the doctor," after encouraging her to be seen gives a double message and seems to present the patient with an alternative to stay home and see how

it goes. Also, if the patient develops an "infected bug bite" again, we want her to call for assessment so we can provide the appropriate advice for that particular situation.

Instructions for aftercare are provided when closing the call. Having received care and advice from the nurse, the patient needs to understand options for further care if necessary. For example, the patient should always be offered the option of calling the triage nurse again if any questions or concerns arise. It is inviting for the nurse to say to the patient, "You can always call us back if you need us. We're here 24 hours a day for you." If this is not the case, the patient should be advised of other options for additional care if needed.

Finally, in order to evaluate the care provided (the last step of the nursing process), it may be sufficient to ask the patient to call back if he or she does not improve. However, there are patients for whom formal follow-up initiated by the nurse will be necessary. If it is foreseeable that the patient won't be able to carry out the plan of care (he or she seems hesitant or the nurse recommends a disposition that might be difficult for him or her to implement) *and* the risk to the patient is high, the nurse should initiate a call back. This risk management concept will be discussed further in Chapter 12.

Collaborating

Collaboration with the patient is critical to the development of an appropriate plan of care. Collaboration is a key element of planning and implementing nursing interventions and closing the call. This phase of the interaction must be given close attention because this is the last chance for the nurse to "get it right" if anything important has been overlooked.

- ***Read the Note Back to Caller.*** In our experience, organizations that compare recorded calls to the written medical record have found that nurses occasionally document information inaccurately, not hearing all the patient has said. Navigating the software can distract the nurse, resulting in ommissions or inaccuracies in data collection. Reading the note back to the caller will provide validation to the patient that the nurse was attending closely. But more importantly, if anything has been misinterpreted or overlooked, the patient has the opportunity to set the record straight before completing the call.

- ***Develop the Plan Collaboratively.*** Collaborating with the patient to develop a plan is necessary because once the patient hangs up the phone, the patient will direct his or her own actions, but the nurse could be held accountable for the outcome. Patient participation in the decision-making process is a key aspect in ensuring both patient satisfaction and patient follow-through with the advice given.[3,20] Ensuring that the patient agrees with the plan increases the likelihood that he or she will actually carry it out.

- ***Ask the Caller to Take Notes.*** Having the patient (or caller) take notes is helpful to improve accuracy of patient instructions and continuity of care.

- ***"Now Tell Me What You Plan to Do."*** Asking the patient what she plans to do will give her the opportunity to verbalize understanding, express her intent to comply (or not), and, together with the nurse, evaluate her ability to follow the plan. Evidence indicates that checking for understanding and acceptance of the advice is one area of the telephone triage encounter to which nurses do not pay enough attention.[6,20,21] A patient with a plan and a means to carry it out is more likely to do so than one who has good intentions but no plan or means. For example, if the caller agrees to take an OTC drug, this is a final opportunity to assure that she has the drug on hand and knows the appropriate dose to take.

- ***"Are You Comfortable With This Plan?"*** The importance of this question can't be overemphasized. It is important to ask this question verbatim and in a tone of voice that makes it apparent that it is acceptable for the patient to disagree with the nurse. Do not assume that because the patient expressed understanding and willingness to comply that he or she is comfortable with the plan. Patients, bowing to the perceived authority of the nurse, may agree to take actions with which they are uncomfortable. Giving the patient "permission" to express discomfort with the plan provides the nurse with an important strategy to determine if something has possibly been overlooked. Generally speaking, if the caller is uncomfortable, the plan should be re-evaluated and possibly upgraded.

- ***Ask for and Answer Additional Questions.*** Ask the caller if he or she has any other questions or if there's anything else you can do for him or her today. We realize that after being on an extended call, it takes courage to ask this question, but as illustrated below, occasionally this is when the nurse might find out the true nature of the patient's concern.

A woman called the telephone triage nurse crying because she had osteoporosis. When asked why she was crying, she replied that it was because now she couldn't work in her garden. Upon inquiring why she wasn't able to work in her garden, she said that her back was hurting her. The nurse interrupted the patient (see Table 1 in this chapter), pointing out that osteoporosis is a painless condition and that if her back were hurting she needed to see her primary care provider. The remainder of the conversation involved developing a disposition for her back pain and providing teaching about osteoporosis. However, the patient continued to cry throughout the encounter. Thirty minutes later, when the patient

finally stopped crying and the nurse was about to close the call, the patient asked the nurse if she had time for "one quick question." The nurse, although ready to conclude the encounter, said she'd be happy to help further to which the patient inquired, "How long do you have to wait after you're exposed to AIDS before you get an HIV drawn?"

Had the nurse not allowed the patient her "one quick question," she would have never known the true reason for the call. It is likely that during the first 30 minutes of the call, the patient was mustering courage to share her secret and evaluating the compassion and professionalism of the nurse to be sure she felt comfortable asking her this very sensitive question. However, had the nurse been a little more sensitive to the patient's angst early in the call, perhaps she would have commented on or inquired about the fact that the patient was so upset. This example illustrates the importance of asking the patient if she has other questions or concerns before you hang up the phone. Failure to do so may deprive the patient of discussing what is really on his or her mind.

- ***Tell the Caller What to Expect.*** The nurse should tell the patient to call back if symptoms change, worsen, new symptoms develop, or the patient has any additional concerns. Then, to the fullest extent possible, the nurse should tell the patient what to expect and the warning signs to watch for in the event of a complication. The nurse should take sufficient time to be sure the patient and/or the family are adequately prepared to identify problems and follow-up as appropriate and necessary.

SUMMARY

In this chapter, we have covered the basic principles and processes regarding the patient interview. In our next chapter, we will consider how to handle challenging situations that arise, in ways that ensure that the quality of the patient interview is maintained.

References

1. Greenberg, M.E., & Schultz, C. (2002). Telephone nursing: Client experiences and perceptions. *Nursing Economic$, 20*(4), 181-187.
2. Hagan, L., Morin, D., & Lepine, R. (2000). Evaluation of telenursing outcomes: Satisfaction, self-care practices, and cost savings. *Public Health Nursing, 17*(4), 305-313.
3. Ström, M., Marklund, B., & Hildingh, C. (2009). Callers' perceptions of receiving advice via a medical care help line. *Scandinavian Journal of Caring Sciences, 23*(4), 682-690.
4. Moscato, S.R., Valanis, B., Gullion, C.M., Tanner, C., Shapiro, S.E., & Izumi, S. (2007). Predictors of patient satisfaction with telephone nursing services. *Clinical Nursing Research, 16*(2), 119-137.
5. Wahlberg, A.C., & Wredling, R. (2001). Telephone advice nursing – callers' experiences. *Journal of Telemedicine and Telecare, 7*(5), 272-276.
6. Derkx, H.P., Rethans, J.J., Maiburg, B.H., Winkens, R.A., Muijtjens, A.M., van Rooij, H., & Knottnerus, J.A. (2009). Quality of communication during telephone triage at Dutch out-of-hours centres. *Patient Education & Counseling, 74*(2), 174-178.
7. Purc-Stephenson, R.J., & Thrasher, C. (2010). Nurses' experiences with telephone triage and advice: A meta-ethnography. *Journal of Advanced Nursing, 66*(3), 482-494.
8. Valsecchi, R., Andersson, M., Smith, C., Sederblad, P., & Mueller, F. (2007, April). *Telenursing: The English and Sweden experiences.* Paper presented at the 25th Annual International Labour Process Conference AIAS Amsterdam. Retrieved from dspace.mah.se:8080/bitstream/handle/2043/5440/ILPC_2007%20Valsecchi%20et%20al_rev_.pdf;jsessionid=F36E781E8FB1C54FA464093848D7CB0B?sequence=1
9. Knowles, E., O'Cathain, A., Morrell, J., Munro, J.F., & Nicholl, J.P. (2002). NHS direct and nurses – opportunity or monotony? *International Journal of Nursing Studies, 39*(8), 857-866.
10. Valanis, B., Moscato, S., Tanner, C., Shapiro, S., Izumi, S., David, M., & Mayo, A. (2003). Making it work: Organization and processes of telephone nursing advice services. *Journal of Nursing Administration, 33*(4), 216-223.
11. Thompson, C., Bucknall, T., Estabrooks, C.A., Hutchinson, A., Fraser, K., de Vos, R., … Saunders, J. (2007). Nurses' critical event risk assessments: A judgement analysis. *Journal of Clinical Nursing, 18*, 601-612. doi:10.1111/j.1365-2702.2007.02191.x
12. Thompson, C., Dalgleish, L. Bucknall, T., Estabrooks, C.A., Hutchinson, A., Fraser, K., … Saunders, J. (2008). The effects of time pressure and experience on nurses' risk assessment decisions. *Nursing Research, 57*(5), 302-311.
13. Pettinari, C.J., & Jessopp, L. (2001). 'Your ears become your eyes': Managing the absence of visibility in NHS direct. *Journal of Advanced Nursing, 36*(5), 668-675.
14. Accor North America, Inc. (2011). *Motel 6 corporate profile.* Retrieved from http://www.motel6.com/about/corpprofile.aspx

15. Levinson, W., Roter, D.L., Mullooly. J.P., Dull, V.T., & Frankel, R.M. (1997). Physician-patient communication. The relationship with malpractice claims among primary care physicians and surgeons. *JAMA, 277*(7), 553-539.
16. Wahlberg, A.C., Cedersund, E., & Wredling, R. (2005). Bases for assessments made by telephone advice nurses. *Journal of Telemedicine & Telecare, 11*(8), 403-407.
17. Espensen, M. (Ed.). (2009). *Telehealth nursing practice essentials.* Pitman, NJ: American Academy of Ambulatory Care Nursing.
18. Greenberg, M.E. (2009). A comprehensive model of the process of telephone nursing. *Journal of Advanced Nursing, 65*(12), 2621-2629.
19. Wheeler, S. (2011). *Telephone triage nursing: Roles, tools and rules.* Comptche, CA: Wild Iris Medical Education, Inc. Retrieved from http://www.nursingceu.com/courses/290/index_nceu.html
20. Valanis, B.G., Gullion, C.M., Moscato, S.R., Tanner, C., Izumi, S., & Shapiro, S.E. (2007). Predicting patient follow-through on telephone nursing advice. *Clinical Nursing Research, 16*(3), 251-269.
21. Leclerc, B., Dunnigan, L., Côté, H., Zunzunegui, M., Hagan, L., & Morin, D. (2003). Callers' ability to understand advice received from a telephone health-line service: Comparison of self-reported and registered data. *Health Services Research, 38*(2), 697-710. doi:10.1111/1475-6773.00140

Chapter 9

Clinical Practice Part II: Dealing With Challenging Situations

Effective communication lies in the hands of the nurse on the telephone. In Chapter 8, we discussed a number of communication principles and techniques in-depth. However, regardless of the skill of the nurse, it is inevitable that telephone triage nurses will have to deal with challenging situations from time to time.

Compassion Fatigue

Compassion fatigue (a form of what was once called "burnout") is a risk for most nurses and results in decreased satisfaction and sense of accomplishment at work. Nurses with compassion fatigue experience decreased empathy and compassion and are sometimes unable to feel satisfaction in dealing with a routine patient,[1] let alone one of those challenging patients discussed later in this chapter. It can be hard to "refuel" when the calls keep coming one after another with several waiting in the queue, or when a nurse feels he or she can't get his or her other work done because the calls won't stop. Also, frequent interactions with poorly motivated or uncooperative patients can make the job feel somewhat futile. However, looking at the interaction from the patient's perspective, trying to walk in his or her shoes, can be a powerful remedy for compassion fatigue. To combat lack of empathy, try to visualize the situation through the patient's eyes. Who among us hasn't been concerned about their own health? Which of us with children haven't been terrified by an illness or injury at one time or another? And sadly, too many of us have lost loved ones and understand firsthand the ravages of grief.

Although we might not recognize each call as a crisis of sorts, it is important to always keep in mind that patients turn to us at their most vulnerable moments and share their most personal information with us. Patients deserve a nurse who is fully engaged, understands the situation, and can make it clear that he or she cares. The American public trusts and respects nurses more than any other profession.[2] We must work continuously to be worthy of that trust. When patients look to the nurse for advice, they often put their lives or the lives of their loved ones in our hands. The nurse must therefore provide care that will assure as safe and effective an outcome as possible. Although for us, this patient might represent just another call during the course of our day, the person on the other end of the phone is experiencing an event that might be fraught with fear, concern, pain, or other physical or emotional discomforts. We must be sensitive to his or her discomfort and perception of the problem. It's helpful to remember why we're here and how blessed we are to have the opportunity to participate in such an intimate and meaningful way in the lives of others.

If unable to restore empathy, there are other strategies to combat compassion fatigue.

- ***Talk About Your Frustrations with a Trusted Friend or Loved One.*** After a difficult interaction or a volley of calls, just getting it "off your chest" can relieve some stress and otherwise be very therapeutic. However, complaining in the workplace only adds to everyone's stress and can create a culture of negativity and increased frustration.
- ***Create a Stress-Free Area at Work, Such as a Pleasant Break Room.*** Taking a short walk outside to see the sun and breathe fresh air is another excellent strategy. It is important for nurses to take regular breaks that involve getting away physically from the workstation for even a few minutes every 3 or 4 hours. These "mini breaks" can work wonders for your physical and emotional health.

- ***Leave Work at Work.*** When you're home, be home and engage in activities you enjoy. One person said she couldn't be a nurse because she wouldn't be able to "turn it off" when she went home. Of course, many of us don't "turn it off" either, but keeping our connection to our patients in proper perspective can make it a good thing, providing gratification and a sense of purpose, rather than adding stress.

- ***Exercise Regularly and Eat Right.*** Sitting at a computer or workstation all day can cause actual injuries. And skipping meals is courting disaster. We know from studying physiology that regular balanced meals are necessary to keep your brain functioning optimally. We know that for many of us eating sugar (such as a candy bar) and working through lunch can cause insulin overshoot followed by rebound hypoglycemia. And when we're hypoglycemic we get irritable and have difficulty processing information. If you can't force yourself to walk away for a meal for your own sake, do it for your patients. They deserve a nurse who isn't cranky and having trouble thinking because of hunger or low blood sugar.

- ***Nurture Relationships with People Who Will Help You Refuel.*** Whether you're a social creature or not, being surrounded by people you care about and who care about you is one of the things that makes life worthwhile. Being with these people can restore your soul and help you put your frustrations at work in proper perspective.

Regardless of the amount of empathy we can muster or how well we manage to treat or avoid compassion fatigue, we will still have those little difficulties we all have to face from time to time. Let's take a constructive look at some of our most challenging situations.

The Angry or Demanding Caller

Dealing with the angry or demanding caller can take patience, commitment to making it right, and skill. It is important to realize that when someone is angry, he believes that he has a legitimate right to that anger. Generally, anger in telephone triage situations results from the patient feeling out of control in a situation that's important to him. The following are a few tips for dealing with a difficult patient.

- ***Remember, They're Sick.*** When a person has to call a health care professional for advice, it's usually because they are having a problem. He or she might be in significant physical or emotional discomfort and seeking a solution to his or her problem. In truth, there are few interactions with the health care system that are really fun, and there are certainly other ways the patient would rather be spending his or her time and money.

- ***Empathize.*** We've all had bad days. Most if not all of us have had a bad experience with a specific business in the past and are not looking forward to having to deal with them again. Perhaps your patients feel the same way about your health care organization. Sometimes we have to work hard to overcome previously established poor impressions. Remember, all it takes is one negative experience to make the patient skeptical about our competence or caring.

- ***Don't Take It Personally.*** When patients are acting out, it's not about *you.* It's about them, or more likely, it's about what they want that they aren't getting. And really, if someone wants health care that badly, don't we want them to have it? In discussing a patient who was using particularly ugly language, one nurse remarked, "No one deserves to be abused." Of course, that's absolutely true, but it is critical to keep in mind that foul or abusive language or behavior doesn't become *abuse* until you *personalize* it.

- ***Defuse.*** Our job is to defuse the situation. However, without meaning to, we often escalate the situation with poorly thought-out strategies such as asking them to "calm down" (remember how you felt the last time someone said that to you?). It is also especially annoying when we fail to accept responsibility for our actions, or more often, the actions of someone else in our organization. If a patient says, "You said you'd call in my prescription, and you didn't!", the worst thing you could respond with would be, "I didn't say I'd call it in." Remember that when the patient is talking about "you," he or she is usually referring to the organization which, for better or worse, you represent. Also, if a patient says, "You didn't call me back!", excuses such as "I just got your message," or "We're short staffed today and doing the best we can," are also not good ideas. If you have a broken system that drops patient messages through the cracks, or if you have a staffing shortage, it's not the patient's problem. A more appropriate response would be to apologize, take ownership of the problem, and make meaningful efforts to resolve the problem to the patient's satisfaction. Remember, they're sick, empathize, and don't take it personally. Anything you can do to validate the caller's concern and make a genuine effort to make it right will be appreciated. Comments such as, "I don't blame you for being upset," "I am so sorry this happened," or "I will look into it right away," make the patient feel heard and valued.

- ***Recognize and Respect the Anger Curve.*** We've all experienced it. First we're mildly annoyed, then the more we think about it (or the longer we have to wait), the angrier we get. As the situation escalates and reaches a peak, judgment and self-control diminish and a really angry person will say or do almost anything. Now the defusion ship has sailed. At this point, often your only hope is to let the patient vent, perhaps over and over again. If this is the case, listen to him or her quietly, and acknowledge her concerns. You might be surprised that with a few well-placed and sincere apologies and offers to make it right, the storm will blow over. Often when patients are allowed to verbalize their concerns (especially when they're angry), the end result will be the patient regaining his or her composure, possibly feeling remorse, and perhaps even apologizing for his or her aggressive or inappropriate behavior. However, if we don't let anger run its course, and we try to interrupt or intervene during the escalation or crisis phase, the result might be nuclear, and then often there's no turning back.

- ***What Are the Consequences of Not Defusing the Patient's Anger?*** Well, for one thing, the patient will likely tell everyone he or she knows how awful your organization is. And the more disturbing the story (or the more he or she embellishes it over time), the more the story will be repeated by others. Before you know it, your organization's name on the street is mud. Also, if there is a bad outcome associated with this situation, you may have bought a ringside seat to a lawsuit. Of course, on the other hand, if you are successful in defusing the patient, especially if you are gracious about it, you will have a friend for life, and everyone will win.

- ***Remember the Golden Rule.*** Almost all advice about patient-centered care can be summed up with the Golden Rule. We may feel it's difficult to empathize with angry or demanding patients because we believe we would "never act that way." But it's likely most of us have, at one time or another, acted that way. And our anger was likely directed at someone over the phone because it's much easier to be angry with a faceless voice than a real "live" person. Be genuine and keep your attitude pure. If you are really concerned and want to help, the caller will recognize and respond to your sincerity. However, if you develop an attitude (even a teensy one), the caller will recognize and react to that as well, and you won't like the results. We all have it in us to do the right thing. We just need to try to walk a few feet in the other guy's shoes.

Third-Party and/or Surrogate Callers

One area that deserves special attention is receipt of calls from someone other than the patient. While it is best to speak directly to the patient whenever possible, there are occasions in which the patient is not available or is otherwise unable to provide a good history. While patients can be "unavailable" in varying degrees, the underlying concern is the same: that the nurse is relying on information from someone other than the patient. This is of course common and accepted in the context of pediatric care, where nurses are accustomed to speaking with a parent or caregiver. However, it is also not an uncommon occurrence with other patients.

For example, a wife might call to discuss her husband's chest pain while he is at work. Or the patient might be physically present but for one reason or another unable to provide a history. Examples of this patient might be a preverbal or very young child, someone who has developmental disabilities, or a patient who is confused or unconscious. The patient might also be generally capable of providing a history under normal circumstances, but due to the present situation (such as in the case of severe pain or vomiting), the patient is unable or unwilling to come to the telephone. Managing a call when the patient isn't present is a controversial area.[3] In a study of the ten most difficult problems for telephone triage nurses, not being able to speak directly to the patient was identified as the second-most difficult problem.[4]

Conventional wisdom leans toward the sentiment that nurses shouldn't triage patients who aren't present. However, refusing to provide care in these situations is not patient-friendly and may lead to a missed opportunity to provide a valuable service. In one study, over half of the calls received from someone other than the caller were regarding men, and the percentage of calls placed on behalf of the patient also increased with advancing age.[5,6] These findings suggest that management of third-party or surrogate calls might be a way to improve health care access for both men and the elderly.[5]

In an adult population, the rate of calls from someone other than the patient has been identified as 14% and this number increases to 40% for adult patients over 80.[6] Obviously, due to the significant number of calls received from someone other than the patient, i.e. "callers" instead of "patients," organizations must have strategies in place to address these calls. While there can be some risk associated with triage under these circumstances, there is no reason not to discuss the caller's concerns with him or her.

It is important to keep in mind that these calls might be significantly longer,[6] especially in cases in which the patient is present but unable to come to the phone and the caller is relaying information back and forth. Often the most meaningful outputs associated with a telephone triage encounter are support, collaboration,[7] and care coordination[8] for the caller. The guiding principles in third-party and/or surrogate calls should be to provide support and collaboration, educate the caller, and help him or her problem-solve; but above all, to do no harm. To this end, the nurse should be certain the caller understands the limitations the nurse is under with third-party and/or surrogate calls. If a nurse talks with a caller when the patient is not present, it should be made clear that the advice is provisional and based on the accuracy of the information provided by the caller. In these cases, the nurse might say, "I'm happy to talk with you, but I need to be sure you understand that the quality and value of the advice I'll be able to give you is equal only to the accuracy and completeness of the information you are able to provide."

When the Patient Won't Comply with Your Recommendations

As referenced briefly in Chapter 4, there is an imbalance of power and authority between the nurse and the patient/caller. The nurse must do everything possible to minimize the negative aspects of that disparity and level the playing field, engaging the patient as a partner in the health care team. Discerning what's important to the patient is a key strategy for collaborative planning. As mentioned in Chapter 8, the nurse should ask the patient at the end of the call if he or she is comfortable with the plan of care, using a tone of voice that conveys "permission" to disagree. Sometimes it is difficult to defer to the patient's wishes because they may be in conflict with the nurse's own values. Also, there are times that the nurse must consider defying the patient's wishes and taking action on his or her behalf when the patient is unable or unwilling to do so, such as in the case with a caller who is suicidal.

When patients are unwilling to follow our suggestions and we feel their safety is at stake, we are faced with an ethical dilemma. The following is a formula the nurse might use in determining whether to defer to the patient and allow him or her to follow his or her own course of action or whether to take definitive measures to protect the patient such as exercising our "duty to terrify"[9] or dialing 911 over the patient's protest.

- *Is the patient competent to refuse care?* While it is not possible for the telephone triage nurse to perform a reliable mental competency exam over the telephone, there are situations in which the patient is clearly not competent to refuse care. Examples of patients who might fall into this category are children; confused patients, whether related to dementia, substance ingestion, or mental illness; women with postpartum depression or psychosis; and patients who are suicidal, homicidal, or otherwise unable to safely care for themselves or others. Also, patients experiencing severe pain, hypoxia, or shock should not be considered competent to refuse care. If in doubt, it is probably best to err on the side of caution, acting in the patient's best interest.

- *Does the patient understand the consequences of his or her decision when refusing care?* Although patients can verbalize their understanding, the real question is, to what extent do people actually recognize that they are making life and death decisions?

A man phoned a call center with classic signs of a myocardial infarction, although he appeared to be hemodynamically stable. When advised to dial 911, the patient refused, at first saying he wanted to wait and see if it got better. After repeated attempts at persuasion by the nurse, he eventually agreed to drive himself to the ED. The nurse advised the patient that he would be taking an unacceptable risk, potentially risking not only his life but the lives of others on the road. To that, the patient responded that he

would ask his wife to drive him to the hospital. The nurse advised the patient that option was still unacceptable, but realizing that time was of the essence, the nurse told the patient that although she was capable of being pretty persistent and could most likely eventually "win" the argument, even if she did, he might "lose" because by the time the ambulance arrived it might be too late. The nurse went on to advise the patient if that was the best he could do, then to do it and do it quickly, but she wanted him to do two things before he left the house.

First, she wanted him to tell his wife if he arrested enroute to the hospital whether he wanted her to pull to the side of the road and do CPR or continue to the closest hospital, because she couldn't do both at the same time. And second, the nurse suggested he might want to kiss his wife goodbye before they left, because if he did arrest enroute to the hospital, it wouldn't matter which option he had chosen (for her to keep driving or to stop and do CPR) because he wouldn't survive in either event. And then, to further emphasize her recommendation, the nurse pointed out that if he arrested in the car, it would be incredibly hard on his wife, and if he couldn't do the right thing for himself, to do it for his wife. Somewhat predictably, the patient called the ambulance.

- *Has the nurse done everything a reasonable, prudent nurse would have done under the same or similar circumstances?* The purpose of the preceding story isn't to encourage the reader to tell patients to "kiss their wife goodbye." Some readers will think the nurse in the preceding example went too far. Others would have taken the same measures, had they been creative enough to think of them. The point is that if called to defend her actions, to the patient's wife, to her employer, to the court, or to the court above, did the nurse feel she had done everything possible to safeguard the patient? Perhaps a good perspective is "better angry than dead."

- *Document everything.* When patients are deemed competent to refuse care, seem to understand the consequences of their actions, and the nurse has done everything within reason to motivate them to seek appropriate care, the nurse should document the call carefully. And in such a situation, quoting the patient is usually a good idea.

An elderly woman called the triage nurse asking if she could turn her oxygen up from 1.5 liters to improve her comfort because she was "having a hard time breathing." The nurse told her it wouldn't be advisable but offered her evaluation in the ED and suggested she call 911. The patient declined and a debate ensued between the nurse and the patient. The nurse wanted the patient to seek care and the patient declined. The nurse told the patient, "I don't believe you understand how grave your situation might be." The patient replied, "Oh no, Honey. I understand you. You just don't understand me. I have end-stage lung disease. My doctor told me what that means. I've got my affairs in order, I've said my goodbyes to my family, and I've made my peace with my Maker. When my time comes, I want to die at home in my own bed instead of in a hospital on a ventilator they can't wean me off of."

In the preceding example, it seemed the patient was competent to make a decision, understood the consequences of her actions, and the nurse had taken strong and direct measures to encourage the patient to go to the hospital. Respecting the patient's wishes, the nurse did inform the doctor and received an order to increase the oxygen. The only thing left was to document the encounter, which the nurse did in quotes, exactly as the patient had said it to her.

The Frequent Caller

Frequent callers provide special challenges for telephone triage nurses. Often, nurses can be annoyed by these frequent calls and complain about them when they happen, but two points are important when considering these frequent callers. First, these patients are high risk and should be reassessed carefully each and every time they call. Just because there were no red flags during their last assessment (even if it was yesterday) doesn't mean they aren't experiencing significant problems today. Second, pause and reflect on what these frequent calls might mean. Is the patient frightened, lonely, or depressed? Or is the patient sick with a previously unrecognized and undiagnosed disease? There is always a good possibility that these patients do have an obscure illness which hasn't yet been identified and are having persistent troublesome symptoms. In reality, we know providers do sometimes fail to diagnose obscure problems, especially if the patient doesn't seem credible or is a poor historian. The telephone triage nurse is in an ideal position to identify and advocate for these patients. Also, if the patient's frequent calls involve drugs potentially associated with abuse, the patient is often labeled a "drug seeker." It is extremely important to keep in mind that patients requesting such drugs as narcotic analgesics are either (a) in pain, (b) possibly addicted, which is itself a disease that must be addressed, or (c) addicted *and* in pain.

Martha called the office on average three times a week complaining of a headache. Her opening line would usually be, "Honey, my head is hurting so bad, I just don't know what to do. I've taken so many aspirin. I'm about to turn into one." If this were the second or third call in a week, and nothing serious had been identified on previous call(s), it was sometimes difficult for the nurses to reassess the patient with the same gusto each time she called. However, just because she didn't have a life-threatening cause of her headache on Monday didn't mean she didn't have a

potentially life-threatening problem today. Being elderly and thus a fall risk and taking a fair amount of salicylates, this patient was always at risk of developing an intracranial bleed or a variety of other potentially serious problems, so she had to be reassessed every time she called.

Eventually, the triage nurses decided to take a more proactive and helpful stance and conducted a team conference to try to establish the cause for Martha's frequent calls. In meeting with Martha's provider and clinic nurse, they learned of her disabled husband's recent death. They had been married for 52 years, and a large part of her adult life had been devoted to caring for the love of her life.

It was not difficult to recognize the possibility that her headaches might be complicated by depression and loneliness. The medical team developed a plan that included an antidepressant and enrollment in an adult daycare center. Because Martha was wait-listed for that program, the telephone triage nurses took turns calling her each morning to check in and let her know they were thinking about her. Her calls to the office decreased dramatically and, after a short time, the headaches were no longer the focus of her calls.

Rather than agonizing over these frequent callers, recognize that their calls are meeting a need for them and thus it is unlikely they will diminish on their own. It is better to just accept that we will have a few frequent callers and value the fact that they rely on us to meet their needs. Consider this touching story.

Jennifer was developmentally disabled with below average intellectual abilities but was able to live alone in a small apartment. Jennifer called her triage nurses frequently for a variety of reasons, some for health care and some for only remotely related reasons. She had a favorite nurse, Madeline. One afternoon, Jennifer called and asked to speak directly with Madeline, who was initially irritated that she had to take yet another "probably unnecessary" call from Jennifer. As it turned out, Jennifer was having her first date ever that evening, and she was cooking dinner for him. She didn't know how to cook spaghetti, so she called Madeline on the triage line to ask for cooking instructions.

While Jennifer's call was clearly an inappropriate use of the triage line, Madeline was reminded by one of her colleagues how lucky she was to be part of such a special event in Jennifer's life. Jennifer didn't call her mother, aunt, or best friend for advice. She called Madeline, her *triage nurse!* We are indeed fortunate to be in a position that potentially allows us to make a difference in so many lives. We should never take for granted or fail to recognize the honor and privilege it is to be the ones our patients turn to when their needs are greatest.

Questioning the Patient's Credibility

Nurses are often annoyed by patients who they believe exaggerate or misrepresent their symptoms in order to get an appointment. Determining the credibility of the caller is "one of the greatest challenges" for telephone nurses (p. 489).[10] Experienced patients often know the key words that seem to get action, such as "lethargic," "chest pain," and "shortness of breath." Then upon presentation to see the provider, they sometimes change their story, ostensibly calling into question the credibility or assessment skills of the nurse. As mentioned in Chapter 3, such behavior often represents problems with the organization's system and, in fact, a patient who is creative enough to circumvent the obstacles placed in his or her path.

An appropriate initial response to a patient who is seeking an appointment would be for the nurse to reassure the patient, prior to taking the history, that she can be seen. A patient who has this sense of confidence that the nurse is "on her side" probably won't feel a need to misrepresent her actual problem. Then, if indicated, the nurse can offer home care advice with the understanding that if the patient doesn't improve (with the appropriate time frame defined), the patient should call back, and the nurse would facilitate an appointment. The patient who is feeling ill and trusts the nurse's motives would probably rather stay at home in bed anyway.

However, if the patient requests an appointment for an obscure reason, and is unable or unwilling to clarify, the nurse should make every effort to get him or her an appointment. If a patient is evasive, there might be a reasonable explanation. There might be problems such as sexual dysfunction, domestic violence, addiction, or a variety of psychiatric illnesses that the patient might not feel comfortable discussing over the phone. As with every phone call, the ability of the nurse to listen and hear the caller's concerns is critical to a successful encounter.

Poor Historians

Not every patient can give a good history, and not every nurse, regardless of his or her skill, will be able to develop a good picture of the patient's situation every time. Examples of patients who might be poor historians would include those with circuitous or tangential speech patterns. Also, patients with poor memories and those who are evasive, misinformed, or uninformed, may prove difficult to extract an accurate history from. Finally, patients who are hearing impaired and patients who don't speak or understand English also pose unique challenges in efforts to provide them with telephone triage services. These patients might be perfectly capable of providing an excellent history but because of their language barrier or lack of proper equipment (such as a TDD/TTY phone for the deaf) are unable to communicate well with the nurse. In both cases, help is just a phone call away with services such as Language Lines for those who don't speak English and Relay Operators for the Deaf. But consider the potential for miscommunication in one of those calls. Because the call is going through an interpreter who is usually not a medical person, the chance for misunderstanding remains great. If the nurse doesn't feel the picture he or she is getting is clear and complete, it is best to refer the patient for evaluation in a face-to-face setting.

Cultural Challenges

Nurses face challenges in trying to understand and be sensitive to the innumerable cultural differences among members of their patient population. The nurse must try, however, to understand cultural concerns and incorporate them, with the patient's assistance, into an individualized plan of care appropriate for that patient. There is nothing wrong with asking the caller outright if there are any cultural, religious, or other practices the nurse should be aware of in order to provide comprehensive care and meaningful teaching. In-service education relating to cultures prevalent within their caller base can only enhance nurses' abilities to provide appropriate care.

The Patient Who Pushes Your Buttons

We all have patient (or people) types we just don't like. Maybe they remind us of an annoying relative or a person with whom we had a negative encounter. Recognizing that patient type and the effect it has on us is the first step toward providing them with appropriate and compassionate care. No one says we have to *like* every patient. We just need to try our best to meet their needs. Occasionally, if the situation is extremely stressful for the nurse (or the patient), passing the call off to a competent colleague might be the best route to take.

COMMUNICATING AND COLLABORATING WITH THE PROVIDER

Telephone triage is nursing practice, and a hallmark of professional practice is collaboration. We have addressed the patient interview and the importance of collaborating and communicating with the caller and the patient in order to provide individualized, high-quality care. In providing nursing care over the telephone, interaction with other members of the health care team is also necessary. One of our most important collaborative relationships is with the patient's physician or mid-level practitioner. In other words, to provide excellent care, we must have a strong, professional, collaborative relationship with the provider. Because nursing and medical education and training are different, and each discipline has a different perspective, situations may arise that could potentially result in misunderstandings and thus require attention and good communication skills for resolution. Here, we want to address a few situations nurses may find challenging.

- Physicians are taught that they are accountable for the health and well-being of their patients. As the Captain of the Ship, they are accustomed to delegating tasks to members of the team they feel are competent to perform them. It is likely that some of our physician colleagues might not understand that state regulations may not allow RNs to recommend OTCs or renew prescriptions without a direct order. They are likely to tell nurses that they're smart and capable of initiating these interventions. But it is the nurse's responsibility to help the physician understand that it's not a matter of competency, but rather it's a matter of licensure. There are plenty of worthy tasks an RN can engage in that don't require the nurse to step outside the boundaries of his or her license.

- A related issue is that both nurses and their physician colleagues must understand that RNs maintain accountability for the actions they take, regardless of the direction given to them by a physician. As professionals, although RNs work *with* physicians as a member of the same team, they don't work *for* physicians. Unless it is clearly understood that the ultimate accountability for nursing care rests with the RN, there are likely to be misunderstandings about what an RN may and may not do.

- Occasionally in the call center setting, or where RNs are otherwise doing telephone triage at night for a particular physician's patient population, nurses are reluctant to awaken the doctor. They occasionally feel, "That's why they hired us." A clearer understanding would be that providers and organizations depend on the telephone triage nurses to provide excellent care to their patients after-hours. Most of the time, the care the patient needs is nursing care, which can be handled by the nurse. However, on occasion, the nurse will need to consult with the physician for clarification or a second opinion, or the patient will need something that is outside of the nurse's scope of practice. On those occasions, the nurse should feel free to call the doctor as appropriate and necessary without fear of reprisal.

- Some organizations require "second-level triage" for those patients who need an ED referral. This means that they expect the nurse to collaborate or get "permission" from the physician prior to sending the patient to the emergency department. These policies can inadvertently result in two unfortunate situations. First, taking the time to call and speak to the physician can result in a delay in care, a common reason for lawsuits when bad outcomes occur. Second, there is always the possibility that the physician will not "authorize" the ED referral. Presumably, in a system requiring second-level triage, the nurse needs an "order" to send the patient to the ED. If the physician declines to provide that order, but the RN believes an ED referral is necessary, it puts the RN in a difficult position. At that point, if unable to negotiate a disposition that is acceptable to both the RN and the provider, the RN is obligated to elevate the concern to the nursing supervisor or medical director, further delaying care to the patient. It is better to avoid this type of policy (i.e., second-level requirement) altogether, and if the organization does require it, they should also require the physician who disagrees with the nurse to call the patient and draw an independent conclusion, based on his or her own assessment of the patient.

- SBAR is a technique that helps organize thought and enhances communication in many areas of nursing, including telephone triage. The acronym stands for Situation, Background, Assessment, and Recommendations. Nurses who utilize this technique are able to present the patient and their thoughts to the provider in a better organized, more expedient, and more professional manner, thereby enhancing the nurse-provider relationship and facilitating effective collaboration.

- Although this will be discussed at greater length in Chapter 15, no discussion of nurse/physician relations would be complete without mention of constructive feedback. Telephone triage nurses should invite timely feedback, either positive or negative, from the providers for whom they are triaging or to whom they are referring patients. Immediate feedback on a good call is gratifying and helps reinforce knowledge. And the nurse who has exercised poor judgment or otherwise mismanaged a patient would be grateful for immediate feedback so he or she could incorporate that information into his or her knowledge base and not repeat the error. These discussions between the provider and the triage nurse also permit the nurse to explain his or her rationale, which is often based on basic telephone triage principles such as erring on the side of caution, of which physicians without special training in telephone triage are often unaware.

SUMMARY

The resolution of challenging situations depends primarily on good communication skills. Communication is a two-way street, and competent telephone triage nurses know how to make necessary adjustments and utilize strategies to enhance care and best meet the needs of their patients. In Chapter 10, we will apply these communication principles to the skill of performing a patient assessment over the telephone.

References

1. Coetzee, S.K., & Klopper, H. C. (2010). Compassion fatigue within nursing practice: A concept analysis. *Nursing & Health Sciences, 12*(2), 235-243. doi:10.1111/j.1442-2018.2010.00526.x
2. Jones, J. (2010). *nurses top honesty and ethics list for 11th year.* Gallup, Inc. Retrieved from http://www.gallup.com/poll/145043/nurses-top-honesty-ethics-list-11-year.aspx#1
3. Koehne, K. (2009). Third party caller. *AAACN Viewpoint, 31*(3), 14-15.
4. Wahlberg, A.C., Cedersond, E., & Wredling, R. (2005). Bases for assessments made by telephone advice nurses. *Journal of Telemedicine & Telecare, 11*(8), 403-407.
5 North, F., Muthu, A., & Varkey, P. (2011). Differences between surrogate telephone triage calls in an adult population and self calls. *Journal of Telemedicine & Telecare, 17*(3), 118-122. doi:10.1258/jtt.2010.100511
6 North, F., & Varkey, P. (2009). A retrospective study of adult telephone triage calls in a US call centre. *Journal of Telemedicine and Telecare, 15*(4), 165-170.
7. Greenberg, M.E. (2009). A comprehensive model of the process of telephone nursing. *Journal of Advanced Nursing, 65*(12), 2621-2629. doi:10.1111/j.1365-2648.2009.05132.x
8 Vinson, M.H., McCallum, R., Thornlow, D.K., & Chanpagne, M.T. (2011). *Design, implementation, and evaluation of population-specific telehealth nursing services. Nursing Economic$, 29*(5), 265-272, 277.
9. Wheeler, S.Q., & Windt, J.H. (1993). *Telephone triage: Theory, practice, & protocol development.* Albany, NY: Delmar Publishers, Inc.
10. Purc-Stephenson, R.J., & Thrasher, C. (2010). Nurses' experience with telephone triage and advice: A meta-ethnography. *Journal of Advanced Nursing, 66*(3), 482-494.

Chapter 10

Clinical Practice Part III: Patient Assessment

In Chapters 8 and 9 we discussed interviewing and communication techniques that help ensure a successful telephone triage call. In this chapter, we present a more specific content-based model that provides a comprehensive, systematic, clinical approach to patient assessment over the telephone. We describe a practical method to quickly identify life-threatening emergencies, collect data that establishes the context, and conduct a meaningful history of the present illness. We also provide you with a process, based on diagnostic reasoning, that encourages and assists the telephone triage nurse to look beyond the obvious to consider other possible etiologies of the patient's problem, thereby decreasing the likelihood of overlooking something significant.

SYSTEMATIC APPROACH TO PATIENT ASSESSMENT OVER THE TELEPHONE

In formal telephone triage settings, a great deal of emphasis is often placed on the use of protocols in patient assessment. In more informal settings, the process of patient assessment over the phone is more often left to the judgment of the individual. In both settings, however, a systematic approach to patient assessment is necessary to ensure appropriate care.[1]

It is essential to keep in mind that due to the very nature of patient assessment over the phone, even the most experienced and thorough nurse might overlook key assessment parameters. Telephone triage nurses must be alert to the potential for the caller's condition to be more complex than initially presented, and thus, a thorough assessment that incorporates the principles of anticipating the worst possible, and erring on the side of caution is a key to successful triage.

Determining the nature and urgency of the patient's call without the benefit of a systematic assessment can result in inappropriate or inaccurate advice. Likewise, although protocols provide structure and evidence-based decision support and are thus an essential part of the process, selecting a protocol without first performing an assessment can result in flawed protocol selection. In this chapter, we present a systematic method for assessment over the telephone that involves a four-step approach: recognizing life-threatening emergencies, establishing patient context, completing a history of the present illness, and looking beyond the obvious, or thinking diagnostically. Decision support tools should be selected and used after the nurse has completed an inital assessment. The use of decision support tools and the documentation of the patient encounter are discussed in Chapter 11.

TRIAGE CATEGORIES

In order to facilitate clear communication and cogent care planning, patients are assigned a triage category that signifies the urgency of the patient's problem. Customarily, in the telephone triage setting, categories are utilized as follows:

- Emergent (see immediately): Life, limb, and/or vision-threatening
- Urgent (see within 24 hours): Potentially life, limb, and/or vision-threatening
- Non-urgent (routine or home care): No threat to life, limb, or vision

Emergent

Patients in the Emergent category are seen at once because without immediate intervention, they are likely to sustain loss of life, limb, or vision. Problems in this category often occur suddenly and are frequently described as severe. While patients with emergent problems may be seen in a variety of settings including ED, UCC, and/or office and may be transported by ambulance or private vehicle, it is probably inadvisable to put a patient with an Emergent problem behind the wheel. Examples of Emergent presentations include stroke, myocardial infarction, shock, sepsis, or a variety of other profound problems involving airway, breathing, circulation, neurologic deficit, or psychiatric emergencies.

Urgent

Patients in the Urgent category have problems that are potentially life, limb, or vision threatening. Thus, they might in fact be gravely ill or conversely have nothing of consequence going on. With these patients, it is imperative that the nurse err on the side of caution. With patients in the Urgent category, their presentation might seem deceptively low acuity. Patients with Urgent problems may complain of a "migraine headache," "pink-eye," "allergies," "constipation," "break-through bleeding with oral contraceptives," a "bruise," or "a fussy baby." However, with closer examination, the very same patients may be found to be experiencing meningitis, glaucoma, congestive heart failure, a bowel obstruction, an ectopic pregnancy, a compartment syndrome, or postpartum depression.

Non-Urgent

Patients with routine problems will be categorized as Non-Urgent. They may receive delayed care in the office or even benefit from home care. Although ill, if care is delayed, the worst-case scenario is that they might get worse before they get better, but their condition would not lead to death or disability.

Betting Their Life

As elucidated in Chapter 7, the approach to patients in each triage category will differ. Generally speaking, Emergent patients are identified with *pattern recognition,* Urgent patients by use of a *focused* assessment, and Non-Urgent patients will usually require *deliberative* problem solving. While Emergent patients are characterized primarily by explicit information, Urgent patients often provide more implicit information and are more difficult to assess. While the Urgent category usually triggers evaluation within 24 hours, it is important for the nurse to evaluate the particulars of each situation, deciding how quickly within that 24-hour period the patient needs to be seen. A good rule of thumb is to get those patients evaluated before bedtime for three reasons. First, patients who are stable during the day may decompensate over night when patients are physiologically at their nadir. Second, resources are sparse at night, with referral sources often being limited. And finally, patients in the Urgent category have problems that might deteriorate, and thus they will be advised to call back "If…". Because of the nature of these "ifs," we want to know as soon as possible if the patient's condition begins to change, and if he or she is sleeping (or if the family is sleeping), the chances of problems being decompensated by the time they're brought to our attention increases. In fact, it's critical to realize that when we delay evaluation and treatment of a patient in the Urgent category until the next day, we are quite literally betting the patient's life that tomorrow will be soon enough.

Julie, who was several weeks postpartum, called her OB-GYN office complaining of a high fever without signs of breast tenderness, urinary symptoms, vaginal discharge, or other localizing signs. The nurse brought her into the office for evaluation because of her fever, which was over 104 degrees. The physician diagnosed Julie with the flu and sent her home with instructions to call back if she got worse. The next day, a call was placed by her husband, who stated that her fever was now just under 100, but she was vomiting and needed something for nausea. The nurse performed a cursory assessment, noting that she had not requested an antiemetic when she was in the office the previous day. She sched-

uled her for an appointment the following day without completing a more thorough assessment. What she didn't know, because she didn't ask, was that Julie was immunosuppressed due to a previous splenectomy. Tragically, this asplenic patient was septic, and for her, there was no tomorrow.

While neither of the nurses inquired about Julie's past medical history, it was less critical for the first nurse to have done so, since she gave Julie an appointment to be seen in the office that day. Of course, had she noted the history of splenectomy, it's likely that either she or the physician would have redirected Julie to the ED instead of bringing her into the office, and they certainly wouldn't have sent her home that afternoon. However, the omission on the part of the second nurse was more grievous because she made the decision to delay Julie's care until the next day without first doing an adequate assessment to determine whether she was stable or not. Of course, the physician overlooked Julie's history of splenectomy as well, but unfortunately, two wrongs don't make a right. Although the physician was remiss in failing to review her past medical history, that didn't relieve the nurses of their responsibility to have done so. The important take-away in this story is that if you are putting a patient off until tomorrow, you'd better be certain that he or she is stable enough to delay the evaluation.

This scenario speaks to why it is important for RNs to do telephone triage and otherwise field calls for same-day appointments. The reason is as follows: Patients in the Emergent category must be seen immediately, in the proper site, via a safe mode of transport. The knowledge, judgment, and patient management skills of the RN will serve the patient well in these situations. Additionally, most patients in the Non-Urgent category will often benefit from home care if offered. RNs are specially qualified to determine which patients could be safely and appropriately cared for at home and to provide adequate patient teaching and discharge instructions to assure safe home care. But the primary reason that telephone triage must be done by RNs is because Emergent and Urgent patients with potentially life, limb, or vision threatening problems must be seen promptly in a facility that is equipped to evaluate, diagnose, and treat their high-risk problem. Once again, some patients with life threatening problems will be obvious, while others may be "Zebras" and sometimes difficult to recognize; if nurses are not looking for them, they are unlikely to find them until it's too late.

RECOGNITION OF LIFE-THREATENING EMERGENCIES

Our discussion of triage categories makes it clear that the first step in any assessment is to rule out life-threatening emergencies. Assessment for any gross abnormalities in respiratory, hemodynamic, and neurologic status will enable the nurse to take immediate life-saving actions when necessary. Conducting an ABCD survey (airway, breathing, circulation, and deficit or depression) is an effective approach used to rule out life, limb, and vision-threatening emergencies.[2] Key words to watch for are "sudden" and "severe," although some serious problems, such as a stroke, may present incipiently and progress slowly.

Airway

In order to assess the patient's airway, it is necessary to speak directly to the patient, regardless of the patient's age or condition. Various forms of airway involvement can be detected using audible cues such as wheezing, stridor, muffled voice, hoarseness, and coughing. However, it is important for the nurse to keep in mind that severe airway obstruction may exist with significantly diminished breath sounds, so the absence of obvious audible cues doesn't mean the patient isn't in respiratory distress. Potential airway obstruction, such as that seen with an allergic reaction; neck, mouth, or throat trauma; or aspiration of a foreign body, might not reveal any abnormal sounds and must thus be assessed carefully by evaluating other respiratory parameters.

Breathing

Because breathing can be audible, the RN might utilize the telephone as a quasi stethoscope. However, some respiratory efforts are inaudible and thus must be assessed utilizing the patient or caller as the nurse's eyes. For example, careful assessment for tachypnea, nasal flaring, pursed lip breathing, and other signs of increased work associated with breathing can reveal respiratory distress. Identification of intercostal, subxyphoid, suprasternal, or supraclavicular retractions is also important in assessing the patient's respiratory status. The competent telephone triage nurse is able to guide the caller verbally in the identification of cyanosis, remembering that words such as "blue" and "dusky" might not be descriptive enough for the inexperienced observer. Likewise, whether the caller is directed to examine nail beds, ear lobes, oral mucosa, or look for circumoral cyanosis is dependent upon patient-specific factors such as skin pigmentation and the presence or absence of nail polish.

Circulation

Assessment of the patient's hemodynamic status requires the nurse to think pathophysiologically because of the wide range of potential manifestations of circulatory compromise. For example, cardiovascular problems might manifest as hemorrhage, shock, arterial occlusion, deep vein thrombosis, disrupted peripheral circulation, loss of vision, or testicular torsion.

Hemorrhage may be manifest in numerous ways. Patients who are bleeding must be queried regarding the amount of bleeding and signs and symptoms of shock. Sources of bleeding might be lacerations, epistaxis, hemoptysis, hematemesis, rectal bleeding in the form of hematochezia or melena, or vaginal bleeding, which can be measured by the number of pads or tampons saturated per hour.

Significant internal bleeding may occur secondary to trauma or spontaneous anatomic events. For example, significant bleeding might occur secondary to a ruptured spleen, lacerated liver, ruptured ectopic pregnancy, dissecting aneurysm, or fracture of long bones.

Although pain will most often be present in the case of internal bleeding, the most important assessment is to rule out signs of shock. While shock is relatively easy to recognize in the face-to-face setting, the competent telephone triage nurse will look for findings such as orthostatic hypotension (manifested by dizziness upon standing), diaphoresis, tachycardia, and altered mental status. It is important to remember that shock is a syndrome which presents in a variety of ways in different patients, and telephone triage nurses must maintain a high index of suspicion with complaints which might represent or be accompanied by shock.

Shock can also occur in situations of hypovolemia not related to bleeding, such as in the case of severe gastroenteritis in which the patient has lost a good deal of fluid due to vomiting, diarrhea, diaphoresis, fever, and mouth breathing and is not able to keep up with the fluid loss via PO intake. Pump failure may result in cardiogenic shock manifested by respiratory distress with frothy sputum production and either normal or excess intravascular volume, unlike hypovolemic shock. Patients with acute or chronic spinal cord injuries occasionally develop neurogenic shock, which might be identified by warm dry skin below the level of the cord injury accompanied by hypotension. Hypertensive crisis may also occur secondary to excess sympathetic activity distal to the injury, resulting in a wide variety of emergent presentations. Anaphylactic shock should always be considered when patients are exposed to known allergens such as insect bites, peanuts, or various medications and in any case in which a patient experiences a rapid onset of facial swelling and airway involvement with or without urticaria. Finally, septic shock must be considered in toxic patients with a history of an infectious process or febrile illness. Occasionally unexpected symptoms might develop such as rash and vomiting, seemingly inconsistent with the patient's underlying disease process. In sepsis, the temperature is an unreliable indicator of pathology, often following an unexpected course from high to low. And it is critical to remember that patients who are immunosuppressed (and thus more likely to become septic) often can't generate a significant fever, with 100.4^0 F or less often being the adjusted fever guideline.

Vascular occlusion might result in changes in color, motion, sensation, and temperature distal to the occlusion and represents an emergency. An arterial occlusion will present as a pale, cold, painful extremity and can occur with or without trauma. Venous occlusions, such as deep vein thromboses (DVT), will be manifested with pain, warmth, swelling, and occasionally discoloration over the affected vein. Due to the potential for emboli, any patient with a suspected DVT must be referred immediately.

Sudden onset of unilateral or bilateral blindness may occur in situations such as temporal arteritis, retinal detachment, and other ocular or vascular emergencies; these warrant immediate evaluation. Testicular torsion is also an emergency, often leading to sterility if not treated promptly.

Finally, it is prudent to keep in mind that most syncope or near syncope is likely cardiogenic in origin rather than neurogenic. With patients complaining of severe dizziness or fainting, the potential for orthostasis or arrhythmia should generally be a primary consideration.

Deficit

Patients with acute neurologic deficits might display a variety of symptoms, ranging from subtle to dramatic. Alteration in level of consciousness, regardless of how slight, may herald significant pathology. For example, children who don't play normally are suspect as well as elderly persons who experience new onset confusion or excessive fatigue. Unilateral changes ranging from weakness to paresthesias and loss of function are cause for prompt evaluation. Bowel and bladder dysfunction including retention or incontinence may represent a neurologic deficit. Suspicious mechanisms of injury should be referred for evaluation, including falls, blows to the face or top of the head, and severe flexion/hyperextention injuries. A key point to remember is that any suspected spinal cord injury must be transported via ambulance with appropriate spinal immobilization.

Depression (Psychiatric Emergencies)

Various psychiatric emergencies require immediate evaluation. Patients with suicidal ideation are at risk and the nurse should remain on the phone with the patient until he or she is in the hands of a responsible adult who understands the risk. Because of the potential ambiguity of the telephone encounter, the nurse should act conservatively, referring the suicidal patient for prompt evaluation even in the absence of a plan or a means to carry out the plan. Patients who admit to homicidal ideation must be dealt with promptly, including alerting the appropriate officials, and any individuals or groups in imminent danger. Finally, patients who are unable to care for themselves or others safely must be referred. Examples of this type of patient might include unsupervised children, confusion in the elderly, patients who are impaired due to substance abuse, women with suspicion of severe postpartum depression, psychosis, or any apparent break with reality that renders the patient or his or her contacts at risk.

ESTABLISHING CONTEXT OR THE 'SO WHAT?'

Once life-threatening emergencies have been ruled out, the nurse moves on to a more comprehensive assessment (Step 2). Individual patient characteristics such as age, gender, baseline health, language barriers, health literacy, and resources must be identified as necessary to support a meaningful patient assessment and care planning. Co-morbidities such as diabetes, immunosuppression, or asthma must be identified, and current medications are relevant in most situations. Other information such as last menstrual period and whether the patient is pregnant or nursing may impact decision making. Additional information relevant to the individual medical specialty may be of interest, such as immunization status, weight, and other factors deemed necessary to establish the significance of various findings.

For example, under most circumstances, an ingrown toenail would be considered a low acuity problem, but in the presence of diabetes or vascular insufficiency, prompt evaluation is indicated. Vaginal bleeding in a woman of childbearing age is usually of little concern unless, for example, the patient is pregnant. A fever of 101^0 F is generally not cause for alarm, but if the patient is immunosuppressed, this otherwise low-grade fever might be a significant finding.

HISTORY OF THE PRESENT ILLNESS (POSHPATE)

The third step in the process is for the telephone triage nurse to determine why the patient has called and get detailed information about the problem, as necessary to make an appropiate disposition and provide care to the patient. Use of the following mnemonic, POSHPATE (Problem, Onset, Symptoms, History, Precipitating factors, Aggravating or Alleviating factors, Timing, Etiology) provides structure and reduces the likelihood of something important being overlooked in the history of the present illness.[1] As discussed in Chapter 8, it is preferable to allow the patient to provide information in his or her own way and at his or her own pace, but the following format provides a method to organize the information collected. If the patient doesn't independently volunteer the following information, tips are provided regarding how questions might be asked to obtain the desired information.

Problem

What is the patient's main problem or chief complaint? While the reason for the patient's call is usually recorded as the "chief complaint," the patient's actual problem might be something different than the patient's identified concern. Because the patient's call might have been prompted by his or her most worrisome associated symptom, it is necessary for the nurse to listen to the patient's story before identifying the presumed problem. For example, a patient calling with a chief complaint of vomiting and fever might turn out to have flank pain consistent with possible pyelonephritis. In this case, while the chief complaints are vomiting and fever, the problem of greatest significance might be the flank pain. Patients sometimes don't understand the significance of their signs and symptoms but place a call to the nurse because of a related concern. For example, the patient with a severe contact dermatitis and associated cellulitis might very well call complaining of "poison ivy" and request a remedy for itching, not even being aware of the presence or significance of the infection.

Onset

How long has the patient had this problem, or when did it start? The duration of an illness can give clues as to whether it is a chronic or acute problem and cue the nurse to ask about previous or recent treatments or other interventions. It can be helpful to ask the patient what he or she was doing when the problem began, or whether it began suddenly or gradually. Sudden onset can herald an acute event such as a bleed or torsion.

Symptoms

Once a patient has verbalized a chief complaint, it is tempting to ask about associated symptoms immediately. For example, if a patient complains of vomiting and fever, it might be natural to want to inquire about diarrhea. However, as a general rule of thumb, the nurse is advised to allow the patient to talk freely, disclosing the information he or she feels is important prior to the nurse initiating a question and answer session. Direct questioning can interrupt the patient's train of thought, making it difficult if not impossible for the patient to recollect his or her thoughts and complete his or her story. Eventually it will be appropriate and necessary for the nurse to ask direct questions and to focus on the symptoms in order to formulate a clear and complete clinical picture. However, in actuality, until the nurse has heard the entire story, it is sometimes difficult to distinguish between the chief complaint and associated symptoms and to determine which information is relevant and which is not.

History

The pertinent history is different than the patient's medical history and is actually related to the history of the present illness. There are two important lines of investigation that might prove fruitful when interviewing a patient or reviewing his or her medical record.

First, it is important to inquire about the patient's recent medical history.

- Has the patient been ill or seen the doctor recently?
  - If the patient reports recent illness, is there a possibility that today's complaint might be related? An example of this might be the child recently diagnosed with strep who has now developed a rash or a woman treated recently for cystitis who is now complaining of flank pain.
  - If the patient has seen the doctor recently, could today's symptoms be related to a recent change in medications or treatment of an acute or chronic illness?
  - Has the patient had any recent therapeutic or diagnostic medical procedures? If so, might today's symptoms be related to that procedure? Examples include the patient with a headache following a lumbar puncture or a patient who has had recent surgery and has now developed pain or another complaint which might be associated with a post-op complication. Another example might be the patient with a cast on his lower extremity who is therefore high risk for a thromboembolic event. Recent medical procedures might also provide insight into any current workups in process. For example, if he has recently had blood drawn, was it routine or related to a specific illness or symptom?

- Is today's problem an old, ongoing problem or a new disease process? If the patient reports she is calling about a previously diagnosed problem, it is important to inquire about how the diagnosis was made. For example, with a patient complaining of a "gallbladder attack," answers might come in a variety of forms:

  - The patient might have done research online and self-diagnosed the problem.
  - The patient might have tried a treatment targeting the problem and assumed the diagnosis due to the therapeutic effect of that treatment. For example, if in the past a family member took a

particular drug (such as hydrocodone) for gall bladder disease and the patient has recently taken that drug with good results, the patient might make a self-diagnosis based on the response to the drug.

- Or the patient might say, "My doctor told me it's my gallbladder." In this case, it's important to ascertain whether the diagnosis was made on the basis of an actual workup or if the patient assumed the diagnosis because the possibility had been discussed with her in the past as part of the differential diagnosis.

Precipitating Factors

Can the patient identify any particular circumstances that precipitated the problem? For example, does the patient get indigestion every time he eats spicy food or every time he shovels snow or otherwise engages in strenuous activities in the cold? Does he develop a wheeze every time he exerts himself, every time he is exposed to a known allergen such as a cat, every time he develops an upper respiratory infection, or every time he ingests a peanut or gets stung by a bee?

Alleviating or Aggravating Factors

What treatments has the patient tried? Did an antacid relieve the indigestion or did an over-the-counter (OTC) analgesic relieve the headache? What about other interventions such as ice or heat? Can the patient identify any activities that make the symptoms better or worse? For example, does the headache get better or worse when the patient goes into a dark room?

Timing

Timing would be related to the clock or the calendar. Questions about timing may provide important clues as to the underlying disease process.

- For example, problems associated with activities of daily living or symptoms related to the patient's occupation might occur daily. Nocturia is something else that might be roughly related to time.

- Weekly events such as house cleaning, gardening, or recreational activities on the weekends might precipitate symptoms related to allergies or activities. Children visiting non-custodial parents might experience symptoms secondary to environmental changes, schedule modifications, or emotional factors.

- Symptoms associated with the patient's menstrual cycle might occur monthly such as premenstrual syndrome (PMS), estrogen withdrawal migraines, mittelschmerz, or changes in the vaginal pH resulting in yeast infection.

- Annual events include seasonal allergies, seasonal affective disorder, bipolar disorder, seasonal (or holiday related) depression, and sentinel events, such as anniversary dates associated with the death of a loved one.

Etiology

By this point, having collected a fairly comprehensive history, an astute nurse will usually have an idea of what is going on with the patient. An experienced RN with a sound background in pathophysiology might begin to see a disease pattern emerge. At this point in the interview, there will likely be a need for the nurse to clarify and verify information, confirming pertinent positives (i.e., meaningful signs or symptoms the patient is experiencing). Additionally, the nurse must also be sure he or she has not overlooked, or otherwise failed to consider, a more obscure but primary cause of the problem. The nurse, before deciding on the probable nature, or etiology, of the patient's problem, must now "think outside the box," looking for the less obvious problems that the patient might be experiencing. This is accomplished by comparing and ruling out pertinent symptoms, being sure all of the important pertinent findings have been considered. A pertinent negative is the absence of a sign or symptom that allows the nurse to eliminate the possibility of a problem or condition under consideration. For example, patients with chest pain must always be asked about the presence or absence of shortness of breath, nausea, and diaphoresis. Positive findings (pertinent positives) would increase the suspicion of a cardiac event. Conversely, when those pertinent findings are absent (pertinent negatives), the likelihood of a cardiac etiology is diminished. It is important for the nurse to ask and document the pertinent negatives in order to (a) record a complete and relevant history and (b) demonstrate critical thinking (i.e., that the nurse is processing information as it is being collected).

To be sure the pertinent findings have been addressed in the history, the nurse must consider less overt etiologies to determine what else, if anything, might be going on with the patient other than the obvious. At this point, a guided thought process, described in the following section, will help the nurse be sure no significant stone has been left unturned.

THINKING DIAGNOSTICALLY OR LOOKING BEYOND THE OBVIOUS (TICOSMO)

Thinking diagnostically or developing a differential diagnosis, the final step in the process, is not a conventional part of nursing practice. However, when dealing with a patient over the telephone, it is an important strategy to assure that vital clues have not been overlooked. At this point, a comprehensive routine for consideration of pertinent findings would be helpful to the nurse. It is important for the nurse to identify significant clinical possibilities and rule out as many as he or she can before deciding on the nature and urgency of the patient's problem and developing a plan of care.

To this end, we suggest a mnemonic tool (TICOSMO) to help nurses tap into their existing knowledge base, jog their memory, or otherwise consider a wide variety of possible, but often unapparent etiologies. TICOSMO stands for Trauma, Infection, Chemical, Organ, Stress, Musculoskeletal, and Other. If the nurse has stereotyped the patient, jumped to a conclusion, or accepted the patient's self-diagnosis, this tool will assist him or her in consideration of other, less obvious problems. Diagnostic reasoning should be utilized with all non-emergent calls to rule out potentially life-threatening emergencies. It is important to note that TICOSMO does not represent yet another set of questions that should be asked, but rather a series of categories used to guide the nurse through potential etiologies that should be considered. This step is the process that forces the nurse to think beyond the obvious. Although lengthy to describe, TICOSMO, being a *thought process,* can actually occur in a matter of seconds. This process represents a quick mental exercise that provides structure and direction to help the nurse identify or rule out potential problems. Using this tool, the nurse can mentally or verbally establish pertinent positives and negatives. This helps assure selection of the appropriate decision support tool and facilitates accurate documentation. The mnemonic itself is not meaningful, the process of considering all reasonable options is, and TICOSMO represents just one way of getting there. (TICOSMO is an anagram for OSMOTIC, which may be easier to remember.)

Trauma

Could trauma be a contributing factor? The patient might have experienced trauma in the form of a fall or a blow to the head that has been forgotten and thus not mentioned unless the nurse queries the patient directly about recent injuries. In addition to obvious blunt or penetrating trauma, the nurse should consider often-unsuspected problems such as a foreign body. Some injuries might seem trivial to patients such as small puncture wounds and bites (animal, insect, marine, and/or human) and thus not mentioned by the patient unless asked directly. Nurses should also consider the possibility of obscure problems such as burns to the eye from watching a welder or inhalation burns when exposed to a fire in an enclosed space.

Infection

Is infection possible? Virtually any part of the body can house an infection and cause a variety of related symptoms. In essentially every triage call, the potential exists for infection to be the cause of or result from the patient's problem. Fever and localized signs of infection should be considered, using a systematic approach, and focusing on the patient's symptoms and their possible causes. In addition to the obvious signs of infection (heat, redness, pain, pus, and swelling), internal organs can be infected and manifest symptoms that are localized to or referred from the infected area. For example, a pulmonary infection might cause a cough with or without purulent sputum production. A urinary tract infection might cause generalized and/or localizing signs. Hepatitis and other forms of infection such as meningitis might be difficult to identify unless the nurse considers the possibility of these high-risk problems. This is also a good time to consider the patient's immunization status and the possibility of acute systemic illness or a chronic infectious process such as AIDS, hepatitis, or chronic bronchitis.

Chemical

Is chemical exposure a possibility? Patients might experience a wide variety of chemical exposures that could be the cause of their symptomatology. Occupational hazards, household chemicals, food additives, and other environmental exposures should be considered as well as fumes and lethal gasses such as carbon monoxide. Prescription, OTC, and recreational drugs should be considered since drug side effects or interactions could cause a full range of symptoms. Don't forget to ask specifically about topicals, patches, drops, and sprays because patients often fail to recognize them as drugs. Similarly, alcohol, nicotine, and caffeine are often overlooked as potent chemicals. Herbals and home remedies should be queried as well as diet pills and nutritional supplements. Accidental or intentional plant ingestion or exposure should also be considered, especially recognizing the number of poisonous house plants that children might encounter. And, of course, use of supplemental oxygen is of significance. Endogenous chemicals such as insulin, catecholamines, thyroid hormones, and sex hormones might explain a variety of symptoms. And, finally, electrolyte imbalances might be the source of the patient's problem.

Organ

What organ or system could be involved? A quick consideration of each organ and system might bring to mind problems that have been otherwise overlooked. In this case, a head-to-toe review will improve the comprehensiveness of the assessment and is an approach most nurses are both comfortable with and accustomed to. And in conducting a mental review of systems, don't forget the integumentary and hematologic systems. While this head-to-toe assessment might be duplicative of problems previously eliminated or identified, it is better to think of a potential problem twice than not at all.

Stress

Is there a possibility that stress is contributing to the problem? It is widely known that stress in its many forms (good or bad) can cause or contribute to illness. Inquiry into the conditions of the patient's life, with special focus on stressors, might provide the nurse with relevant information. However, in questioning the patient about stress, it is important to avoid the appearance of dismissing the patient's problem because it's "related to stress." Stress-induced illness is real, whether physiologic or psychologic, and often needs real attention from the appropriate health care professional.

Gastric hyperacidity, tension headache, irritable bowel syndrome, menstrual cramps, and low back pain are among the problems that might be caused or exacerbated by stress. Although some patients do experience psychosomatic complaints, it is impossible to differentiate them from actual physiologic disease over the telephone, so the patient should always be given the benefit of the doubt. And finally, post-traumatic stress disorder should be a consideration, especially if the patient is verbalizing emotional or psychiatric concerns.

Musculoskeletal

Have musculoskeletal problems been overlooked? Although the musculoskeletal system will often be considered during the head-to-toe organ and system review, musculoskeletal concerns are so common and so accurately mimic serious disease that they deserve special consideration. Problems with the muscles, bones, and connective tissue may be localized, referred, or generalized and be either a primary source of illness or the direct result of illness or injury. Fibromyalgia and other systemic illnesses such as rheumatoid arthritis, autoimmune diseases, and connective tissue disorders should be considered. While evaluation to this extent is not within the traditional role of the RN, keeping a high index of suspicion regarding generalized illness might precipitate an evaluation by the primary care practitioner sooner instead of later. Localized conditions such as temporomandibular joint (TMJ) dysfunction can also obscure the cause of symptoms such as persistent toothache, headache, earache, and facial pain. Because many patients live with chronic musculoskeletal pain, other illnesses might be inappropriately attributed to the chronic condition and subsequently overlooked.

Other

Is there anything else you need to consider? While almost any other consideration could be included in one or more of the previous categories, "other" is included to encourage the nurse to free associate and see if anything else comes to mind. Examples of "other" concerns might include dehydration, altitude sickness, and problems related to prostheses such as dentures or eyeglasses. Congenital or genetic problems (such as pyloric stenosis), endocrine (such as thyroid), and hematologic (such as sickle cell crisis) should be considered. Every patient should be queried about immunosuppression or diabetes because of the potentially profound effect of either of these chronic conditions if overlooked. Invasive medical procedures and problems related to vectors (such as mosquitoes or ticks) might not cause local problems but rather be manifested systemically. Inquiry about the patient's recent travel history or known exposures could also be revealing. Consideration of more obscure problems, such as alcohol or substance abuse or withdrawal, and rare diseases, such as Reye's syndrome, might also be considered if supported by the patient's history.

CLINICAL APPLICATION EXEMPLAR

To illustrate how this diagnostic reasoning strategy is applied, we will use the following example. Please note that the interview strategies discussed in Chapter 8 will only be mentioned here in passing. The focus of this example is critical thinking and diagnostic reasoning, and thus, the systematic assessment scheme previously discussed is applied. To that end, let's consider the example of a patient with a headache. The information collected and the associated documentation are possibly in excess of what you would observe in an actual encounter, but in order to have teaching value, the following assessment and critical thought processes are fully fleshed out.

Chief Complaint

Your patient has a chief complaint of "migraine headache."

ABCD Assessment

When you speak to her, your first order of business is to rule out any life-threatening emergencies. In speaking with the patient, you notice her breathing (AB) sounds unlabored and she is able to speak clearly in complete sentences. From a circulatory and neurologic (CD) perspective, you want to quickly rule out signs of a stroke. So you ask the patient to smile in a mirror, looking for asymmetry; to raise her arms, looking for problems with function and proprioception; and to speak a simple sentence, looking for slurred speech, dysphasia, and/or gross problems with cognitive ability. You would also note any complaints of visual disturbance, paresthesias, unilateral weakness, or other troublesome symptoms that might be associated with a stroke. Finding no immediate indication of a life-threatening emergency, you proceed by allowing the patient to provide her history, prompting and encouraging her only as necessary.

Context

The patient is a 55-year-old female who calls at 3:30 on Friday afternoon complaining of a "migraine headache." She is generally healthy; however, she does have a history of migraine headaches. Her only medications are Premarin® and a multivitamin, and she takes Excedrin Migraine® and Imitrex® as needed. She denies use of other OTCs, herbals, supplements, or other drugs. Her past medical history is negative with the exception of migraine headaches, and specifically she is neither diabetic nor immunosuppressed. She is menopausal, with her last menstrual period having been about 2 years ago. Of course, then, she is neither pregnant nor nursing a baby. She drinks socially, is a non-smoker, and uses no recreational drugs. She travels for work, as a sales representative for a national cellular phone company, and has just returned to town from domestic business travel. She has not been seen in your practice for 14 months, and she is requesting a refill on her Imitrex. She is unable to come to the clinic because she is leaving town again on Sunday.

History of the Present Illness (POSHPATE)

Keep in mind that the nurse is not advised to ask these questions in this particular order. Rather, the nurse should listen for information that addresses each category. When the patient is finished providing her history, the nurse may then ask direct questions to complete the assessment. The following history is provided by the patient, in no particular order. However, the nurse documents the information by category, creating a logical flow and sequence to facilitate decision making.

- ***Problem.*** She describes her headache as periorbital, unilateral, dull, throbbing, constant, non-radiating (although it is causing some "shoulder tension"), and she rates the pain as "manageable" at a 3/10. She states she can "tolerate" the pain but just doesn't want it to "get any worse."

- ***Onset.*** The headache came on gradually yesterday afternoon and has not abated since that time.

- ***Associated Symptoms.*** She complains of accompanying photophobia, irritability, and is somewhat "sick to (her) stomach." She denies other systemic or neurological symptoms, stating, "This is pretty much like my usual migraines." Other than the mild-to-moderate headache and the associated symptoms described, the patient feels fine.

- ***Pertinent History.*** The patient has been generally healthy but admits to having had a "cold" a "couple of weeks ago" and that she had taken most of the pills the doctor had given her for it. She denies any other recent visits to the doctor or any recent medical procedures. She has been diagnosed with migraines by a neurologist several years ago, at which time her MRI was negative. Since that time, she has been followed for her headaches by her primary care provider.

- ***Precipitate.*** She is unaware of any precipitating factors. Years ago her headaches were often precipitated by ingestion of red wine, but she states, "I never touch the stuff anymore," so she's unsure what precipitated this headache.

- ***Aggravating and Alleviating.*** The patient states that bright lights make her headache worse as do sounds and maybe movement. Going into a dark room and lying down seems to help the pain. The headache usually responds to Excedrin if she takes it soon enough, but the Excedrin she took yesterday and this morning "didn't work." She states her migraines "always respond to Imitrex."

- ***Timing.*** Her headaches used to occur every month during the week of her period, but being menopausal, that is no longer an issue. She also reports that in the past, her headaches primarily occurred on Saturday mornings, the only day of the week she was ever able to sleep late. She says her doctor attributed the Saturday morning headaches to caffeine withdrawal accompanied by hypoglycemia.

To maximize the benefit of this teaching example, it would be helpful to review the history and determine other questions you would like to have answered. Although the patient has identified this headache as a migraine, caution is necessary to be sure she hasn't inaccurately self-diagnosed the problem. In taking the patient's history, has anything been overlooked? Were there signs in her history that would raise a question about the certainty of a migraine? Were there red flags in the history that should make the nurse skeptical about this self-diagnosis? For example, the patient says the headaches "used to be caused by red wine, but I never touch the stuff anymore." Also, she referenced a recent "cold" and alluded to the fact that she hadn't completed her course of therapy. Were the pills antibiotics, and is she experiencing a treatment failure manifested by a sinus headache? And finally, she said that Excedrin "usually works" but didn't this time. There are enough inconsistencies in this clinical picture that it is worth looking further and "thinking outside the box." Although in the next chapter we will demonstrate the use of decision support tools, at this point, the nurse is conducting a focused assessment based upon his or her clinical judgment, education, and experience.

Thinking Diagnostically (TICOSMO)

Remember, this does not represent another set of questions to ask the patient but rather a *thought process* the nurse might use to be sure nothing important has been overlooked before selecting the appropriate decision support tool.

- ***Trauma.*** Could this headache be caused by trauma? Has the patient experienced a fall or a blow to the head or been in an accident recently?

- ***Infection.*** What infections might be causing this headache? Meningitis? Sinusitis? Systemic illness? Are there localizing or systemic signs or symptoms of infection such as fever, nuchal rigidity, sore throat, sinus pain or pressure, purulent nasal discharge, or other evidence of infection such as pus, malaise, redness, or swelling?

- ***Chemical.*** What chemical or chemical influences might be causing the headache? Has she had caffeine today? Has she eaten? What medications has she taken lately that might cause a rebound headache? Has she been exposed to any environmental toxins or fumes recently? What about the possibility of carbon monoxide exposure?

- ***Organ.*** What organs and organ systems could be involved? We've already considered the brain (stroke or meningitis) and ENT (sore throat or sinuses). Is she having any problems with her eyes or teeth? Any swollen glands? What about symptoms associated with hepatitis such as clay-colored stools or tea-colored urine? Any signs of skin involvement such as cellulitis or lesions associated with shingles?

- ***Stress.*** To what extent, if any, could stress be causing or aggravating this headache? Was her recent travel uneventful? Does she have any other known stressors?

- ***Musculoskeletal.*** Has she experienced any musculoskeletal challenges such as sleeping on the airplane or sleeping on a strange bed or pillow? Does she grind her teeth at night or does her jaw pop or lock? Does she have any neck injuries or known degenerative joint disease of the spine?

- ***Other.*** Has she had any recent changes in her glasses or dentures? What about temporal and/or jaw pain associated with temporal arteritis? Where is she calling from? Is altitude sickness a possibility?

Findings

No slurred speech or confusion is noted and patient does not sound to be in much distress. The patient denies facial asymmetry or difficulty swallowing.

Reference Decision Support Tool

Satisfied that a headache is indeed the patient's primary problem, the nurse would now review the decision support tool for headache to see what, if anything, she might have overlooked and to help determine the appropriate disposition.

SUMMARY

Although this comprehensive, systematic approach to patient assessment might appear to be excessively lengthy and time consuming, the nurse should be able to complete the call within a reasonable period of time, once he or she is familiar with the approach and the decision support tool. A systematic, comprehensive approach should be based on the nursing process and include:

- Recognition of life-threatening emergencies (ABCD assessment)
- Context (determination of meaningful patient characteristics)
- History of the present illness (POSHPATE)
- Thinking outside the box (TICOSMO)
- Objective findings
- Review of the appropiate decision support tool

Use of this or a similar system such as SAVED, SCHOLAR, and PAMPER[3] will help the nurse ensure that a comprehensive assessment has been conducted. This systematic approach will in turn reduce the likelihood of anything significant being overlooked while maintaining the integrity of the nurse's critical thinking process.

The patient assessment serves as the basis for decision making in telephone triage. Use of decision support tools and a medical record template provide additional structure to assure that a comprehensive assessment has been conducted and to assure the quality of the telephone triage encounter. Use of decision support tools and documentation is discussed in Chapter 11.

References

1. Rutenberg, C. (2000). Telephone triage: When the only thing connecting you to your patient is the telephone. *American Journal of Nursing, 100*(3), 77-78, 80-81.
2. Rutenberg, C. (2008). How to recognize life threatening emergencies over the phone. *Nursing 2008, 38*(2), 56hn1-2, 56hn4.
3. Wheeler, S.Q., & Windt, J.H. (1993). *Telephone triage: Theory, practice, & protocol development.* Albany, NY: Delmar Publishers, Inc.

Chapter 11

Clinical Practice Part IV: Use of Decision Support Tools and Documentation

Decision support tools are most valuable once the nurse has completed a thorough assessment. During the assessment, the nurse is processing information to determine the nature and urgency of the problem and plan an appropriate intervention. Prior to making that determination, a decision support tool should be consulted. In this chapter, we discuss both the use of decision support tools and telephone triage documentation.

Use of Decision Support Tools

Decision support tools (often also referred to as protocols or guidelines) are just that — tools to support nurse decision making. Utilized in both formal and informal triage settings, decision support tools represent more or less structured forms of artificial intelligence. Well-designed decision support tools are evidence based and predicated on biophysical data regarding the average patient. Decision support tools are aids rather than a substitute for critical thinking. Because decision support tools don't incorporate individualized factors, the critical thinking process is the primary strategy used to determine the nature and urgency of the patient's problem, and the appropriate disposition.[1,2]

Types of Decision Support Tools

Various types of decision support tools exist in the marketplace and are available in both paper and electronic formats. They can be homegrown (developed by your organization) or purchased from a book publisher or software developer. They can have various levels of sophistication, ranging from extremes of simple locally developed tools listing elements to consider in decision making, to fully developed scripts designed to control and direct the nurse/patient interaction.

There has been a long-standing debate about use of the terms "guideline," "protocol," "standing order," and "algorithm." While guidelines are developed to "guide" the nurse's thought process, protocols and standing orders are generally considered to be a little more prescriptive, and algorithms actually dictate the path to be followed. We believe that for the most part, these are merely issues of semantics. Applied properly, these tools should be used to support rather than to dictate thinking; as decision *support* tools rather than decision *making* tools. Thus, to avoid the semantic debate and provide clarity, we prefer to refer to all of these as "decision support tools," indicating that the desired purpose of each of them, regardless of their design, is to support decision making. We do, however, throughout the course of this book, use the terms "protocols" and "decision support tools" interchangeably.

Whether purchased commercially or developed by your organization, decision support tools should be customized to fit the needs of your patient population and your practice. While all protocols have an assessment component, some may include a treatment component as well. The assessment component specifies parameters which should be considered but applied as appropriate to each clinical situation. Decision support tools might also specify treatment options that reflect organizational policy and/or physician preferences. Specifically, assessment parameters for a child with a headache should be consistent from nurse to nurse, but options for evaluation and treatment might vary based on the preferences of the physician and the capabilities of the organization. For example, some pediatricians direct cases of suspected meningitis to the emergency department (ED) for evaluation while others would prefer to evaluate the child in the office first. Likewise, if a patient presents with a suspected acute abdomen (or persistent unrelenting abdominal pain), the protocol should suggest office evaluation if the office has lab and x-ray capabilities. If the office does not have those resources, the protocol should suggest urgent care or ED as the appropriate referral source. The general point is that protocols should be customized for the organization and the community. Also, in states in which recommendation of medications is permitted by the Nurse Practice Act, the "treatment" section of the protocol could specify medication interventions that may be implemented by the nurse.

The Purpose and Value of Decision Support Tools

At present, the use of decision support tools represents the standard of care and they should ideally be used with every telephone triage call. Their purpose is to decrease the likelihood of the nurse overlooking critical assessment parameters, to suggest an appropriate disposition, and to standardize practice throughout the organization. Although use of decision support tools represents the standard of care, organizational policy and the nurses' training in their use may either augment or interfere with clinical judgment and independent thinking. Clearly, they are best utilized as an adjunct to clinical judgment and critical thinking rather than as a substitute for them.

Perhaps the greatest value of decision support tools is to serve as a checklist to assure that important elements have not been overlooked during the assessment. One might equate them to the preoperative checklist utilized to prepare a patient for the operating room (OR). Any experienced nurse knows the measures that must be taken prior to sending the patient to the OR, but failure to utilize the checklist may result in one of the many requirements being inadvertently overlooked. Likewise, "pencil-whipping" the pre-op checklist (checking off items to complete the form rather than giving careful consideration to each item) is another form of misuse. One can surely see the parallels between this example and use of decision support tools in telephone triage.

Another good example might be the pre-flight checklist. A passenger hopes the pilot knows a lot more about what's going on with the plane than the few things on the checklist, but one also hopes the pilot doesn't take off until he or she has actually checked each item on that list. A direct correlation may be made between this analogy and use of decision support tools in telephone triage. The nurse better know a lot more about what's going on with the patient than the relatively few elements included in the protocol (thus explaining the need for a thorough assessment); however, the nurse should not hang up the phone until he or she has actually referred to the protocol. A common comment from experienced pediatric nurses is, "We use the protocols with the exception of vomiting, rash, and fever, but we know those by heart and don't need to look at them." The surgical nurse probably knows the pre-op checklist by heart as well, but knowing it well doesn't assure that something important won't be overlooked.

Proper Use of Decision Support Tools

Although protocols are essential to the process of telephone triage, an adequate patient assessment is still required before we decide which one to use.[3] There is some evidence to suggest that nurses who have access to protocols are less likely to use the nursing process than those who do not.[4] Failure to use the nursing process and overreliance on protocols can be dangerous and interfere with critical thinking. Greatbatch et al., in a study of the role of protocols in telephone triage, conclude "...rule based expert systems capture only part of what 'experts' do." (p. 802).[5] Thus, while protocols are a necessary part of the process, the essence of safe and effective telephone triage is found in the area of professional judgment and critical thinking. Improper use of decision support tools often precludes consideration of significant contextual factors and patient preferences and may stymie the triage process.

A few general rules to enhance the use of decision support tools include:

- It is generally best if you don't open the protocol until you have completed the assessment. Settling on the wrong protocol prematurely might interfere with your ability to listen with an open mind.

- Apply the knowledge you have acquired during the assessment to determine which questions in the protocol might still need to be asked.

- Paraphrase questions in such a way that it is individualized to the patient. Don't read the question verbatim. Think about what information you are trying to elicit rather than just seeking a "yes" or "no" response.

- If the patient has three complaints (such as vomiting, diarrhea, and fever), assess the patient once and then quickly scan all three protocols, selecting the highest level disposition among the three.

"In 1996 the American Nurses Association (ANA) made the following statement. It remains true today: "The use of new technologies has also allowed the increased use of protocols for triage, consultation and advice by telephone or computer. The use of protocols, standardized guidelines or computerized algorithms cannot be allowed to substitute for the independent assessment and judgment of registered nurses, who extend the assessment process to obtain contextual and situational information and will determine whether a particular guideline fits a specific patient's conditions and needs" (p. 11).[6]

- If you plan to deviate from a recommended disposition, be certain that you can justify your decision.

- If no protocol exists for the problem, use clinical judgment supported by general nursing knowledge and/or authoritative references.

Deviation from Protocols

Organizational policies dictating protocol use range in structure and formality from nurses simply using protocols as an adjunct to clinical judgment, to nurses being required to read and follow the script precisely. In most settings, nurses are permitted to deviate from the decision support tool as long as the departure results in an upgrade (taking a more conservative approach than dictated by the protocol). For example, an upgraded disposition might result in a nurse sending a patient to the ED even though the decision support tool recommends an office visit. Conventional wisdom dictates that nurses should not "downgrade" protocols, or recommend a lower, less conservative disposition. The argument in support of this restriction is that if a nurse downgrades a disposition and the patient later experiences a bad outcome, the nurse is in an indefensible position in court. However, if a nurses fails to exercise sound clinical judgment and thus recommends a disposition that results in a bad outcome, the nurse's actions will be difficult to defend, regardless of whether the protocol was followed or not.

One call center manager selected algorithmic decision support tools which required clear-cut "yes" or "no" responses that led the triage nurses directly through a decision tree. When the fact that this tool precluded nursing judgment ("thinking") was brought to her attention, her response was, "I don't want them to use judgment. If they use judgment, they can make mistakes. If they follow the protocols, they can't."

What a misguided statement! Critical thinking and clinical judgment are the most important tools available to a nurse in safeguarding his or her patient and in defending his or her actions. Research supports that a process is at work that transcends the use of protocols.[5,7,8,9,10] Nurses should be supported in deviating from protocol, either up or down, when the patient's specific situation indicates that deviation is appropriate and there is a compelling reason to do so. For example, a decision support tool would appropriately recommend 911 transport to the ED for a patient with a sudden-onset neurologic deficit. However, if the nurse discovers that although the problem was of sudden onset, that onset was a week ago and the patient has been stable since that time, transport by ambulance is probably not necessary unless the patient has significant co-morbid conditions or no other form of transportation. The triage process requires (for a multitude of reasons) nurses to inquire about situational elements.[11,12] This is illustrated in the following case.

A call center in a southern state didn't have enough volume to justify staffing a nurse during the night shift, and consequently, they outsourced their nighttime calls to a call center in a distant state. Their agreement was for the call center to answer the phone with the name of the local program so the service would appear seamless and callers wouldn't be aware that they were calling outside of their own community.

One night, a father called the local hospital call center (or so he thought) seeking advice for his 2-year-old son who had fallen and burned his hand on a floor register. The criteria for referral, according to the decision support tool, included a blister the size of a quarter on the palm of his hand. The child met this criterion and was thus referred to the ED for evaluation. The father's response was "Right now?!" to which the nurse responded, "Yes, right now!" Assuming this was a potentially non-compliant caller, she went on to "guilt" the father into taking his son to the ED, citing the potential for pain, infection, and long-term problems such as contractures as reasons he shouldn't delay. The father, following the instructions of the nurse as an authority, bundled his child up, buckled him into the car, and headed out over 35 miles of two-

lane blacktop in the middle of the worst ice storm they had experienced in his region in over 10 years. Of course, the ED physician was livid when the patient presented to the ED, upset that the father had taken the risk of driving on the ice when public service announcements all day had been urging people to stay home. Both the physician and the father subsequently filed a complaint with the local call center.

This is an example of a situation in which the nurse had a compelling reason to downgrade the protocol, but failed to do so because (a) she was prohibited to do so by policy and (b) she misinterpreted the cue "Right NOW?" Instead of investigating the reason for his reluctance, it is evident that she assumed the father was unwilling to go to the hospital for reasons of cost or convenience. Had the nurse taking the call from out of state clarified the father's concern, she would have been aware of the extenuating circumstances related to the weather. Perhaps she would have advised him to seek care as soon as it was safe to do so, providing interim home care instructions to use in the meantime.

Although many organizations prohibit downgrading protocols, the evidence indicates that nurses find ways to deviate, even when they are forbidden to do so by policy.[13,14] To punctuate this finding, call center nurses who are using computerized protocols will often admit they frequently determine the best disposition for a patient and then go "shopping" for a protocol to support their decision making. This approach allows the nurse to select a more appropriate disposition without placing himself or herself in a position that necessitates deviation from the protocol. This is also evidence acknowledging that triage nurses indirectly deviate from the protocol by the way they ask the questions, interpret the answers, and couch their recommendations.[5,15] Given that nurses will find a way to deviate if they are not permitted to do so openly, a safer and better approach should be adopted to allow deviation based on clinical judgment, providing there is a compelling reason to do so. Rather than selecting the wrong protocol in order to get to the desired disposition, wouldn't it be more desirable for nurses to refer to the right protocol, assure they haven't overlooked anything of significance, and then deviate if indicated, acknowledging their deviation, and documenting their rationale? In our experience, it's not deivation from protocol that results in difficulty defending nurses involved in poor telephone triage outcomes, but rather failure to use sound clinical judgment and the nursing process, which makes them most vulnerable in a lawsuit.

A Word About Decision Support Tools for Specialty Practices

Specialty organizations or practices frequently seek decision support tools designed for their own specialty. Although specialty protocols do exist for primary care (adult, pediatric, and obstetrics), only a limited number of decision support tools exist for other specialties. Although most telephone triage protocols are geared toward primary care, that doesn't restrict their use to primary care practices.

It is important to realize that triage is triage regardless of the practice setting. If a patient has chest pain, shortness of breath, fever, palpitations, etc., she needs to be triaged the same regardless of whether she called her primary care provider or her cardiologist. That is to say, although a patient might be seeing a cardiologist, there is no assurance that her shortness of breath is cardiovascular in origin. The patient's shortness of breath must be evaluated with an open mind, first ruling out life-threatening emergencies and then determining the appropriate disposition. The evaluation of the patient must be based on the patient's current problem as manifested by her current symptoms, rather than purely on the basis of a preexisting diagnosis. In other words, just because a patient has a history of congestive heart failure (CHF), it doesn't assure that any problem associated with shortness of breath will be cardiovascular. And more to the point, it would not be appropriate or necessary to have a set of "cardiology" protocols to triage the patient's symptom(s). Such specialty protocols would erroneously imply that the patient's underlying problem is related to the particular specialty, thus limiting the nurse's thinking in considering other options.

Beyond basic *triage* protocols, however, a specialty practice might want to develop some *treatment* protocols that address specific problems in patients once the patient has been assessed and a problem has been identified. For example, patients with known CHF might complain of shortness of breath. Once the nurse, using a *triage* protocol, has determined the problem is likely CHF and not primarily respiratory or metabolic, the *treatment* protocol specific for CHF could be implemented, possibly triggering an extra dose of diuretic.

Summary

Protocols are valuable in numerous ways. They serve as a memory aid and complement and stimulate the nurse's existing knowledge base.[16] They support nursing judgment and decision making by giving nurses a "touchstone" to confirm their rational and reasoning. Nurses rely on the protocol for information when they encounter a problem with which they are not familiar. Protocols may also communicate and document physician preferences such as evaluation and treatment options and medication recommendations where permitted by the Nurse Practice Act. And finally, they serve as a checklist to assure that nothing important has been overlooked.

Application of a Decision Support Tool: An Exemplar

As discussed previously, patients often call with their "most worrisome associated symptom" instead of their primary problem. However, upon completion of the patient assessment, having ruled out life-threatening emergencies, collected data to establish context, conducted a history of the present illness, and run through a mental checklist of other potential problems, the nurse should have identified the actual problem with relative certainty. It is now time for the nurse to select the appropriate decision support tool and review it as a checklist to be sure nothing has been overlooked.

"The decision-making processes required for priority-setting and the provision of advice have been found to be complex and multifaceted. Conceptualization of this valuable patient care activity as a linear 'triage' function serves to make invisible the nursing care provided" (p.160).[17]

Using the example of the patient with the headache in Chapter 10 and one page of a decision support tool for headache[18] (shown in Figure 1), we will demonstrate how use of the protocol augments the patient assessment and enhances quality of care. (Of note: the Headache protocol page used here is page 2 of an 8-page protocol. Although not shown, the protocol does include additional dispositions and recommendations for "Planning," "Intervention," and "Evaluation," as well as clinical information about headaches.) For each of the dispositions listed in the protocol, the *Consider* column lists corresponding considerations to help the nurse think diagnostically and consider other symptoms besides those explicitly listed in the decision support tool. Guided and supported by the decision support tool, the nurse would select the most appropriate disposition based on his or her assessment of the patient's needs, associated contextual factors, and patient preference.

In Figure 1, the top section of the protocol "See Immediately – Consider 911" category includes ABCD questions such as unresponsiveness, seizure activity, markedly decreased level of consciousness, disorientation, sudden onset headache with neurologic deficit, and weakness or loss of function on one side of the body. If the patient is experiencing any of these problems, he should be seen immediately in the ED (this is indicated by the "Y" for "yes" in the *ED* column). In all likelihood, if the patient is experiencing any of these

Figure 1.
Decision Support Tool for Headache

Headache — **Adult-Peds**

Step 2	**Diagnosis/Urgency**						
➤ (*A=Airway/B=Breathing/C=Circulation/D=Deficit*)	**Consider**	**HC**	**OV**	**UC**	**ED**	DR	TR
SEE IMMEDIATELY — CONSIDER "911"							
A/B/C/D Convulsing activity, unresponsive					Y		
C/D Difficult to arouse, unsteady, disoriented					Y		
D New, severe, sudden onset; neurological deficit	Aneurysm, CVA				Y		
D Weakness on one side of body					Y		
SEE IMMEDIATELY							
B/C/D Headache after inhalation of fumes	Poison Control		+/-	+/-	Y		
B/C/D Headache after plant or chemical ingestion	Poison Control		+/-	+/-	Y		
D Cluster headache with diagnosed Hx	Pain		Y	Y	Y		
D Hit head prior; vomits 3 x or more	See "Trauma: Head"		Y	Y	Y		
D Headache with persistent vomiting	Meningitis, Injury		+/-	+/-	Y		
D Headache with change in mental status			+/-	+/-	Y		
D "Worst headache of life"	Aneurysm		+/-	+/-	Y		
D Stiff neck, chin to chest or shoulder difficult; fever, irritable	Meningitis		+/-	+/-	Y		
D Severe pain increases with movement, jarring, bumps	Sinus, Meningitis		Y	Y	Y		
D Temporal headache, vision change, jaw pain - > age 50	Temporal Arteritis		Y	Y	Y		
D Severe headache with Hx	Migraine, Cluster		Y	Y	Y		
SEE TODAY							
Pain same or increasing after home care	Migraine		Y	Y	Y		
Earache progresses into headache	Meningitis		Y	Y	Y		
New onset in elderly	Evaluation		Y	Y	Y		
SEE SAME DAY/NEXT DAY							
Children < 5 yrs (seldom have headache complaint) 1. Wakes from sleep, or occurs in morning 2. Vomiting with no nausea 3. Pain with change from prone to supine to erect	Sinus, Cold		Y	+/-			
Interferes with activity- missing work, school, etc.	Migraine		Y	+/-			
Headache > 12 hrs, no other symptoms	Reason, Sinus		Y	+/-			
Pain located on one side of head	Sinus, Migraine		Y				
Headache periodic > 2 days			Y				
No relief with home treatment			Y				

problems, the nurse has already instructed him to call 911, and the decision support tool will not need to be consulted for decision making. Recognition of the significance of these findings should be a part of the basic skill set for any RN.

The "See Immediately" category in the featured protocol has a list of questions that should be addressed. Because many of these questions have already been explored in the course of the patient assessment (covered in detail in Chapter 10), some of the elements of this "checklist" may remain unspoken.

- *Did the headache occur after inhalation of fumes?* In our patient assessment, we have already explored the possibility of fumes, so we mentally check this question off the list and move on *or* we might choose to revisit this question asking specifically about such things as household chemicals or occupational exposures. If the patient responds "yes" to this question, the protocol recommends immediate referral to poison control or the ED, based on the nurse's judgment. The +/- in the *OV* (office visit) and *UC* (urgent care) columns means that in some circumstances, based on contextual factors and the nurse's judgment, these might be appropriate referral sources.
- *Has the patient ingested a plant or chemical?* Here, the nurse should use judgment, assessing the likelihood that the patient might have ingested plants or chemicals. If the patient is a child, these would be important questions, especially due to the prevalence of accidental poisoning in this age group and the wide range of toxic house plants. A proper way to phrase the question might be, "Do you think there is any chance he's gotten into anything such as a household chemical?" or, "Do you think he might have been munching on any plants inside or outside? The reason I ask is that some plants are poisonous and kids his age can be very curious." The patient in our example is an adult, so one might choose to skip this question. However, without a compelling reason not to do so, the question should probably be

asked. If the patient's response here is "yes," based upon the nurse's assessment of the situation, the patient might be referred to Poison Control or the ED, or for an office visit.

In one case a nurse took a call from a Russian immigrant who had harvested mushrooms in the forest in Oregon and then became quite ill after cooking and eating them. The nurse had enough contextual information to know to ask about ingestion of plants. The patient was advised to proceed to the ED and take the mushrooms with her. The ED physician later credited the RN with saving the patient's life.

- *Does the patient have a diagnosed history of cluster headaches?* In this case, the patient didn't mention such a history, and the description of the headache doesn't resemble a cluster headache. However, it would be perfectly fine for the nurse to ask the patient if she has ever been told she was having cluster headaches. If the response is "yes," the patient should be directed to proceed immediately to the appropriate level of care for evaluation and pain management.

- *Has the patient hit her head and vomited three times or more?* Although the patient has already denied trauma, it wouldn't hurt to ask again. Also, she mentioned being "sick to (her) stomach," but to her, does that mean just nausea or could it also mean vomiting? Perhaps verification and clarification are necessary here. This question is worth revisiting because vomiting associated with a headache following trauma could be (worst case scenario) increased intracranial pressure. A positive response to both elements of this question would prompt an immediate evaluation in office, UCC, or ED.

- *Is the patient experiencing persistent vomiting?* Vomiting was ruled out in the previous question, so we will not ask about vomiting again as it would be redundant and might lead the patient to believe the nurse wasn't listening to her.

- *Is the patient experiencing any change at all in mental status?* With this question, it is important to compare her current state to baseline. Of course, you could ask her directly, but if there is family present, this would be a good time to consult with a family member or friend to see if she is acting normally. If there seems to be a change in her mental status, the nurse should refer the patient for immediate evaluation to the proper location as indicated on the decision support tool and determined by the nurse's judgment, considering the patient's particular situation.

- *Is this the worst headache of her life?* Of course, as we know (and as is listed as a consideration in this protocol), this complaint is often associated with an aneurysm. The patient has already described her headache as a 3/10, saying she could tolerate the pain. If this is the worst headache of her life, it is certainly not the type of headache associated with an intracranial bleed. The nurse may want to use judgment in asking this question. Again, a "yes" response would prompt immediate referral to the ED or other suitable referral location.

- *Does the patient have a stiff neck, fever, or irritability?* Although she admitted to a "little irritability," she has already denied fever and nuchal rigidity, so this question has been asked and answered and thus immediate evaluation to rule out meningitis isn't indicated for this patient.

- *Does the pain increase with movement, jarring, or bumps?* This question prompts us to ask a question that has not previously come up. It serves as a reminder to ask something we otherwise might have overlooked. An appropriate way to assess this might be to say, "I want to ask you to do a little test for me. Please stand up, go up on your toes, and then drop down sharply and tell me if that increases your pain." If the response is "yes," the protocol tells us to consider sinusitis or meningitis, and refer the patient for immediate evaluation to rule out the worse-case scenario. In this case, her response was negative. Although it is not our job to diagnose, nurses do know the symptoms associated with sinus infections and meningitis and here is an example of thinking diagnostically. At this point, if the patient had responded "yes," the nurse might have asked again about facial pain, purulent nasal discharge, or nuchal rigidity. Because the patient has already responded negatively to these questions, if asking the question a second time, the nurse should phrase it differently. For example, instead of asking again about a stiff neck, the nurse might ask the patient to put her chin on her chest and tell the nurse if it's painful, and if so, where.

- *Is this a temporal headache with vision change or jaw pain in a woman over the age of 50?* This question, of course, refers to temporal arteritis, which can potentially lead to blindness or stroke. Because of the potential seriousness of this condition, the nurse might choose to clarify by saying, "You mentioned that your headache is 'periorbital.' What exactly do you mean by that term?" If the patient responds with something that sounds temporal, or the nurse is able to elicit other symptoms associated with temporal arteritis, such as jaw claudication, the nurse would refer the patient for immediate evaluation in the office, UCC, or ED as indicated.

- *Is this a severe headache with a history of the same (such as a history of migraines)?* Although the patient does have a history of migraines, she didn't describe the headache as "severe," which would prompt an immediate evaluation for pain management. In fact, she called it "manageable" and said she could "tolerate it," and thus it is not necessary to *ask* if the pain is "severe." That question has already been answered.

Having ruled out all reasons for a "See Immediately" disposition as listed in the protocol, the nurse would now move on to the "See

Today" section. The questions in this section include:

- *Is the pain severe or increasing after home treatment?*
- *Does the patient have an earache that is progressing into a headache?*
- *Is this a new onset headache in an elderly person?*

At this point, it would be appropriate to say, "I just want to verify: Is the pain increasing at all? And, do you feel that this began as an earache?" Let's say for discussion, the patient responds negatively to those questions. The question about whether or not she's an elderly person has been answered in the data collected. If the answer were "yes" to any of these questions, the patient would be advised (or scheduled) to see a provider today, go to urgent care, or if neither were available, perhaps to proceed to the ED.

Having ruled out all the indications for a "See Today" appointment, the nurse moves on to the next set of questions in the "See Same Day/Next Day" section.

- *The first question deals with a child under the age of 5,* and would thus be ignored.
- *Does the headache interfere with the patient's activities?* We need to ask her this question because it hasn't yet been covered.
- *Has she had the headache for more than 12 hours?* YES! We finally got to our disposition (although in reality, it probably wouldn't have taken more than a minute to run through this list of questions). This "yes" precipitates a recommendation for an appointment in the office today or tomorrow.

However, the contextual factors must be considered in developing a plan of care for this patient. Because today is Friday, the patient cannot be seen in the office, as suggested by the protocol, so the nurse might suggest that she be seen in the UCC today or tomorrow.

On the other hand, if fairly confident that this is her typical migraine, the nurse might seek an order for the refill, advising the patient to proceed directly to UCC or the ED if the headache does not respond promptly to the Imitrex, or if her symptoms worsen or change. Remembering the patient said Imitrex "always works," a dose of Imitrex might confirm or rule out the probability of a migraine. Because of the particular circumstances (the patient hasn't been seen in 14 months, but it is late Friday afternoon), the nurse must be certain that the patient is comfortable with and will comply with the plan to seek further evaluation and treatment if the headache doesn't respond to Imitrex as usual. If, based on discussion with the patient, the nurse feels it is necessary, the nurse might explain her rationale for the need for further evaluation if the Imitrex isn't effective, pointing out that the treatment failure would strongly indicate the possibility of another cause for the headache.

SUMMARY

Although this process took several pages to describe, many of these elements can be processed by an experienced nurse in the blink of an eye. With a little practice, conducting a comprehensive, systematic assessment (see Chapter 10) enhanced by the appropriate decision support tool should be well within your reach. All that's left now, before closing the call, is the documentation. As we all know, the job's not over until the paperwork's done.

DOCUMENTATION OF THE PATIENT ENCOUNTER

If it's not documented, it didn't happen. Well, maybe...But one thing's for sure: If you didn't document it, you can't *prove* it happened!

In many programs, documentation is directed by the decision support software or electronic health record. In any case, the nurses need to complete existing fields, whether they are documenting on paper or electronically. However, documentation should be tailored and appropriate to the individual patient encounter. Therefore, it is important that the documentation tool be designed to support professional practice, not interfere with it.

Charting by exception, that is, only documenting the pertinent positives, has been said to be a plaintiff attorney's dream and a defense attorney's nightmare. It is important to remember that although the medical record is a legal document, it is first and foremost a communication tool. In a study comparing patient perceptions of advice given to the nurse's documentation of the advice, researchers found a significant discrepancy between what was documented by the nurse and what was reported by the patient.[19] Whether representing an underlying problem with the nurse/patient communication or with nurse documentation, these results suggest the need for careful and accurate documentation of the patient encounter. A well-designed tool will help the nurse organize information and thoughts in such a way as to facilitate critical thinking and problem solving. Although it is tempting to say "all previous protocol questions negative," that's not advisable for several reasons. First, unless the reader of the medical record (e.g., the provider) has memorized all of the questions contained in each protocol, this statement is essentially meaningless. Second, without documentation of the pertinent negatives (those specific important signs and symptoms that the patient *doesn't* have), there is limited evidence of critical thinking. Third, did you *really* ask "all previous questions?" As we illustrated in the preceding exemplar, some questions are not asked directly because the information is self-evident. For example, if you are talking to the patient, it's pretty obvious she is not unconscious, choking, or having a seizure. Gender-specific or age-specific questions will only be considered with the proper populations. And sometimes, in the nurse's judgment, some questions just aren't relevant. To say "*all* previous protocol questions negative" might be misrepresenting the nurse's actual actions.

What to Document

So, what is important to document in the telephone nursing encounter? As mentioned briefly in Chapter 7, the amount and nature of the documentation that is appropriate and necessary depends in part upon the type of decision making the call requires. For example, spending time asking the patient who is experiencing respiratory distress if he or she has any allergies doesn't make sense unless the nurse believes an allergic reaction might be the cause of the respiratory involvement. But even then, taking a complete medication history under those circumstances might represent a costly delay in care.

With calls representing life-threatening emergencies, it is generally necessary to document only the information that is relevant to the disposition. For example, the subjective and/or objective assessment that triggers the disposition should be documented, along with any instructions given, such as "get your medications together," "have another adult drive," or "unlock the front door and lie down on the sofa until the ambulance arrives." It is also necessary to document such information as "patient verbalizes understanding," "expresses intent to comply," and "patient states he/she is comfortable with this plan." If, however, this life-threatening emergency represents a call in which the patient refuses to seek care, the nurse must document the particulars of the conversation he or she had with the patient as well as the patient's response, often verbatim. Some information, even if it represents a field on the documentation tool, does not need to be collected with these patients, and in fact, taking the time to collect this information might even be contraindicated.[7,20]

With patients who are seen because of *potentially* life-threatening problems, documentation must include the rationale for having chosen the particular disposition (e.g., time frame and location) and mode of transport. There should also be documentation supporting why the patient is being seen today instead of tomorrow or next week. While current medications, allergies, and past medical history may not be particularly relevant, recognition and documentation of diabetes and/or immunosuppression is usually essential. As described previously, the same closing statements will be necessary with every call. As discussed in Chapter 7, the history taken from the patient will likely be focused on the patient's immediate problem and thus documentation of the pertinent positives and negatives is a must.

Patients who receive home care or delayed care because of nonurgent or low acuity health problems will require the most documentation.[7] Not only will the nurse have more pertinent negatives and other information to discuss with the patient, but there will probably be more considerations relevant to planning, continuity, and home care to discuss and document as well. A plan for follow-up may also need to be documented. Additionally, with low-acuity patients, it is likely that all chronic illnesses, medications, and allergies will need to be recorded (or reviewed, if auto-populated in the medical record). Because a more holistic approach is likely to be taken with these patients, social elements such as their support system and other resources may also need to be queried and documented.

Documenting to Paint a Picture

Regardless of the type of decision making or the nature of the patient's problem, the telephone triage nurse should always endeavor to document in such a way that it "paints a picture." For example, if the patient is complaining of vomiting, it is not only important to describe the nature of the emesis, but also the parameters indicating the patient's hydration status in such a way that the reader can essentially "see" the patient. Consider the difference in the following two descriptions of the same patient.

- ***"Patient has vomited x 6 and voided x 3 in the past 24 hours."***
- ***"Patient has vomited x 6 in past 24 hours; emesis described as copious amounts of watery clear fluid streaked with mucus; lips are dry and cracking, her oral mucosa is tacky, skin is warm and dry, urine output is concentrated and scant, voiding about 'a quarter of a cup' every 8-12 hours, and is she drowsy, nodding off easily and sleeping at intervals."***

It is easy to see that, although both examples seem to include some quantitative information, the second note paints a very clear picture of the patient and the impact of the vomiting on her hydration status. A simple "SOAPIE" format documents use of the nursing process and complies with the standard of care. Other contextual factors must also be documented to justify or explain the actions taken.

A sample form[21] (see Figure 2) illustrates the data that should be considered routinely, and documented as appropriate and necessary for each patient. Although electronic health records are now the norm, this medical record encounter form is depicted in its one-page paper format for ease in reading. Please note that the layout includes sections for each part of the nursing process and could easily be converted to an electronic form compatible with the electronic health record (EHR). A simple "SOAPIE" format documents use of the nursing process and complies with the standard of care. Other contextual factors must also be documented to justify or explain the actions taken.

SOAPIE

- ***S*** *Subjective: Assessment based on the history*
- ***O*** *Objective: Assessment of objective findings audible to the nurse or reported by the patient*
- ***A*** *Assessment: Diagnosis of urgency and identification of associated problems*
- ***P*** *Plan: Plan of care, based on identified goals, with evidence of collaboration*
- ***I*** *Intervention: What will be done, including attention to continuity of care*
- ***E*** *Evaluation: How the nurse will know if the patient doesn't get better*

Elements of the Medical Record

Demographic Data. Basic demographic information such as name, gender, date of birth, address, and phone number should be recorded as dictated by organizational policy. While some smaller doctors' offices and clinics still use paper charts, most health care organizations now use EHRs, in which such basic patient information is auto-populated, or provided electronically. For example, once the proper identifier is entered, the record containing the demographic information appears. If provided, this information should be reviewed with the patient and updated as appropriate and necessary. If lacking, it should be completed. If clerical personnel answer the phones and take messages, they may collect the basic demographic information.

Figure 2.
Telephone Triage Encounter Form

__FYI Only __URGENT

Date	Provider	Patient Name	Gender M F	DOB/Age
Time	Home Phone	Patient Number	Last Seen	Next Appt
Caller	Work Phone	Pharmacy	Insurance	

ASSESSMENT

P	**CC:**	**ONSET:** S G	Wt T	**Caller Request:** Appt Rx Reassur Educ Ref
O				
S	**SUBJECTIVE/OBJECTIVE:**			Occupation:
H	Associated Symptoms			Exposure:
P				Other Hx:
A	Denies (Pertinent Negatives)			
T				
E	Pertinent History			
t				
i	Precipitated by			
c	Aggravated by			
o	Alleviated by			
s	Timing			
m	T I C O S M O			
o	**Medical Hx/Chronic Illnesses:**			Diabetic
				Immunosup
				Preg / Nsg / LMP
	Meds: Rx OTC Herb Vit OCP Depo HRT			Tobacco
				ETOH Other
				See med flow sheet
	Allergies:			Non drug
				See attached allergies

CONCLUSION / PRIMARY PROBLEM	PROTOCOL(S) CONSULTED	TRIAGE CATEGORY
		Emerg (Immed) Urg (24 hr) Non-Urg Non-Triage

PLAN / INTERVENTION

ER UC Office H C Other:	____Caller's questions answered	
911 / Car driven by: Report to:	____Verbalizes understanding	
Permission to fax record to:	____Caller will / will not comply	
Pt agrees with plan -- Yes No	____Caller comfortable with plan	
Upgrade / Downgrade Disposition	Time Call Completed	Sig:
____Pt request ____Ngs Judgment ____Other		Advised speaking to RN / LPN / UAP — Provider

EVALUATION / FOLLOW-UP

FU call: at: by:	____Call if worse	Advised to call back if:
Rx called to: at: by:	____Call if sx change	
Pt Notified at: at: by:	____Call if not better by:	

Form # XYZ

White Copy-Chart Yellow Copy-Triage Pink Copy-QA

C Rutenberg, 1999; Revised 2011

Baseline Medical Information. Additional information may help establish context, such as the date of the patient's last and next scheduled appointments. Elements that are sometimes more or less static include the patient's past medical and surgical history, current medications, and allergy list. This information may need to be updated as well, with special attention to medication reconciliation. It is important to keep in mind, however, that getting an accurate medication history may be very difficult, given the frequent discrepancies between how drugs are prescribed and how patients actually take them. Your organization may decide that medication reconciliation is best done in the face-to-face setting and that in a telephone encounter, knowing the names of the patient's drugs is generally sufficient. And as mentioned previously, there are occasions when, based on the patient's condition, updating this information would be unnecessary and even inappropriate.[20] Special attention should always be given to recognition of patients with Type I diabetes and patients who are immunosuppressed because of the potential impact each of these conditions might have on establishment of acuity and/or development of the plan of care.

Your organization may choose to collect other information, based on your patient population and services offered. For example, immunization status would usually be important in the pediatric and geriatric populations, but shouldn't be neglected in patients in the middle-age range. However, depending upon the nature of the call, attention to the immunization status may either be significant or of little or no concern. Last menstrual period and whether the patient is pregnant, postpartum, and/or nursing a baby would be of significance in any woman of childbearing age, but of special relevance to obstetrics and gynecology practices. Social habits such as tobacco, alcohol, and caffeine may also be a part of the medical record.

Assessment (Subjective/Objective)

Why Did the Patient Call? With each call, a few baseline elements must be identified and documented. The nurse must record the patient's chief complaint as well as the patient's agenda (what he or she wants to do about it). Asking the patient, "What can I help you decide today?" will usually elicit this information.

Informant. It is necessary to document the name and/or relationship of the informant. If you believe for one reason or another that the person providing the history is unreliable or you're otherwise suspicious of the accuracy of the information, it is probably a good idea to note "poor historian" and then make arrangements to evaluate the patient promptly in the face-to-face setting.

As a related issue, it is desirable to specify *who* the caller is. Nurses seem to vacillate among "patient," "caller," and "client" when referring to the person on the other end of the telephone. Our suggestion is that when you are referring to the person who is sick or otherwise in need of health care, that is the *patient.* When speaking with someone other than the patient, that is the *caller,* and it is appropriate to specify relationship (e.g., spouse, parent, caregiver, etc.).

Chief Complaint and History of the Present Illness. Recording the patient's chief complaint, sometimes in his or her own words, is a helpful way to begin the note. Having a template (such as POSH-PATE) that allows the nurse to document information in a systematic manner and as it is received, will help the nurse organize the information and provide a visual indicator of what information still needs to be collected. The value of TICOSMO is in helping the nurse identify pertinent negatives that need to be documented as well as to identify any significant problems that might have been overlooked. The pertinent negatives gleaned from thinking through TICOSMO and during review of the decision support tool should generally be documented in the same area as the associated symptoms. A note is much more meaningful when it contains a series of "patient complains of..." followed by a series of "patient denies..." rather than a variable series of "complains of / denies / complains of / denies..."

Diagnosis (Assessment). As the nurse identifies the nature and urgency of the patient's problem and associated nursing needs, this is documented as the "problem" and/or "protocol consulted," along with a comment about the urgency of the patient's problem. While the nurse doesn't formulate medical diagnoses, a chief complaint of "chest pain" which indicates review of "chest pain and musculoskeletal" decision support tools with a triage category of "non urgent" will give the reader a very different idea than a patient with a chief complaint of "chest pain," review of the "chest pain" decision support tool and a triage category of "emergent." And, of course, the documentation in both of these cases should support the triage category by addressing pertinent positives and negatives. If the nurse upgrades or downgrades the disposition, this should be noted first with the protocol-recommended disposition and then an indication of whether the deviation is due to nursing judgment, patient preference, or physician consultation. If the reason is nursing judgment, the nurse should have a field in which to elaborate, such as "patient seems very sick," or "patient seems unduly concerned," or "situation complicated by co-morbid conditions." It is important to note "physician consultation" is only an acceptable option if the nurse agrees with the recommendation of the physician. As discussed previously, the nurse maintains accountability for his or her actions and thus may not carry out an order that he or she feels is contraindicated. If the nurse disagrees with the physician and is unable to achieve resolution, the call must be taken up the chain of command.

Plan (P). In documenting the plan of care, the nurse should note the disposition, including where the patient is being referred, when, and by what means of transport if specified. If the patient is instructed to have another adult drive to the physician's office, UCC, or ED, that should be documented as well. Basic information should also be documented including:

- Caller verbalizes understanding (if not, keep trying until he or she does).

- Caller is willing to comply (if not, either negotiate an acceptable plan or document in *detail* what you said to the patient and his or her response).

- Caller is comfortable with the plan of care (if not, ask him or her to come into the office).

Intervention (I). Documented interventions might include the referral (e.g., office, UCC, ED), patient education about home care, assisting the patient with problem solving about transportation, calling report, and faxing or emailing a note summary to the patient's physician or local ED. Intervention could also include making an appointment for a patient who is unlikely or unable to do it for him or herself. Often the primary intervention will be patient teaching (which may include reassurance and support), and this should be documented as a record of what transpired. It also provides other members of the health care team content they can reinforce, should the need present itself.

Evaluation (E). A specific plan should be documented regarding what the patient should do if he or she doesn't get better, if he or she gets worse (and what worse looks like), if symptoms change unexpectedly, or if he or she develops any additional concerns. Sometimes, the nurse might plan to make a follow-up phone call to evaluate the patient, and this plan should be documented in the patient's medical record. As noted in the Greenberg Model of Telephone Nursing Practice, hanging up the phone doesn't always mean the encounter is complete. There might be additional interventions needed by the nurse, in which case an addendum should be made, if possible, to the original note.

SUMMARY

Because the nurse can't see the patient, documentation of the encounter in the medical record takes on added significance. Documentation should be systematic, thorough, and descriptive enough to paint a picture. In the next chapter, we will explore risk management principles and common pitfalls in the practice of telephone triage.

References

1. Collin-Jacques, C., & Smith, C. (2005). Nursing on the line: Experiences from England and Quebec (Canada). *Human Relations, 58*(1), 5-32.
2. Purc-Stephenson, R., & Thrasher, C. (2010). Nurses' experiences with telephone triage and advice: A meta-ethnography. *Journal of Advanced Nursing, 66*(3), 482-494. doi:10.1111/j.1365-2648.2010.05275.x
3. Rutenberg, C. (2009). Telephone triage: Timely tips. *AAACN Viewpoint, 31*(5), 4-6.
4. Mayo, A.M., Chang, B.L., & Omery, A. (2002). Use of protocols and guidelines by telephone nurses. *Clinical Nursing Research, 11*(2), 204-219.
5. Greatbatch, D., Hanlon, G., Goode, J., O'Cathain, A., Strangleman, T., & Luff, D. (2005). Telephone triage, expert systems and clinical expertise. *Sociology of Health & Illness, 27*(6), 802-830.
6. American Nurses Association (ANA). (1996). Telehealth: Issues for nursing. In *Nursing Trends & Issues, ANA Policy Series.* Washington, DC: Author.
7. Leprohon, J., & Patel, V.L. (1995). Decision-making strategies for telephone triage in emergency medical services. *Medical Decision Making, 15*(3), 240-253.
8. Edwards, B. (1994). Telephone triage: How experienced nurses reach decisions. *Journal of Advanced Nursing, 19*, 717-724.
9. Greenberg, M.E. (2009). A comprehensive model of the process of telephone nursing. *Journal of Advanced Nursing, 65*(12), 2621-2629. doi:10.1111/j.1365-2648.2009.05132.x
10. Valanis, B., Moscato, S., Tanner, C., Shapiro, S., Izumi, S. David, M., & Mayo, A. (2003). Making it work: Organization and processes of telephone nursing advice services. *Journal of Nursing Administration, 33*(4), 216-223.
11. Derkx, H.P., Rethans, J.J., Maiburg, B.H., Winkens, R.A., Muijtjens, A.M., van Rooij, H., & Knottnerus, J.A. (2009). Quality of communication during telephone triage at Dutch out-of-hours centres. *Patient Education & Counseling, 74*(2), 174-178.
12. Ström, M., Marklund, B., & Hildingh, C. (2009). Callers' perceptions of receiving advice via a medical care help line. *Scandinavian Journal of Caring Sciences, 23*(4), 682-690. doi:10.1111/j.1471-6712.2008.00661.x
13. Dowding, D., Mitchell, N., Randell, R., Foster, R., Lattimer, V., & Thompson, C. (2009). Nurses' use of computerised clinical decision support systems: A case site analysis. *Journal of Clinical Nursing, 18*(8), 1159-1167. doi:10.1111/j.1365-2702.2008.02607.x
14. Hanlon, G., Strangleman, T., Goode, J., Luff, D., O'Cathian, A., & Greatbatch, D. (2005). Knowledge, technology and nursing: The case of NHS direct. *Human Relations, 58*(2), 147-171.
15. Holmström, I. (2007). Decision aid software programs in telenursing: Not used as intended? Experiences of Swedish telenurses. *Nursing & Health Sciences, 9*(1), 23-28.

16. Ernesäter, A., Holmström, I., & Engström, M. (2009). Telenurses' experiences of working with computerized decision support: Supporting, inhibiting and quality improving. *Journal of Advanced Nursing, 65*(5), 1074-1083. doi:10.1111/j.1365-2648.2009.04966.x
17. Wilson, R., & Hubert, J. (2002). Resurfacing the care in nursing by telephone: lessons from ambulatory oncology. *Nursing Outlook, 50*(4), 160-164.
18. Woodke, D. (2005). *Telephone triage decision support tools for nurses: Guidelines for ambulatory care.* Indianapolis, IN: Ambulatory Innovations, Inc.
19. Leclerc, B., Dunnigan, L., Côté, H., Zunzunegui, M., Hagan, L., & Morin, D. (2003). Callers' ability to understand advice received from a telephone health-line service: Comparison of self-reported and registered data. *Health Services Research, 38*(2), 697-710. doi:10.1111/1475-6773.00140
20. Schmitt, B.D., & Thompson, D.A. (2005). Triage documentation: Setting a best practice. *Answerstat.* Retrieved from http://www.answerstat.com/articles/5/42.html
21. Rutenberg, C. (2011). *Telephone triage encounter form #6 in customizable telephone triage policy book/how-to manual on CD.* Hot Springs, AR: Telephone Triage Consulting, Inc.

Chapter 12

Risk Management and Common Pitfalls in Telephone Triage

COMMON PITFALLS AND PERILS

Telephone triage done right can make a difference. Done wrong, it can lead to disaster.

Elsewhere in this book, we discussed the "minimum skill set" necessary for the practice of telephone triage. This skill set includes an extensive clinical knowledge base and a clear understanding of this practice. The telephone triage nurse needs excellent interpersonal and communication skills, the ability to do deductive and inductive reasoning, strong analytical skills including the ability to think diagnostically, and the ability to gather and utilize all relevant information in developing the plan of care. Specific skills and principles of which telephone triage nurses must be aware are also referenced in literature.[1,2,3] Other "truths," or principles of care, are illustrated in the form of pitfalls which must be avoided. Some of the stories in this chapter have been shared by nursing colleagues, and others are based on the authors' experience in serving as expert witnesses in cases relevant to telephone triage and ambulatory care nursing.

Telephone triage nurses are zebra hunters extraordinaire!

Health care professionals might recognize the saying, "If you hear hoof beats, you should look for horses, not zebras." However, in the potentially nebulous world of telephone triage, if the nurse isn't *looking* for zebras, an entire herd might thunder by without notice. In other words, the nurse must remember to look "outside the box" for unanticipated problems. It is critical for the nurse to realize that, although rare, outliers do exist. The nurse will never recognize them unless he or she makes a point to look for them in an effort to rule them out.

Our health care system is designed in such a way that, if one person makes a mistake, mechanisms are in place to compensate. When something goes wrong, in most cases, multiple individual or system errors have been made. However, that is not always the case in telephone triage, where the encounter is usually limited to the nurse and the caller. As a consequence, the smallest oversight by the telephone triage nurse can lead to the worst possible outcome, as many of the examples in this chapter will illustrate.

It is essential to keep in mind that due to the very nature of patient assessment over the phone, even the most experienced and thorough nurse might overlook key assessment parameters or fail to recognize the significance of obscure symptoms. Telephone triage nurses must be alert to the potential for the caller's problem to be more complex than initially stated. Thus, performing a thorough assessment, developing a habit of anticipating worst possible, and consistently erring on the side of caution when in doubt are critical to successful telephone triage.

Failure to assure sound program design is another area of concern. Chapters 14 and 15 are devoted entirely to this important issue because of the significant impact poor program design can have on the quality of care. Program design problems, coupled with failure to apply the principles and use the tools described in this book, can lead to poor outcomes. This chapter addresses a number of practice errors, or pitfalls, that can result in bad outcomes.

Our discussion of pitfalls is illustrated by multiple clinical examples, almost all of which include failure to conduct an adequate assessment and/or failure to utilize critical thinking. Although most stories represent multiple clinical pitfalls, each story has been selected for its usefulness in highlighting one particular problem.

The patient scenarios described in this chapter come from a variety of sources. Some represent lawsuits and some do not. Some resulted in bad outcomes and some were near misses. Some are from call centers, some from doctors' offices; some deal with pediatric populations, others with adults. Some of the nurses used protocols and others did not. However, the truths illustrated in these reports are universal and can be applied to almost any telephone triage situation. The pitfalls are listed here in the order they are discussed in this chapter.

1. Accepting patient self-diagnosis
2. Jumping to a conclusion
3. Stereotyping the patient
4. The frequent caller
5. Failure to speak directly with the patient
6. Fatigue and haste
7. Knowledge deficit
8. Failure to reassess
9. Failure to perform an adequate assessment
10. Failure to use critical thinking and exercise clinical judgment
11. Failure to LISTEN and THINK
12. Failure to err on the side of caution
13. Failure to anticipate worst possible
14. Over-reliance on protocols
15. Failure to use protocols
16. Failure to facilitate continuity of care
17. Failure to advocate for the patient
18. Failure to document pertinent negatives
19. Failure to follow-up
20. Fear of "crying wolf" and being labeled an "over-reactor"
21. Initial triage by unqualified personnel
22. Failure to formalize telephone triage within the organization
23. Functioning outside of scope of practice

1. Accepting Patient Self-Diagnosis

Perhaps the most insidious of all telephone triage pitfalls is accepting patient self-diagnosis. Nurses fall into this trap time and time again, usually without realizing it. Many patients already have a pretty good idea what is wrong with them or at least what they *think* is wrong with them. Most adults probably don't like the idea of having a problem and not knowing what it is, so they do research, talk to friends and relatives, and give it their best shot in trying to identify the etiology of the problem. And they can do an uncanny job of painting a picture to support their hypothesis, especially if they access the Internet, or a well-meaning friend or relative helps them make the initial "diagnosis." Because of the insidious nature of this pitfall, several examples are offered. Consider the following three self-diagnosed cases of "pinkeye," all three of which, if mishandled, could have had disastrous results.

The mother of 12-year-old Stacey called stating her daughter had pinkeye. Mom knew this was pinkeye because Stacey's 8-year-old sister was just getting over a bout of pinkeye. Furthermore, because they were on vacation, they didn't have a local doctor and she wasn't going to "spend the day in the ER for them to just give me the medicine I already have." The mother went on to express her understanding that she wasn't supposed to use one child's eye drops on another but stated she had "kept the tip sterile" and does this "all the time." She said the reason she had called was to find out if she could allow Stacey to go swimming because it was such an important part of her vacation.

The nurse, understanding the mother wasn't going to seek care for her daughter, explained that although she probably shouldn't let her daughter go in the pool, if she did, the child should wear tight-fitting goggles that would keep the chlorinated water out of

her eyes. The nurse went on to do some good teaching about hand washing and cross contamination with hand towels and the like. Learning that the child wore contacts, she advised the mother to have her wear her glasses instead of her contacts until the infection cleared up. The mother replied that Stacey had left her glasses at home but was wearing her prescription sunglasses, even indoors. That information raised a red flag for the nurse who wondered why a 12-year-old would be wearing sunglasses indoors. So the nurse investigated further, learning that the girl was wearing them because "the light hurts her eyes, even indoors." The nurse, not knowing what was wrong with the child, but knowing it wasn't conjunctivitis, urged the mother to take her daughter to the ED for evaluation. When the nurse followed up later that afternoon, she learned that the patient had sustained a deep corneal ulcer secondary to over-wearing her contact lenses.

The advice to have the child wear glasses until the infection cleared up indicated a knowledge deficit on the part of the nurse. In actuality, contact wearers who have pink or painful eyes should be evaluated promptly. It was only a coincidence that the mother mentioned the sunglasses, alerting the nurse to the photophobia. Additionally, the possibility of an error could have been avoided if instead of handling this question as a "health information" call, the nurse recognized it as a triage call, conducted a proper assessment, and used the appropriate decision support tool.

A young man called complaining of "pinkeye" and requesting an appointment for evaluation. The patient's history was negative with the exception of red uncomfortable eyes. The nurse gave him an appointment, but just before hanging up mentally reviewed TICOSMO (see Chapter 10) for the patient. She considered the possibility of eye trauma because conjunctivitis just didn't seem to fit, in that he was a young, single blue-collar worker who lived alone. Her first thought was foreign body, but she ruled that out because it was bilateral. She next thought of a chemical splash and ruled that out. She then thought of welding burn and asked, "You haven't been watching a welder lately, have you?" The patient replied to the affirmative, astonished that the nurse had figured that out. When asking the nurse what made her look further, she said, "It didn't make sense. Given his demographic, the facts that he hadn't been around children, hadn't been sick, and didn't know anyone who had been sick, nothing about his situation would logically explain conjunctivitis."

This example illustrates the importance of assessing a patient adequately, and consulting a protocol, prior to assigning a disposition (such as giving him an appointment). Given that his problem was likely a welding burn, the patient was referred to an ophthalmologist for prompt evaluation.

A final example of a patient's misdiagnosis of conjunctivitis is illustrated by a woman who called her primary care physician's (PCP) office requesting a prescription for "pinkeye." She stated her co-worker had just been diagnosed and now she had it, so it must be "going around the office." The triage policy for conjunctivitis allowed telephone treatment of conjunctivitis in a family member or close associate of someone with a positive diagnosis, so following the treatment protocol, the RN was going to initiate a prescription for the recommended ophthalmic antibiotic drops. Unfortunately, the nurse had not used a protocol or considered other etiologies of the pink eye, accepting the logic of the patient's self-diagnosis. When she asked the patient for her pharmacy information, the patient asked that they deliver the prescription to her because "when I went out for lunch, the light hurt my eyes." Fortunately, the nurse heard the patient and realized the photophobia was not consistent with conjunctivitis. The fact that her colleague had "pinkeye" was merely a coincidence. In reality, the patient had iritis requiring a prompt evaluation by an ophthalmologist.

Here again the nurse and the patient were fortunate that light sensitivity was mentioned before treatment for the wrong disease was initiated. Patient diagnosis may well be the most tricky and dangerous pitfall nurses face because of the apparent validity of the patient's assumption. Without a high index of suspicion, even a conscientious nurse might miss important cues. The triage nurse must keep an open and clear mind and utilize decision support tools and clinical knowledge in order to recognize symptoms that fit the pattern of an unanticipated problem. Each and every patient, regardless of his or her perception of the reason for the call, deserves an adequate, open-minded, and fresh assessment to identify the nature and urgency of the problem accurately.

2. Jumping to a Conclusion

Just as in the case of patient self-diagnosis, nurses may jump to a conclusion by not looking beyond the obvious. For example, the patient who complains of "indigestion" might automatically be regarded as suffering from gastro-esophageal reflux disease (GERD). In the following case, the zebra was not far from view, but the nurse fell short of discovering the most significant finding of all.

An elderly gentleman visited an UCC for evaluation and treatment of gout, for which he was placed on indomethacin. He took his first dose that evening and his second the next morning. Shortly thereafter, he began vomiting and called the UCC to inquire about what he should do. The nurse, assuming the problem might have been related to the indomethacin, asked him if he had eaten breakfast before taking his morning dose, which he had not. Assuming the patient's GI upset was related to indomethacin, she advised the patient that indomethacin can be hard on the stomach and to be sure to eat before he took his next dose. He then inquired about what he should do for the associated pain in his throat, for which the nurse recommended acetaminophen, once again assuming the throat pain was related to the vomiting. The patient was dead 1 hour later secondary to an anaphylactic reaction to indomethacin.

While this seems to be a somewhat obscure presentation for anaphylaxis, if the nurse had simply asked the patient, "Is there anything else going on?" he most certainly would have reported that his face was "all swollen," as he had reported to his wife. It is essential for the nurse on the phone to look beyond the obvious and avoid jumping to a conclusion. We are not accustomed to asking such basic questions as "Is your face swollen" because in the face-to-face setting, those types of findings are self-evident. The telephone triage nurse must be dedicated to looking for the zebras which might be lurking in every call.

3. Stereotyping the Patient

Stereotyping patients also puts the nurse at high risk of overlooking the real problem. It is often tempting for the nurse to assume the obvious, potentially overlooking a life-threatening cause of the patient's symptom(s). For example, the nurse might stereotype the patient, reaching a conclusion based on nothing more than the patient's demographics. Patients in this category might include the following faulty stereotypes:

- Women don't have heart attacks.
- Young people don't have strokes.
- Middle-aged businessmen don't abuse street drugs.
- White, middle-class women don't abuse their children.
- Ministers or doctors don't drink too much.
- The elderly are often forgetful or confused.
- RNs don't need home care instructions for their children.

It's not difficult to see the fallacy in the preceding examples, but many stereotypes are subtle, often occurring on a subconscious level.[4] Nurses are trained to avoid these stereotypes and recognize and respect each patient as an individual, but because their influence can be so subtle, telephone triage nurses must remain ever vigilant to avoid allowing stereotypes to affect care delivery. The old saying "You can't judge a book by its cover" applies to telephone triage as much if not more than any other form of nursing practice.

Julie, a young professional, called the nurse late Saturday night complaining of tingling in her right hand. She was obviously upset, crying, and seemed to be hyperventilating. She had just had a fight with her husband. She told the nurse she had been yelling and crying hard. Now that the fight was over she had a bad headache, was having trouble catching her breath, and the fingers in her right hand were tingling. She reported having a glass of wine to calm her nerves and felt a little off-balance and lightheaded. When asked, Julie told the nurse she "kind of felt like this once before" when she "had a panic attack." The nurse, assuming this was a panic attack, failed to inquire about history of smoking and birth control pills and instead followed the anxiety protocol. Assuming it unlikely that this young woman was having a stroke and thus minimizing the significance of the neurologic symptoms, the nurse followed the anxiety protocol disposition and advised Julie to seek care within 24 hours if her symptoms didn't resolve promptly. Julie later presented to the UCC and was immediately redirected to the ED where she was diagnosed with a stroke.

Had the patient not been so young, the nurse would most likely have focused more on the neurologic symptoms. However, it is likely that because of this patient's youthfulness, the nurse failed to consider what would otherwise have been of significant concern.

4. The Frequent Caller

An especially risky patient is the one who is well-known to the staff. Frequent callers are often regarded as troublesome patients. If the patient has multiple and/or obscure symptoms, the likelihood is increased that the nurse might disregard or minimize the patient's complaints. We sometimes fail to recognize that patients probably have more enjoyable ways to spend their time and money than frequenting the doctor's office in person or by phone.

Among these frequent callers may be patients who are addicted to a substance, and thus their calls represent drug-seeking behavior. Additionally, there are rare patients, like those with Munchausen syndrome, who might not be suffering from a physiologic disease in spite of their persistent complaints. However, it is important to remember three things about these patients. First, they might be misdiagnosed and have neither a substance abuse problem nor Munchausen syndrome. Second, both addiction and Munchausen syndrome represent legitimate illness and these patients are in need of appropriate treatment and compassion. And finally, even addicts and patients with Munchausen syndrome can become physiologically ill. Unfortunately, having psychological or emotional problems doesn't exempt a patient from being legitimately ill with a physical disease. Good policy dictates that if a patient *says* he is hurting, he is hurting! If a patient *says* she is sick, she is sick! Second-guessing a patient, especially over the telephone, is courting disaster.

Two very different scenarios illustrate the pitfalls associated with making assumptions about frequent callers.

Experiencing a relatively severe headache, Mark made an appointment to see his PCP. Having previously been diagnosed with chronic sinusitis, he was seen, and because of a subtle difference in the headache, the provider ordered a CT. Unfortunately, both

of the CT scanners in the community were non-functional for the remainder of the week and the nurse advised Mark she would call him when his CT was scheduled. He called later in the week, complaining about the headache, and the nurse advised him progress was being made on the scanners and she should be able to schedule him soon. He called again on Friday, when his own PCP was out of the office, and another physician was taking call. The nurse advised the on-call physician that the patient was a frequent caller, had already been seen earlier that week and was being scheduled for a CT. The nurse felt the patient was being impatient and expressed frustration about the frequent calls. The on-call physician, not wanting to ignore the patient's complaint, prescribed a narcotic analgesic. Unfortunately, over the weekend, Mark experienced a catastrophic bleed, which eventually resulted in his death.

Had Mark not been a "frequent caller," perhaps the nurse would have been more discriminating in her assessment of the nature of his problem and less likely to minimize his complaints to the on-call physician. To assure patient safety, telephone triage nurses must assess patients every time they call, regardless of the frequency and interval that they were last evaluated over the phone or face-to-face. In Mark's case, presence of documented chronic sinusitis did not preclude the possibility of other, potentially more serious, causes of the patient's headache.

Another case of knowing the caller too well illustrates the same principles.

Irma was a 67-year-old widow who called almost daily around 6:00 p.m. When Irma first began calling, the nurses were vigilant about completing an assessment, and physical problems were ruled out repeatedly. Over time the nurses learned Irma's son had passed away within the past year and Irma had a cocktail (and sometimes more than one) every day around 6:00 p.m. Irma showed signs of depression and was urged to see her doctor. She was given information on available resources about how medication could help make a difference. However, it seemed Irma was more interested in telling, and retelling, her story, and eventually the calls turned into more of a lengthy social chat than the provision of professional nursing care.

Fortunately, Irma's call was eventually taken by a nurse new to the system who performed a complete assessment. She noted the slightly slurred speech and the "tipsy behavior" but instead of attributing it to the evening cocktail, she investigated further. The nurse discovered that Irma had listened to the information she received from the nurses about the benefits of taking antidepressants and had been taking the Lexapro® she found in the medicine cabinet that had been prescribed for her son. Recognizing that Irma's behavior represented an alteration in level of consciousness, the nurse referred her to the ED for evaluation. Irma was subsequently hospitalized with the potentially fatal serotonin syndrome.

In this case the patient was not well-served by nurses who, although kind and compassionate, knew her "too well." Irma was lucky to have eventually had her call taken by a nurse who viewed her situation with a "fresh set of eyes" and looked beyond the obvious.

5. Failure to Speak Directly with the Patient

Often, there are legitimate reasons someone other than the patient is making the call to the triage nurse. Perhaps it's a parent calling for their child. It could be a wife calling for a husband who is reluctant to make the call or prefers that his wife interact with the nurse. The patient might be confused, developmentally disabled, or otherwise unable to provide an accurate history, and thus the call is initiated by a caregiver. Often of greatest difficulty is the situation in which the caller prefers that the patient not know about the call to the nurse. When a call is placed by a non-patient, after speaking with the caller, the nurse should always make an effort to speak directly with the patient (see Chapter 9, "Third-Party Calls").

There are several important reasons to ask the caller to put the patient directly on the telephone.

- The patient often has information the caller doesn't have, and speaking directly with the patient increases the potential for accurate and complete information gathering.
- Even if the family calls with a thorough history in mind, it is almost inevitable that questions will arise for which the caller has limited or no knowledge.
- Assessment of the patient's respiratory and neurologic status can be accomplished in part by talking directly to the patient.
- Sometimes, issues such as sexual activity, symptoms of STDs, cigarette smoking, drug or alcohol use, and other sensitive topics may not have been revealed to the caller, especially with children or adolescents.

- Likewise, psychiatric problems such as depression, delusions, or suicidal ideation might not be disclosed if the patient isn't the direct historian.

The reader can probably think of multiple other situations in which information might be skewed or incomplete if the nurse does not speak with the patient. An important rule of thumb is to *always* speak directly with the patient, even if that seems to be difficult or impossible because of the patient's age, as with an infant, or with a patient who has impaired neurologic status, such as developmental disabilities or dementia. Every nurse knows the importance of assessing the character of the patient's respirations, so failure of the nurse to ask the caller to at least hold the phone near the patient's mouth might result in an inadequate assessment. And with the suicidal patient, the reluctant patient, or the patient with symptoms that are not evident to the caller, often the only way to discover the truth is to ask the patient directly. Consider the following two examples of patients with suicidal ideation in which the calls were mismanaged due to failure to speak with the patient.

A husband called a triage nurse asking for advice for his wife, who was being treated for anxiety and depression, presumably related to menopause. He stated, "I have always heard that women going through the change sometimes act crazy, and boy-oh-boy, is my wife acting crazy!" He wanted her to have an appointment with the doctor so they could "see if her female hormones need to be adjusted." The nurse failed to speak directly with the patient. The nurse scheduled the patient for the first available appointment, which was the following week. Before the appointment date arrived, the wife committed suicide.

In this situation, the husband's "self-diagnosis" coupled with the nurse's failure to speak with the patient and to anticipate worst possible led the nurse to overlook the patient's frankly psychotic behavior.

In another case, a wife called to talk to the nurse because her husband was depressed. She told the nurse she didn't want him to know she had called. The nurse failed to insist on speaking with the patient and instead conducted an assessment through the wife, documenting that the patient "has no suicidal ideation." The patient committed suicide later that evening.

The nurse's position was indefensible because it is impossible to know whether a patient is having suicidal thoughts without asking him directly.

The following case further illustrates the importance of talking directly with the patient.

A wife placed a call to her husband's call center, complaining that her husband had the "flu" accompanied by a high fever which was not responding to Tylenol®. The nurse gave the patient an appointment that same day. The patient was seen and diagnosed with seasonal flu.

The wife called the next day, complaining that the patient had a "pounding headache and stiff neck." He was once again given an appointment in which the history and physical conducted by the physician were unremarkable.

Day 3, the wife called again, stating that her husband had been diagnosed with the flu and she was "very concerned about his fever

of 102.9 that isn't coming down with Tylenol." The nurse did a cursory assessment, asking if the patient had a stiff neck and if he had been prescribed medication during his last visit to the doctor. The nurse was provided misinformation by the wife that (a) his neck was not stiff (but it was), and (b) he had not been prescribed any medication the preceding day (but he had been given cefaclor).

The nurse, having failed to assess the patient but believing she had accurate information, advised the wife as follows: "It sometimes takes 10 days for this to go away. We just treat the symptoms. The fever is fighting infection. Have him drink lots of cool water and call us back if his fever gets to 103."

This is an example of inadequate assessment based on failure to talk to the patient and a lack clinical judgment. Had the nurse talked to the patient, the additional information would likely have triggered a more appropriate recommendation by the nurse. In addition, the nurse should have recognized a fever of 102.9° F as being essentially the same as 103°, the level at which the patient should have been referred. Perhaps the nurse failed to grasp the significance of repeat phone calls for the same problem, or perhaps the fact that the patient had been seen and evaluated in the office the 2 preceding days gave her false reassurance that there was nothing significantly wrong with the patient. Regardless, this patient did have meningitis (perhaps having developed it on day 3), and he subsequently suffered a significant neurological event which left him in a persistent vegetative state. The settlement in favor of the plaintiff was considerable, covering loss of wages, loss of consortium, and sufficient money to provide around-the-clock nursing care to prevent problems associated with long-term immobility. When organizations say they can't afford to put RNs on the phone, this case serves as an example of why they can't afford not to. Only well-prepared and qualified RNs will do.

What Lessons Can Be Learned from this Case?

Red Flags

- *Repeat calls for the same problem*
- *Concerned wife*
- *Symptoms associated with a serious medical condition*
- *Recurrent symptoms not responding to treatment*

Risk Management Principles

- *Always speak to the patient.*
- *Reassess patients each time they call.*
- *Listen to concerned patients and callers.*
- *Do not over-rely on protocols; use your judgment.*
- *Err on the side of caution.*
- *Communicate with the providers.*

6. Fatigue and Haste

Nurses have become accustomed to working in situations in which it feels like there is too much to do and too little time to accomplish all of the important tasks of the day. However, the telephone triage nurse must carefully guard against fatigue because it can lead to dangerous oversights during the patient assessment and result in faulty judgment. Fatigue and haste, especially unrecognized, can also lead a nurse to take potentially dangerous shortcuts that might result in a bad outcome. An assessment of the mental acuity of nurses working in programs with 10 or 12-hour shifts may be in order, especially toward the end of long shifts. Some call centers employ ergonomically sound design to lessen physical fatigue, but nurses must remain alert to their own physical, mental, and emotional states as they have the potential to impact the quality of care being delivered.[5]

And while we're on the subject of taking care of ourselves, we must keep in mind that adequate nutrition is critical to mental acuity. Many of us have experienced the mid-afternoon slump that occurs in the wake of a heavy lunch, or worse, the reactive hypoglycemia that follows on the heels of a quick candy bar or other snack high in refined sugar. Regular breaks and reasonable meals facilitate the clear mind that is necessary for complex cognitive functions.[6] It is up to each of us to be aware of and address our own physical, mental, and emotional needs in order to provide safe quality care over the telephone. It is entirely possible that the following scenario would have had a different outcome if the call had not been handled at the end of a long day.

Two-year-old Jason had been seen in the office that morning. He was diagnosed with tonsillitis, given an antibiotic, and sent home. The mother called later in the day, about 4:00 p.m., and said she was concerned about his breathing. The secretary sent a note to the office nurse, and the call was returned at 4:55, 5 minutes before the office was to close. Although this is a high-risk chief complaint, the nurse's note simply said, "Called parent. Advised if respiratory gets worse to go to ER or the local urgent care center, it's open 24 hours."

Unfortunately, that was the note the nurse wrote before she learned 2 weeks later that the child had died at home that night. The following are bolded excerpts from her late entry 2 weeks later.

Chief Complaint: "Mother said his breathing *seemed* difficult." The nurse evidently minimized the seriousness of the problem; however, the patient was dead hours later.

Assessment: "...he was *up*" Up what? Up playing normally or up supporting himself in a tripod position so he could catch his breath? And when asked if his color was abnormal, the nurse documented "**the mother stated, 'Not really'.**" Clearly, implicit information was inherent in that answer.

Advice: Nurse advised the mother that the office was closing in 5 minutes and that, **"if there was any difficulty breathing or what she is seeing now gets worse," she should take him to the UCC or ED "because they are open 24 hours."**

Closing: In closing, the nurse noted, **"She thanked me and we hung up."** Was the nurse trying to imply that the mother was satisfied? According to the mother's deposition, she wasn't satisfied, and in fact, she was extremely concerned. She consulted her home medical references, called her sister, and then (upon her sister's suggestion) gave her son a puff of albuterol (with neither spacer nor instruction, so it's unlikely that he got any medication at all). And then she sat down to watch him.

Given nothing more than the knowledge that the child was seen that morning and treated for tonsillitis, what occurs to you in regards to what might be going on? Obviously, there was concern about swelling and airway obstruction. Nurses thinking diagnostically might recognize the possibility of epiglottitis, peritonsillar abscess, anaphylaxis, or choking. However, it is important to point out that in such a case, "thinking diagnostically" is not necessary. Recognizing the possibility of an airway obstruction should be enough to guide the nurse's decision making.

The reader might ask why the mother didn't take her child to the ED for evaluation, but with her untrained eye, even though his condition was deteriorating, she thought he was getting better. Throughout the evening, as is often the case with patients who are hypoxic, he went from struggling to catch his breath to simply appearing calm (so lethargic and exhausted that all he could do was lie down and go to sleep). Mother, herself, was eventually able to lie down and take a nap because she was so relieved that he was "doing better." Both parents were present when Jason got out of bed and arrested. Of course, as is so often the case, the mother, referring to the nurse, commented in deposition, "I trusted her."

What Lessons Can Be Learned from this Case?

Red Flags

- *Call at the end of day (not getting better or getting sicker)*
- *Mother's concern*
- *Symptoms inconsistent with presumed diagnosis*

Risk Management Principles

- *Use extreme caution when rushed (end of day).*
- *Listen to mom.*
- *Use protocols (and sound nursing judgment).*
- *Err on the side of caution.*
- *Be sure the caller knows what worse looks like.*

7. Knowledge Deficit

There are two kinds of "not knowing" in telephone triage. The first is the clinical knowledge deficit discussed previously. The second is related to lack of training specific to the practice of telephone triage. This section deals with lack of clinical knowledge.

We all have clinical knowledge deficits. In fact, often the more experience we have the more aware we become of our knowledge deficits. In other words, the more we know, the more we know what we *don't* know. We also have areas of clinical strength in which our knowledge excels. Nurses who are specialists in one area, while possessing an impressing depth of information in that specialty, don't always have a broad knowledge base. This makes them especially vulnerable to overlooking clinical entities that are outside of their specialty area. On the other end of the spectrum are generalists. These nurses often have a great breadth of knowledge without particularly specialized knowledge in any one area.

Ideally, the telephone triage nurse has experience (thus has "been there and done that") in a wide variety of clinical areas. To whatever extent possible, it is best if the telephone triage nurse is a "jack of all trades, and a master of them all," so to speak. Emergency department nurses, unless overwhelmingly invested in the psychomotor aspects of nursing, can be great telephone triage nurses because of their experience with triage and exposure to a wide variety of medical and surgical presentations, both chronic and acute.

There are also relatively inexperienced nurses who either don't yet know what they don't know or may be overly aware of how much they don't know. The relatively new nurse has limited clinical knowledge and experience from which to draw. This limited knowledge base creates fertile ground for errors. On the other hand, it often causes them to be relatively cautious, which is the ideal default position in telephone triage. If in doubt, the telephone triage nurse should always err on the side of caution.

Take for example the following illustration of how both specialized knowledge and a knowledge deficit can impact decision making.

A father of a week-old infant called the advice nurse because his infant was "blue around his lips." The nurse appropriately queried the father about other symptoms and learned that there was no further evidence of cyanosis, the child was "eating ok," and "seemed as alert as usual." Objective assessment conducted by the father as coached by the nurse revealed that there was no nasal flaring or retractions. On audible exam (holding the child to the phone), there were no wheezes or grunts.

The nurse, believing the baby was probably ok because he was acting ok, also realized cyanosis could be a sign of something seriously wrong with the baby. Erring on the side of caution, she sent the child to the ED. The father was reluctant to go, but the nurse convinced him it was in his child's best interest to do so.

Later that day, the call center director received a call from an aggravated ED physician who informed her that circumoral cyanosis is a normal finding in a newborn and that referral to the ED was inappropriate. The call center manager patiently explained to the physician that knowing cyanosis could also indicate a significant problem, the nurse appropriately erred on the side of caution.

Augmenting the physician's concern was the fact the nurse had sent the infant by ambulance in spite of all other findings being normal. This probably was the result of a knowledge deficit on the part of the nurse, that circumoral cyanosis can be a normal finding in newborns. However, the nurse appropriately followed the axiom, "if in doubt, send them out."

This scenario represents a paradox. Although circumoral cyanosis can be a normal finding in newborns, even physicians can vary widely in their description and interpretation.[7] Circumoral (or peripheral) cyanosis can be a normal finding in infants, but it can also be associated with serious problems. The nurse erred on the side of caution, acting in what she thought was the best interest of the patient. However, in retrospect, the result was an unnecessary 911 transport and ED admission. The primary point here is that instead of "playing the odds" that the infant was just experiencing normal peripheral cyanosis, the RN appropriately erred on the side of caution, sending the baby for evaluation. The more experienced pediatric nurse might not have considered the child to have a problem, knowing that circumoral cyanosis is a normal finding in infants, and overlooked the possibility of significant pathology. This is an example of how both a knowledge deficit and knowing the topic too well can potentially present problems.

8. Failure to Reassess

When patients who have either called earlier in the week or have been seen in the office or ED then call the nurse for the same reason, it is often tempting to handle the patient based on the previous encounter, especially if a diagnosis had been offered. However, when patients call, they call for a *reason!* If the first encounter (whether over the phone or face to face) had adequately resolved the problem, there would most likely not be any additional calls. Diseases do evolve and patients do occasionally develop complications. Without an appropriate reassessment, these complications might be overlooked. Finally, however infrequent, doctors do occasionally misdiagnose patients' problems and thus the repeat caller always deserves a fresh look.

Linda's presenting complaint was, "I called this morning and they told me I have food poisoning. I've been vomiting all day and my urine is so concentrated it's almost pink. I'm having pain around my belly button, and I'm aching all over, especially in my back." The nurse, although quite experienced, must have quit listening closely after the patient mentioned "...they told me I have food poisoning" because she immediately accessed the vomiting protocol and was about to recommend the BRAT (bananas, rice, applesauce, and toast) diet to the patient. Fortunately, her call was being monitored by a colleague who motioned for her to put the call on hold and reviewed the history with her (pink urine [blood tinged?], abdominal pain, back pain). The nurse taking the call exclaimed, "Oh, I didn't hear that!"

The nurse's reliance on the earlier "diagnosis" may have contributed to her failure to hear that the patient had just described classic symptoms of pyelonephritis. However, the overarching clinical concern was her failure to reassess the patient, which if done, would most likely have led to an appropriate disposition.

9. Failure to Perform an Adequate Assessment

At the root of almost all of the pitfalls discussed is failure to perform an adequate assessment. Sometimes this occurs secondary to another problem, such as failure to speak to the patient, accepting patient self-diagnosis, or jumping to a conclusion, but occasionally it is just failure to do the job right. Consider the following example from labor and delivery.

A labor and delivery nurse was expected to field calls from the public while maintaining a patient load in the hospital. On one such occasion, the nurse took a call and performed an inadequate assessment. She asked about signs and symptoms of labor, but failed to inquire about high-risk obstetric indicators. She learned that the woman was having mild contractions and had vomited once, basing her plan of care on this limited information. She failed to complete her assessment and thus was unaware that the patient was hypertensive and diabetic. Based on an inadequate assessment, the nurse gave faulty advice (to stay home and take an antacid). The pre-eclamptic woman followed the nurse's advice and, as a result, experienced a bad outcome. The nurse, in her own defense, pointed out that the patients she had in the hospital were her first priority. Unfortunately, however, in this case, the patient on the phone was more than likely the nurse's most high-risk patient at the time.

Although nurses are often challenged by situations that represent less than ideal circumstances (such as short staffing), there is no excuse for failing to perform an adequate assessment. Regardless of the challenges, we have a duty to meet the standard of care.

10. Failure to Use Critical Thinking and Exercise Clinical Judgment

Occasionally, by virtue of training or organizational policy, telephone triage nurses over-focus on the protocols to the exclusion of using their critical thinking skills, or they simply fail to apply clinical judgment to the situation. In fact, several examples in this chapter have at their roots, simple failure to think.

A family called requesting an ambulance for their 19 year old with abdominal pain. The call had initially gone to EMS dispatch, but having not met the criteria for emergency transport, the call was transferred to a telephone triage nurse in a call center. The task before her was to determine the appropriate disposition for the patient.

Within the first 90 seconds, the nurse was provided with the following information:

- *Patient is 19 years old.*
- *Chief complaint: abdominal pain*
- *Patient is now rolling on floor, kicking in pain, pleading for an ambulance.*
- *Patient has chronic kidney disease.*
- *Discharged from hospital 2 days ago, seen in ED last night for "swelling."*
- *Patient is heard in the background crying out in pain, "Oh please!" and "Help me!"*
- *Patient and family are requesting 911.*

Within the next 45 seconds, the nurse learned that his pain onset (described as 10/10) was 30 minutes ago accompanied by three episodes of vomiting. When asked, "Can he get up and stand and walk to the bathroom?" the caller replied, "I don't believe so. He's on the floor kicking because he's in so much pain." The nurse asked a second time, "He can't stand?" The caller's second response was, "If he stands, he may double over because he keeps kicking and begging for help…and begging for an ambulance." However, the RN, apparently adhering strictly to the protocols, was on the phone for over 8 minutes, asking questions, such as presence of allergies, medication history, exact location of his pain ("middle, upper, or lower?"), and then continued to follow the protocol questions (is he having chest pain, does he have a history of seizures, is he choking, etc.) long after she should have called an ambulance.

All together, she queried onset of pain three times, assessed the level of the pain twice, asked if he were able to stand three times, and evidently ignored the background noises. Long after the ambulance should have been dispatched, she continued to ask high-priority questions regarding history of an abdominal aortic aneurysm, trauma, hematemesis, toxic or caustic ingestion, and abdominal distention.

After completing her data collection, the nurse advised the family to drive the young man to the hospital by private vehicle. The family asked, "Can you hear the kid hollering?!" and insisted on an ambulance. When the nurse acquiesced and was providing interim home care instructions, she mentioned keeping him on his side and "Have his airway open, especially if he's vomiting." The caller's response was, "...we've done the best we can because his face is all swollen..."

There are obviously multiple problems with this call, the primary being that the nurse followed her documentation tool (e.g., asking about allergies and medications) and protocol precisely instead of listening to the information provided and making a prompt decision based on clinical judgment. It is likely that the organizational policy or the nurse's telephone triage education (or both), dictated the approach of strict adherence to the protocols. And because the call was being tape-recorded, perhaps the nurse was even more reluctant to deviate from the prescribed process than she might have been under different circumstances. Besides failure to use critical thinking and exercise clinical judgment, this vignette is a clear example of overreliance on the protocols.

11. Failure to LISTEN and THINK

As has been demonstrated, preoccupation with decision support and/or documentation software can interfere with the nurse's thought processes. Although the following call didn't result in a bad outcome, it is an interesting study in failing to really listen to what is said and use clinical judgment.

Mom, obviously frustrated, called complaining of her infant having an immunization reaction. Mom stated, "She has a temperature of 101.2, she screams every time I touch her leg, and she's spitting up everywhere! ... I've had it! My face hurts, my head hurts, and my back hurts." The experienced pediatric call center nurse appropriately started her interview with a question about the location of the child because there was no audible crying in the background. The mom responded that she had enlisted the help of her mother because of her frustration. Assured that the infant was safe, the nurse began her assessment.

Consulting the immunization protocol, the painful injection site was to be expected and the temperature of 101.2° in this 6-month-old infant was of no concern. The nurse was about to advise acetaminophen for fever and pain when a colleague who was monitoring the call asked the nurse to put the caller on hold. She pointed out that the mother had said the baby was "spitting up everywhere," not generally regarded as a symptom of an immu-

nization reaction. The nurse returned to the mother and reviewed the vomiting protocol with her, followed by the fever protocol. She was again about to terminate the call when the colleague pointed out something that would never be reflected in the protocols — the mother was also symptomatic. Putting the patient's and her mother's symptoms together, a pattern began to emerge. A vomiting, irritable, febrile infant plus a mother with head and back pain deserved evaluation to rule out a more serious etiology than immunization reaction, such as meningitis. Additionally, the nurse needed to fully explore the mother's frustration, coping skills, and resources to be sure the immunization reaction wouldn't evolve into a volatile situation resulting in an injured baby.

Perhaps if the nurse had consulted the "crying baby" protocol, some of these questions might have been raised. However, regardless of the decision support tool used, the nurse must be sure to listen to what's said (verbally and non-verbally) and think about what it might mean with its associated implications. Picking one particular protocol prematurely can lead the nurse down a very narrow path and lead to oversight of more significant problems.

12. Failure to Err on the Side of Caution

Although truly high-acuity calls may be few and far between, it is important that the nurse maintain a high index of suspicion on every call. It has been said that if you don't find it often, you often don't find it. Therefore nurses must go out of their way to look for, and rule out, the uncommon and worst case scenarios, often referred to as high-risk, low-volume problems.

A patient had a same-day appendectomy and was sent home the afternoon of the surgery in stable condition. She called a nurse later that day, complaining of increasing pain and emesis. Since the patient was post-op abdominal surgery earlier that day, the nurse evidently assumed the patient's problems were routine events associated with her procedure and reassured the patient that she would feel better if she took her pain medication and her antiemetic. The patient also complained of being "very weak and tired," but the nurse failed to pick up on these significant symptoms, being convinced that this was a routine case. Unfortunately, this patient was experiencing a significant complication in that she had ruptured her appendical stump and was leaking fecal material into her abdominal cavity. This failure to recognize the potential seriousness of the patient's condition was thought to have contributed to her eventual death from sepsis.

It would have been impossible for the nurse to know that the patient was experiencing such an unexpected but significant complication. However, the patient's complaints of being "weak and tired" were both red flags in the decision support tool she was using and should have gotten her attention. In reviewing the other stories in this chapter, you will find that in many cases with bad outcomes, the nurse failed to "listen," and to err on the side of caution. Additionally in this case, as with others, if the nurse had consulted the decision support tool closely, it would have alerted her that this was not a routine call.

13. Failure to Anticipate Worst Possible

As mentioned previously, if we don't look for worst possible, when it comes along, we might not recognize it.

A teenager was diagnosed with the flu earlier in the week but was improving. Her mother let her go out to an indoor sporting event one evening, admonishing her to not get overheated and to come home as soon as the game was over. The teen went to the game and stayed up late watching TV with her boyfriend after they got home. The next day was Saturday, and the patient was worse, but the mother considered that a "relapse," blaming it on her having "overdone it" the night before. The next day she was sicker still.

Mom placed a call to the call center Sunday morning because her daughter was having chest pain. The nurse assessed her, finding no indication for referral, but she connected the mother to the physician nonetheless because the mother was concerned. The physician assessed the teenager, identifying no need for concern at that time, but advised the mother to take her daughter to the ED should she develop any shortness of breath. Although she didn't develop shortness of breath, the mother remained concerned, so she took her daughter to the ED, where they X-rayed her chest, read it as normal, diagnosed her with pharyngitis, and discharged her to home with an antibiotic. On her way out of the ED, she started vomiting, so they brought her back to the treatment area and gave her a prescription for a PO antiemetic. However, the reason for the vomiting wasn't evaluated.

When the child returned home, she kept vomiting and eventually was so weak that her father had to carry her to the bath-

room to void. Another call was placed to the call center with a complaint of persistent vomiting, and the nurse transferred the mother to the physician again. He prescribed a suppository to stop the vomiting, giving the mother instructions to call back if the vomiting didn't get better. Unfortunately, neither the nurse nor the physician assessed the hydration status of a patient who was too weak to walk to the bathroom. Assessment and documentation should have been made regarding her mucous membranes, her urine output, and her level of consciousness at a minimum. The nurse did note that the girl had voided within the past 12 hours. (However, this nurse should realize that unless kidneys are completely shut down, there is a 30 ml per hour obligatory urine output. Reason thus dictates that the character of the urine is more important than the frequency of voiding in this teenager since, for those with bladder control, frequency of voiding is often a matter of choice.)

The girl's vomiting did respond to the antiemetic. However, a third and final call to the nurse was placed to ask, "What's a normal temperature?" By this time, the teen's temperature was 96° axillary. The nurse, unsure about how to answer the question, but in an organization that placed high value on protocol use, consulted the frostbite protocol, even though there had been no environmental exposure. She used that protocol to assess the teen and advise the mother, telling her to put her daughter in a warm bathtub to warm her up, to take her temperature under both arms, and to call back if her temperature fell below 95° axillary. It is noteworthy that the reason the nurse suggested axillary temperatures is because the protocol advised if the vomiting child is sleeping, don't awaken her because sleeping helps the stomach

empty. It is unlikely that these instructions were meant to apply to a teenager as sick as this girl.

Following instructions precisely, the parents concluded that their two thermometers were broken because they "weren't registering anything," so dad went to the store to buy a third thermometer. While he was gone, the 15 year old asked her mother if she were going to die, to which her mother replied that she just had to weather the storm today, and she would be better tomorrow. Within minutes, the girl arrested, her death likely related to septic shock and dehydration.

This is a tragic story indeed. The mother *knew* her daughter was very ill, but thought she and her husband were being "worry warts." All this mother needed was the nod to take her daughter back to the ED for evaluation, but the third nurse, concluding that she was "getting better" said, "I thought we could watch her." The attorney replied, "Are you aware that's what the mother did…? Watch her daughter die in her arms!" The nurse clearly did not use critical thinking, was over-reliant on the protocols, and failed to consider worse possible scenarios, a fatal trifecta.

It's impossible to read or hear that story without your heart going out to the parents. They were totally compliant, having taken their daughter to the doctor, visited the ED once, talked to the doctor twice, and called the nurse three times, dutifully checking her temperature under both arms as instructed. The only thing the parents did "wrong" was to trust the nurses. There are several possible lessons associated with this case study, but perhaps the most poignant of all is recognition that the mother would have most certainly taken her daughter back to the hospital, given the slightest prompt to do so by the nurse.

What Lessons Can Be Learned from this Case?

Red Flags

- ***Repeated calls (three in 24 hours)***
- ***Symptoms inconsistent with diagnosis of flu***
- ***Too weak to walk***
- ***Mother's concern***
- ***Hypothermia***

Risk Management Principles

- ***Err on the side of caution.***
- ***Listen to the parents; they know their kids!***
- ***Use critical thinking and clinical judgment if there's no protocol (and use the right one if there is).***

14. Over-Reliance on Protocols

The examples associated with Pitfalls 8, 10, 11, and 13 likely involved over-reliance on protocols, but the following case is a particularly vivid illustration of this problem. This example is also especially disturbing because the patient was a registered nurse who probably knew the right action to take but was depending on her triage nurse for validation she never got. Consider the following case involving three calls to the triage nurse over a period of 10 days.

Betty had been experiencing peculiar headaches with unusual associated sensations for about 10 days. She reported having had an episode she described as a sudden onset of light headedness accompanied by a "terrible pain in the top of my head and down the back of my neck." That episode had resulted in a call to the triage nurse who had sent her to the ED where she was diagnosed with sinusitis.

The patient's headaches persisted, and about 9 days later, she developed polyuria during the night. She had once again consulted

a triage nurse who had sent her back to the ED for evaluation, where they had ruled out a urinary tract infection and changed her antibiotic for her sinusitis.

But upon return from the ED that morning, Betty had experienced what she described as "feeling like someone pulled a rubber band back and shot it right at my brain." She reported associated nausea, reiterating that she had "felt this 'ping' in my head and it was very painful ... and I felt like I was going to throw up for a minute..."

Although the symptoms subsided, Betty had placed her third call to a triage nurse, concerned about whether she had received an appropriate evaluation in the ED that morning. She repeatedly expressed a wish that she had pushed for a consultation with a neurologist, expressing regret that she had not done so.

As the patient provided her history, the nurse systematically accessed three protocols. She first referred to the Headache protocol, and finding no current neurologic symptoms, was unable to justify an immediate referral to a health care provider. She next reviewed the Sinus protocol, followed by the Urinary Symptoms protocol with similar results. It is likely that the nurse was uncomfortable with the story and with Betty's concern, but without a protocol-driven disposition to send the patient back to the ED or consult a physician, the nurse was evidently reluctant to do so and advised Betty, "Maybe you should go back to the ER tomorrow if it's not better."

Of course, Betty's instincts were good and she had a superior knowledge base, having worked on a neurologic unit in the past. She was aware of the unusual nature of the symptoms but needed collaboration and support to return to the ED or call a neurologist. Unfortunately, Betty's aneurysm ruptured the next morning while she was getting dressed to return to the ED.

The nurse in this case evidently over-relied on the protocols, thereby failing to utilize nursing judgment and allowing the protocols to make her decision for her, despite her probable discomfort with the situation. The call lasted over 20 minutes, with the nurse most likely looking for any "excuse" to send the patient back to the ED. Protocols aside, the patient was describing disturbing recurrent neurologic symptoms. The addition of the polyuria, most certainly representing syndrome of inappropriate antidiuretic hormone (SIADH), further raised the question of a significant neurologic event. Unfortunately, evidently no one clarified that the complaint of polyuria did not represent symptoms of a UTI but rather unexplained excessive urine output. It is critical for telephone triage nurses to not wholly depend on decision support tools or allow them to interfere with or obscure their decision making.

One final note: If a patient describes something that sounds extremely unusual or unlikely to the nurse, it's a good idea to have the patient evaluated. Unfortunately, not many patients live to describe the sensation associated with leaking or rupture of their cerebral aneurysms or many other rare but fatal conditions.

15. Failure to Use Protocols

Multiple examples of over-reliance on protocols have been presented but there are also cases in which nurses fail to use protocols when they should. We have seen in prior examples (Pitfalls 1 & 6) how failure to use protocols, combined with other factors, can contribute to poor outcomes. In this case, failure to use protocols was clearly a central problem.

One Sunday afternoon, a nurse received a call from a 55-year-old woman who was experiencing mid-scapular back pain. The patient explained it as a "strain" related to quilting, which involved leaning over a table all morning. The nurse, being unable to locate the patient's medical record in the database, inquired as to

whether the patient had been seen by that organization in the past. The patient replied that she was an old patient, having not been in to see the doctor in 12 years. The nurse, recognizing the patient as not having been conscientious about routine health maintenance, remarked that the patient should make an appointment to obtain a Pap smear. Then the patient said she was also experiencing "a little indigestion" to which the nurse responded, "There are some things you can do for that." First she suggested that the woman avoid tight waistbands, saying, "Sometimes elastic waistbands are best for women our age." Next she told her that there were some foods that aggravated indigestion including coffee, chocolate, and peppermint, stating peppermint was possibly the worst trigger, so she should avoid peppermint. So, by this time, the nurse, focusing on health education, had recommended that the patient get a Pap smear, wear elastic waistbands, and avoid peppermint.

At this point, the patient's husband, with some apparent frustration, took the phone, asking the nurse if she thought it could be his wife's "heart." The nurse sounding a little exasperated replied, "She said it was indigestion. Put her back on the phone." Once again speaking to the patient, she said, "You're not having any trouble breathing, are you?" to which the patient replied, "Not really, but I do get a little winded when I walk up stairs." The nurse next asked, "You're not sweating, are you?" to which the patient replied, "Well, I'm a little damp, but it's warm here today." The nurse went on to ask about family history, learning that one parent had experienced a sudden death at 55 and the other parent had gotten a stent placed at 58.

The nurse then consulted the physician, reporting the associated symptoms and positive family history. However, preceding that information the nurse made a comment to the effect of, "I have this woman on the phone, but I don't think it's much of anything." The physician, recognizing the significance of the associated symptoms and positive family history but also being respectful of the nurse's opinion, countered with, "I think there's enough going on here that she deserves an evaluation, but I guess she doesn't really need to go by ambulance."

The nurse continued her call with the patient, telling her, "The doctor thought it would be a good idea to get your back pain checked out, so you should probably have your husband take you to the hospital this afternoon" (specifying a hospital that was within the patient's insurance network). Because the nurse didn't express any urgency, the patient made her bed, did her dishes, took a shower, and straightened her house before her husband drove her to the hospital.

Unfortunately, the patient arrested enroute. Being in front of a hospital (but not the one to which she had been referred, which was farther away), her husband pulled into their ED parking lot. The patient was resuscitated, but not before sustaining significant brain damage which left her with short and long-term memory loss and paranoid delusions. She is now unable to be left alone at all, thus dramatically impacting not only the quality of her life, but the quality of her husband's life as well.

Of interest is the fact that in speaking with the physician, the nurse said, "I hate these protocols!" The Back Pain, Indigestion, Chest Pain, and Atypical Chest Pain protocols that should have been used, all said "911 to the ED," which was evidently counter-intuitive to what the nurse thought was indicated. Had the patient been transported promptly by ambulance, her arrest might have been averted, or at the very least, she would have been in the hospital, rather than her family car, when she arrested.

16. Failure to Facilitate Continuity of Care

Although telephone triage represents episodic care, there is no doubt that facilitation of continuity of care is the responsibility of the telephone triage nurse. The following case represents a surprising twist, and contradicts a long-held belief of many nurses regarding our ongoing responsibility for our patients.

A man's wife called requesting an appointment for him to be seen for "leg pain." The telephone triage nurse pursued his complaint by using the Leg Pain protocol. When she asked, "Is he having chest pain?" (attempting to rule out a pulmonary embolism), the wife's response was a hesitant, "No...not today. But he had chest pain last week." The nurse, hearing "no," went through the rest of the protocol questions, identifying nothing of particular concern, and thus sent a message to the appointment clerk asking her to schedule the patient for an appointment. However, of significance, no clinical information was shared with the physician. The request for the appointment was the endpoint of the nurse's interaction. The patient kept his appointment, but the question of chest pain never came up. The doctor didn't ask and the patient didn't offer. He was discharged home and suffered a lethal cardiac arrest a week later. The wife sued.

There was an illusion that the nurse was protected since she had referred the patient into the hands of the physician. However, the attorney contended that the nurse was responsible because she had access to critical health information relevant to the care of the patient, but she failed to share it with the physician or anyone else who could do something about it.

This argument presents an interesting premise, punctuating the ongoing accountability of the triage nurse for his or her own actions. Thinking of the inpatient setting, for which most readers have a frame of reference, an analogy (although far fetched) would be a patient reporting chest pain during bedtime rounds but the nurse not documenting it, knowing the doctor would be making rounds in the morning and that he would discover the history of chest pain then. Ridiculous, right? From a nursing accountability perspective, this is roughly equivalent to either (a) failure to document or (b) failure to provide relevant information to the physician responsible for the patient's care. The nurse should have alerted the physician to the history of chest tightness. Not having done so, she shared in the responsibility when the patient suffered a poor outcome.

17. Failure to Advocate for the Patient

Telephone triage often puts the nurse in the position of being the sole history taker, occasionally requiring the physician to make treatment decisions on the basis of the nurse's history. This is fertile ground for putting the nurse in a potentially precarious position. Consider the following example.

Nancy called complaining that her 8-year-old son, Dylan, was "still very sick," reporting a high fever, sore throat, cough, headache, "lethargy," anorexia, and significant weight loss in the past 10 days. Nancy reported that he coughed to the point of gagging and throwing up, and when he coughed, he held his head because it hurt. The nurse documented that the mother was "unsure whether to bring him in or not" and sent the note to the physician for disposition. It is unclear whether the nurse sent the information to the physician because she was unsure what course to take or whether office policy dictated that she do so. The physician, after reading the nurse's note, prescribed an antibiotic and rec-

ommended an office visit if he was not better in 3 days. Unfortunately, Dylan did not improve, and he was subsequently admitted to the hospital with necrotizing putrefying pneumonia and complications related to sepsis.

On deposition, the nurse contended that she had argued with the mother to bring the child in, which seemed to contradict her comment that "mother was unsure whether to bring him in or not." She went on to say that she didn't believe the disposition was appropriate, thereby putting herself in a gray zone. Although whether or not to prescribe an antibiotic isn't within the scope of practice of an RN, it is clear that RNs may not carry out an order they believe is inappropriate. Unfortunately, the nurse had indeed carried out the order in spite of the fact that on deposition, she stated that if it had been her child, she would have gotten him seen and, furthermore, she strongly suspected that the child had pneumonia. Evidently, her legal strategy was to divest herself of any responsibility for the bad outcome, placing all of the blame on the physician's decision making.

However, as soon as she made her position clear (that she thought the physician had acted in error), the attorney asked her if she was familiar with her organization's chain of command policy that required her to question and elevate orders through the chain of command if she thought they were inappropriate or not in the best interests of the patient. Nurses are expected to serve as patient advocates and to exercise clinical judgment. Because RNs maintain professional accountability for their actions, carrying out an order that the nurse believes is contraindicated, puts him or her in an indefensible position.

Nurses are put in a very similar situation when they are *required* to facilitate "second level triage" (consult with the provider) prior to assigning a disposition. Although second-level triage might seem to improve safety, it sets up a potentially untenable situation for the nurse, should he or she disagree with the decision of the provider. However difficult, patient advocacy is our professional duty. See Chapter 15 for additional discussion of the chain of command policy.

18. Failure to Document Pertinent Negatives

Some nurses have been taught that only the positive responses to protocol questions need to be documented. That is to say, to document only what the patient *has,* not what he or she *doesn't have.* This "charting by exception" approach assumes that all protocol questions are asked in order, from the top to the bottom, and is meant to indicate that all questions asked prior to the first "positive" response were negative. As discussed in Chapter 11, documentation of pertinent negatives is critical to clear communication and to provide evidence of critical thinking. Additionally, as demonstrated below, it will serve a nurse well if he or she ever has to defend his or her actions in court.

A mother called the after-hours triage nurse for her pediatrician's office with a complaint that her 11-year-old daughter, Lilli "has been experiencing intermittent bouts of dizziness and headache." She also had some questionable difficulty concentrating and frequently seemed to be distracted. However, the mother attributed her daughter's behavior to being a "normal pre-teen." She was also having a little trouble reading and her mother thought perhaps she needed glasses.

The nurse, presumably following the protocol, advised the mother to make an appointment to have the child seen in the office the next day. Lilli was seen by the physician, asymptomatic at the time, and was diagnosed with possible migraines. Several days later, Lilli died of a ruptured aneurysm.

The mother sued the practice, naming the physician for failure to diagnose and the nurse for delay in treatment. Based on the wording of the nurse's note, her attorney argued that the symptoms were being reported in the past tense instead of the present, thus making the next day referral appropriate. And based on the nurse's decision to delay evaluation until the next day, it appeared unlikely that the child was experiencing symptoms at the time of the call. However, the plaintiff's attorney argued that the child was symptomatic when the mother called the nurse and that immediate evaluation had been indicated.

Unfortunately the nurse had no independent recollection of the event due to the time lapse, and thus the dispute had to be decided purely on the basis of the documentation. Because the nurse hadn't documented the pertinent negatives, it called into question what her documentation, "has been experiencing," meant exactly. It was clear that Lilli had been having the symptoms, but what was unclear was whether or not she was symptomatic at the time of the call. Had she been symptomatic when the mother called, the appropriate disposition would have been immediate evaluation in the ED, which, in the presence of active symptoms, would have increased the chances of the aneurysm being diagnosed. And the fact that the mother called after hours instead of during the day also reinforced the likelihood that Lilli was symptomatic at the time of the call. Otherwise, why would the mother have called the after-hours nurse rather than waiting until the next day to call the office to make an appointment for ongoing symptoms? This example vividly demonstrates the value of clearly documenting pertinent negatives.

19. Failure to Follow-Up

There are occasions in which, based on nursing judgment, the situation requires a follow-up call.

Mr. Carson, an elderly gentleman with dementia, was losing his vision, and his wife called the telephone triage nurse to ask for advice. The nurse, recognizing this as an emergency, recommended that the patient see the ophthalmologist that day. The nurse reportedly did everything "right." She stressed the importance of being seen "today," confirmed that the wife understood, was comfortable with the plan of care, and would carry it out.

The wife called the ophthalmologist's office requesting an appointment, but because the ophthalmologist was out of town, her husband was given an appointment for 2 weeks later. Mr. Carson kept that appointment and when he was seen, he was then totally and irrevocably blind.

So who do you think was responsible in ths situation?

Let's look at each party individually. First, the patient, or his wife as his proxy, certainly had a responsibility. She was instructed to have him seen today, verbalized understanding, and expressed an intent to comply. Although the patient and his wife had a responsibility, that didn't relieve the health care professionals of their responsibility to the patient. Thus, this case illustrates the adage that "two wrongs don't make a right."

Let's imagine, for the sake of teaching value, that the wife contacted the ophthalmologist's office, asked for a today appointment, and was reassured by the secretary that the delayed appointment would be satisfactory. Who is the wife to trust? Although the wife was speaking with a secretary in the ophthalmologist's office, is it possible she assumed she was speaking to a nurse? And not just *any* nurse. She was the *specialist's* "nurse," to whom the telephone triage nurse had evidently deferred. And before you judge the wife as being "non-compliant," please be aware that she *did* comply with the instructions of the specialist's "nurse."

Further, the ophthalmologist probably had a responsibility because he had an unlicensed person making a decision that superseded the plan of care developed by an RN. In other words, based on the secretary's judgment, it was decided that the patient could wait to be seen, and the wife had no reason to doubt her advice.

But what about the nurse? It's already been pointed out that she "did everything right," and yet the patient outcome was unacceptable. What could the nurse have done differently to increase the likelihood of a good outcome? She could have either followed up with the patient or made the appointment herself via a conference call or "warm transfer" to the ophthalmologist's office. This would have enabled the nurse, who maintained responsibility for the outcomes of her actions, to discover that the ophthalmologist was out of town and thus refer the patient directly to the ED.

Although following up or making the appointment for each patient you refer is not always indicated, there are patients for whom this extra time and effort will be necessary. A good rule of thumb to use in identifying patients who require this extra step is to determine (a) the likelihood the patient won't be able to carry out the plan of care and (b) the risk to the patient if he or she does not. Generally speaking, these will be judgment calls on the part of the nurse, based on evaluation of the specific circumstances of each situation.

For example, in this case, there were two reasons the nurse might have predicted the patient/wife's inability to carry out the plan. First, the chances of securing a same-day appointment with a specialist are often slim to none. Second, the wife was elderly, representing a demographic that is not always able to advocate well for themselves in our complex health care system.[8] And, of course, the risk to the patient was huge.

20. Fear of "Crying Wolf" and Being Labeled as an "Over-Reactor"

Most of us learned in childhood about the parable of the little boy who "cried wolf," with the clear message being that "crying wolf" isn't a good thing. However, as telephone triage nurses charged with the responsibility of looking for worst possible and erring on the side of caution, we must become comfortable making referrals as we deem necessary, understanding that while appearing to "cry wolf," we are actually acting in the best interest of our patient.

It is not unusual for nurses to be reluctant to send patients back to the ED after they have already been evaluated and sent home (see Pitfall 14 describing the patient with unusual neurological symptoms). We are often concerned that once our credibility suffers (because of failure to read our crystal ball properly), we won't be taken seriously in the future. However, we must walk a fine line in realizing that sometimes, in advocating for our patients, we must send them back again (and sometimes again).

The following scenario is one to which many telephone triage nurses can probably relate.

A nurse was going home for Christmas and her father said that her mother wasn't "acting herself," describing weakness and a somewhat altered level of consciousness. These symptoms could have indicated infection or dehydration, so the RN urged her father to take her mother to the ED for evaluation. Later that day, she got a call from home, with her father telling her that the ED had evaluated her mother and had said that there was nothing they could do for her. Presumably they had assumed this was her baseline, given her advanced age. The RN felt that response was unacceptable and urged her father to take her mother back to the ED. He resisted, reiterating that the doctor had said there was

nothing they could do. Upon the daughter's insistence, he finally took his wife back to the ED because by that time, the daughter was on her way home and threatened to take her mother to the ED herself if he did not do so.

In the meantime, the daughter called the charge nurse in the ED, asking her to see what evaluation had been done the day before. They discovered that a urinalysis (UA) had not been performed, so the ED nurse pledged to be certain that a UA would be done upon the patient's return. The daughter arrived at the hospital just as they were discharging her mother home on an antibiotic. During the ride home, her mother began vomiting, and the daughter made a U-turn to take her back to the ED, recognizing that she was likely too sick to respond promptly to oral antibiotics. However, the mother refused to return, saying, "Tomorrow is Christmas Eve, and I'm going to be at home with my family!" The daughter acquiesced, against her better judgment, telling her mother that if she weren't better in the morning, or if she got worse during the night, they were going back to the ED for re-evaluation.

The next morning, the patient was sicker still, almost lethargic, and having difficulty sitting up straight. The daughter once again insisted that they return to the ED, but both parents refused, saying they had not yet given the antibiotics time to work. Over their protests, the daughter finally coaxed them into letting her drive her mother back to the ED. As they were sitting in triage, they heard a loud male voice in the back saying, "Three visits in 3 days! In my book, that's an ... automatic admission!" Imagine the RN-daughter's relief. Her mother wasn't being sent home again. That ED visit resulted in a hospitalization of several days for urosepsis and pneumonia, but had the daughter not been insistent in advocating for her mother, that Christmas might have been her last.

Of course, most readers will understand that on the repeat visits to the ED, while nurses don't wish their patients any harm, they are almost *hoping* that the problem is really emergent. Otherwise, a visit to the ED three times in 3 days would appear to be inappropriate use of resources or incompetence on the part of the nurse. This illusion could potentially result in embarrassment and loss of credibility for the nurse. In this case, had the daughter failed to act aggressively, hoping to maintain credibility for the "next time," perhaps there would have been no next time.

This example illustrates the importance of advocating for the patient, even if the nurse feels like he or she is "swimming upstream" against the patient, their family, other health care professionals, or the "system." Remember, although just "another call" to the nurse, the patient is someone's mother, father, sister, brother, spouse, or child, and he or she is depending on *you* to help them make the right decision.

SYSTEM FAILURE

Telephone triage nurses need to be aware of certain principles for safe practice. We have reviewed 20 pitfalls that demonstrate tragic outcomes and near misses when nurses have failed to attend to these principles. However, the best efforts of the nurse, regardless of how competent or cautious he or she is, can all be for naught if the system isn't designed to allow him or her to succeed. Chapters 14 and 15 are devoted to critical program design issues, but here we provide a few examples to illustrate pitfalls that result from flaws in program design. Specifically, we address three of the most common system errors: initial triage by unqualified personnel, failure to formalize telephone triage within the organization, and nurses functioning outside their scope of practice.

21. Initial Triage by Unqualified Personnel

The following three calls were managed by intake clerks or customer service representatives who made initial triage decisions with potentially dangerous results.

An 82-year-old patient called the triage number, and reaching a clerk, presented with the following complaint. "I'm very upset. I was in to see my doctor and they put me on medicine for my urine infection. I didn't know I had an infection, but now I'm sick from the medicine. I can't sleep, I'm having indigestion, and I just don't feel well..." The patient understandably blamed her symptoms on her new medication, an antibiotic to treat an asymptomatic urinary tract infection. A note was subsequently sent by the clerk to the doctor asking if the patient could "change her medication because she's not tolerating it well."

Because the call was handled by a clerk, who was trying to be helpful, no one had an opportunity to assess the patient. Taking the note at face value, the physician might have simply changed the antibiotic. However, upon closer scrutiny, an RN might have discovered that the patient's sleeping difficulty was related to orthopnea and nocturia. While the nausea *could* have been related to the medication, other problems should have been considered and ruled out before labeling the symptoms a drug side effect. And if asked, this patient might admit to dizziness, which she hadn't mentioned because she thought it was related to lack of sleep. Get the picture?

Consider the following call, once again fielded by a clerk.

A husband called complaining that his wife's "Dramamine®" was making her sleep "all the time" and that she had just slept through a deposition. The clerk, who was charged with the responsibility of screening and routing calls, noted from the record that the patient was taking meclizine. Knowing both drugs can be used for prevention of motion sickness, the clerk assumed the "Dramamine" the husband was referring to was actually meclizine. The clerk announced to the husband, "All calls about current meds have to be handled by the pharmacy," and transferred him to the pharmacy line.

Nurses know that while Dramamine® (dimenhydrinate) can cause drowsiness, meclizine (dispensed OTC as Bonine® and Dramamine Less Drowsy Formula®) generally does not. So, several questions were left unanswered. First, if she really was taking Dramamine, why? Second, if she's not taking Dramamine, what was the cause of her somnolence? And third, was she perhaps taking both Dramamine and meclizine? The result of this call was that a patient with an altered level of consciousness of unknown etiology received no assessment and there wasn't even any documentation that the call had occurred.

A third and final example of a potentially dangerous situation being overlooked by a clerk is a patient who called with a chief complaint of "bump on my leg," accompanied by nausea and not feeling well. What little history was given to the clerk could have represented a spider bite, cellulitis, or a DVT. Unfortunately, the

potential seriousness of this problem was not recognized by the clerk, who scheduled the patient for an appointment later in the week. Again, there was no documentation of the call and no assessment of a patient with a potentially significant problem.

While quite possibly the outcomes in these cases would have been ok, these three calls are indicative of the organization "playing the odds." Would you want to play with these odds if you or your loved one were the patient? Many organizations utilize clerical personnel to screen, route, or otherwise "front end" calls, even though this practice can be fraught with problems as we will discuss further in Chapter 15.

22. Failure to Formalize Telephone Triage within the Organization

The importance of formalizing the practice of telephone triage within the organization can't be overemphasized. Tools such as policies, decision support tools, a documentation template, and other organizational factors are discussed in Chapter 15. However, as discussed in Chapter 14, careful consideration must also be given to selection, training, and proper assignment of competent nursing staff to manage patients over the telephone. Nurses who are multitasked with various telephone and non-telephone responsibilities may not give the required attention to their practice of telephone triage because of distractions or conflicting responsibilities. Conditions such as these, along with failure to provide specialized training to nurses who will be managing patients over the telephone, are a recipe for disaster, as is demonstrated in the following example.

Nine-year-old Jonathan had a same-day procedure for a routine ENT problem. Post-operatively, the surgeon wrote a prescription for a narcotic analgesic, which was subsequently filled incorrectly by the pharmacy. The liquid medication was ordered in milliliters but the prescription was filled in teaspoons, resulting in an administered dose 5 times that which was ordered.

After Jonathan's second dose of narcotic analgesic, his mother became concerned about symptoms he was having, most specifically that he seemed to be having problems with his equilibrium and was having trouble sitting upright without support. Mom was concerned but had been told the same-day surgery nurse would be calling the next day to check on Jonathan, so she decided to wait for that call to discuss her concerns with the nurse. As instructed, she gave her son his bedtime dose of antibiotic and pain medication, and put him to bed. Also as instructed, she woke him up twice during the night to force fluids. He drank water on both occasions but was aggravated with his mother for having awakened him the second time.

The next morning, the nurse from same-day surgery called to conduct her routine post-op check on her patient, screening him for such parameters as pain, bleeding, infection, dehydration, and other possible post-op issues. After listening to the mother's concerns, the nurse advised her to call the surgeon's office, which the mother did immediately.

The call was put through to the ENT nurse (an RN). The mother claimed to have advised the nurse that Jonathan was having equilibrium problems, was excessively tired, having a little trouble breathing, and was experiencing increased nausea. The nurse doc-

umented, "Mother called worried about son being tired and nausea increasing. Mother advised to push clear liquids and that sometimes the antibiotic and pain med could be hard on the stomach. She should call back if any other questions or problems occur." Unfortunately, only the nausea and fatigue were documented, but the documentation was suspect due to the fact the nurse had taken the call in the morning but didn't document the call until mid-day.

Jonathan's mother, being reassured that his symptoms were to be expected, continued to medicate her son throughout the day. She didn't call back because his symptoms, while still of concern to her, weren't appreciably different (he didn't develop any new symptoms), and those which she had already reported did not appear to be of concern to the nurse. Jonathan's mother did go to his room that night to arouse him, but he was sleeping soundly, and remembering that he was upset about being awakened the previous night, she decided to let him sleep. When she went to his room to awaken him the next morning, he was pulseless and apneic and efforts to resuscitate him were unsuccessful.

Jonathan's mother, on deposition, says she tried her best to impress upon the nurse that she was extremely concerned about her son but stated that she didn't feel the nurse was listening to her. There is some disagreement about what the mother actually reported to the nurse, but if the nurse had performed an adequate assessment, she would have realized that some of the symptoms reported (equilibrium problems, excessive fatigue, trouble breathing) were not consistent with a routine post-op course and warranted follow-up. This scenario also begs the question of how many implicit cues did the nurse fail to pick up? Given the fact that the autopsy reported the cause of death as a narcotic overdose and aspiration pneumonia superimposed upon laryngeal and tracheal edema, there is little doubt that Jonathan's condition at the time of the call warranted immediate evaluation.

In this situation, as with most cases which result in lawsuits, several factors apparently contributed to this tragedy. Although this was obviously the pharmacy's error, and they settled out of court for an undisclosed sum, this case illustrates how the telephone triage nurse was in a position to either prevent or compound the error.

Jonathan's case highlights several important principles of telephone triage, including the importance of performing an adequate assessment and exercising sound clinical judgment. Also, considering every call life threatening until proven otherwise would have created the proper mindset for the nurse to hear the mother's plea for help. Likewise, erring on the side of caution, if for no reason other than the mother's concern, would have at the very least resulted in a same-day appointment. While the narcotic overdose may not have been readily identified as the source of the problem, it would have been evident that Jonathan's condition was not consistent with what one would expect to see after an uncomplicated routine procedure. And as a postscript, this vignette stresses the importance of verifying how the patient is taking medications, whether prescription or OTC. Some research suggests that prescribing errors are the leading causes of medication errors in the outpatient setting.[9] Others say patient errors are the most common.[10] And still others report that labeling errors are among the most common causes of medication errors.[11] Regardless, the telephone triage nurse has a critical role in medication assessment, education, and communication.

Unfortunately, the RN in this ENT office had received no training in telephone triage and thus was unaware of her duty to heed the concerns of the mother, speak directly to the patient, err on the side of caution, and look for "zebras." Specialized training, protocols, and a documentation template would have armed the nurse to handle this call more competently, perhaps averting the bad outcome.

- The mother's deposition included phrases such as:
  - "He was having difficulty walking."
  - "He walked into the kitchen and just kind of bounced...he was hitting things."
  - "He was having problems breathing, just slumping over on me complaining of the shortness of breath."
  - "He did not have enough strength or balance to sit up without being strapped in."
  - "He was acting very tired...very drugged."
  - "I felt very urgent in the conversation."
  - "I felt like I wasn't being listened to. I felt like I was doing all the talking and she was just saying push liquids."
  - "I was trying to make her understand whether I did it the right way or not."
  - "I was scared. I guess I trusted what she was telling me."
  - "I thought I was following the directions."
- The nurse's deposition included phrases like:
  - "What I was *hearing* over the phone as far as the symptoms are perfectly normal symptoms..."
  - "I don't think there was a level of pain or anything *given* to me at that time."
  - "I was not *given* any information that would *have lead me* to do that."

- "There were no red flags *given* me that day..."
- "With the information I *received*, there was no reason to (notify the doctor)."

Notice all the passive verbs used by the RN? Evidently she didn't realize whose job it was to know what information is needed in order to perform an adequate assessment. It is the nurse's job to anticipate and obtain the necessary information. It is not the caller's job to know what information is relevant and what is not.

This is a perfect example that if we are going to provide care over the telephone, we'd better do it right. The mother *knew* her child was very ill but allowed herself to be inappropriately reassured by the RN. The responsibility for telephone triage is awesome and, occasionally, truly a matter of life and death.

23. Functioning Outside of Scope of Practice

In Chapter 5, we discussed scope of practice issues that present common challenges to telephone triage nurses. The following scenario represents an extreme example of liberties sometimes taken in the office setting in situations in which the nurse and physician have a close working relationship.

An LPN working in an orthopedic surgeon's office was given the responsibility of carrying the physician's beeper at night and "taking call" for him, handling what she could and alerting him when his advanced knowledge and expertise were needed. One night, she got a call from a patient who was 10 days post-op following a knee surgery, specifically, an anterior cruciate ligament repair. The patient was requesting a refill on his analgesic, his third such request in the past 4 days. One doesn't have to be an orthopedic nurse to understand that at 10 days post-op, if all is well, the pain should be

decreasing rather than increasing. In addition to the red flag of increasing/persistent pain, the patient said he also told her about "redness and swelling" in his knee. However, instead of recognizing and addressing a possible septic joint, the nurse (without a doctor's order) picked up the phone and called in a prescription for hydrocodone. It was 2 days later when the patient finally sought care in an ED for his infected joint, and by that time, it was too late. He wound up with osteomyelitis, eventually losing his patella, and was thereafter unable to walk without a splint or a brace, sharply curtailing the activities of this otherwise healthy young man.

The most surprising thing about this case was that neither the nurse nor the physician had any idea that they had done anything wrong. The nurse, on deposition, was asked, "Why did you do that?" and her response was, "Because the doctor told me I could." And at the physician's deposition, when asked if he had really authorized such actions, he replied, "Yes, she's a good nurse and knows my pain protocols." Of course, "knowing" was not the issue. The LPN was clearly exceeding her scope of practice, which is established by the Nurse Practice Act of the state in question, not the physician by whom she is employed.

WE MORE OFTEN GET IT 'RIGHT'!

By this point in the chapter, the reader might be wondering if all telephone triage calls are disasters. Hopefully, the reader can see the value in learning from the mistakes of others, and that such occurrences can be prevented.

To end on a positive note, let's look at a couple of good "saves" that were accomplished by nurses in well-designed programs. At least one, if not both, of the following calls saved a life.

A woman called with a chief complaint of a "cold." As the nurse took her history, the patient reported watery eyes, runny nose, and a cough. The nurse investigated further and the patient admitted to shortness of breath and chest tightness. The patient was referred to the ED and subsequently diagnosed with an acute MI. One might ask, "What were the cold symptoms about?" There are two logical explanations. First, the patient might have had a cold when she had her MI and perhaps it was the combination of all the symptoms that made her pick up the phone and call the nurse. Second, the patient might have suspected there was more going on than an upper-respiratory infection, but was seeking reassurance that it was "only a cold." Of course, delay in seeking treatment is a major contributing factor to death and disability for those experiencing heart attacks, so the possibility of a patient with an MI immediately recognizing, accepting, and acting upon the symptoms are slim.[12] Although not always the case, if a patient accepts the fact that she is possibly having an MI, she is likely to be proceeding to the ED rather than calling the triage nurse for reassurance.

This nurse, rather than accepting the patient's self-diagnosis, looked beyond the obvious to rule out worst possible. She utilized the prescribed system for patient assessment and use of decision support tools, and discovered that the patient was experiencing a potentially life-threatening event.

The following is another example of the nurse looking beyond the obvious.

Diagnosed with acute sinusitis in the office on Friday, a patient called early Monday morning complaining of a severe headache. He had been given an antibiotic and a decongestant, but this morning he was asking for "a pain pill for this headache." The telephone triage nurse, being specially trained and armed with good decision support tools, asked (among other things) when his headache had started, if it had come on suddenly or gradually, and if he were having any visual difficulties. The patient responded that the headache had started suddenly this morning, and said, "It's funny you should mention the vision thing. I've seen double a couple of times this morning." The nurse, recognizing these symptoms as being inconsistent with a benign sinus headache, had to argue with the patient for almost 30 minutes before getting him to agree to allow a colleague to drive him to the hospital, where he got a CT of his head. He had an intracranial bleed that probably developed that morning during a paroxysm of coughing. Subsequently, the nurse got flowers from him every year on her birthday because the patient thought she had saved his life, and she probably had.

This call shows the effectiveness of having dedicated (non-multitasked) nurses who know how to use decision support tools properly, think outside the box, and advocate for the patient (even against himself if necessary).

SUMMARY

Understanding of and attention to the pitfalls discussed in this chapter represent elements of a minimum skill set for telephone triage nurses. Application of the principles illustrated in the vignettes presented will help ensure patient safety in the provision of care over the telephone.

In the next chapter, we will look at quality management principles that focus on practices to help assure quality care. This is followed by chapters on program design and implementation. The vital information in these chapters can help ensure the preceding disastrous calls don't happen to you.

References

1. Canadian Nurses Association. (2007). *Telehealth: The role of the nurse.* Position Statement. Ottawa, Canada: Author.
2. Mitchell, J.K. (2010). Telephone triage. *ONS Connect, 25*(9), 8-11.
3. Wheeler, S. (2011). *Telephone triage nursing: Roles, tools and rules.* Wild Iris Medical Education, Inc. Retrieved from http://www.nursingceu.com/courses/290/index_nceu.html
4. Judd, C.M., Blair, I.V., & Chapleau, K.M. (2004). Automatic stereotypes vs. automatic prejudice: Sorting out the possibilities in the Payne (2001) weapon paradigm. *Journal of Experimental Social Psychology, 40*, 75-81.
5. Tabone, S. (2004). Nurse fatigue: The human factor. *Texas Nursing, 78*(5), 8-10.
6. Witkoski, A., & Dickson, V. (2010). Hospital staff nurses' work hours, meal periods, and rest breaks: A review from an occupational health nurse perspective. *AAOHN Journal, 58*(11), 489-497. doi:10.3928/08910162-20101027-02
7. Kamp, G., Heymans, H., & Breederveld, C. (1989). [Is circumoral cyanosis a sign of peripheral or of central cyanosis?]. *Nederlands Tijdschrift Voor Geneeskunde, 133*(27), 1360-1364.
8. MacCracken, L., Pickens, G., & Wells, M. (2009). *Matching the market: Using generational insights to attract and retain consumers.* Retrieved from http://www. health carestrategy.com/usermedia/TSHW-185A_BRIEF_generational_0109.pdf
9. Gandhi, T.K., Weingart, S.N., Seger, A.C., Borus, J., Burdick, E., Poon, E.G., & ... Bates, D.W. (2005). Outpatient prescribing errors and the impact of computerized prescribing. *JGIM: Journal of General Internal Medicine, 20*(9), 837-841. doi:10.1111/j.1525-1497.2005.0194.x
10. Balkrishnan, R., Foss, C.E., Pawaskar, M., Uhas, A.A., & Feldman, S.R. (2009). Monitoring for medication errors in outpatient settings. *Journal of Dermatological Treatment*, 20(4), 229-232. doi:10.1080/09546630802607487
11. Jeetu, G., & Girish T. (2010). Prescription drug labeling medication errors: A big deal for pharmacists. *Journal of Young Pharmacists, 2*(1),107-111. doi:10.4103/0975-1483.62218
12. Moser, D., Kimble, L., Alberts, M., Alonzo, A., Croft, J., Dracup, K., & Zerwic, J. (2007). Reducing delay in seeking treatment by patients with acute coronary syndrome and stroke: A scientific statement from the American Heart Association Council on Cardiovascular Nursing and Stroke Council. *Journal of Cardiovascular Nursing, 22*(4), 326-343.

Chapter 13

Quality in Telephone Triage

We have written a great deal about how to deliver quality care over the telephone, but how is quality best defined, measured, and assured? Although a great deal of effort has been devoted to quality measurement in telephone triage settings, few of the measures focus specifically on the practice of nursing. In this chapter, we will address forces and misconceptions that have most often guided quality assurance in the telephone triage arena. We will also propose new strategies for optimizing quality in the provision of nursing care over the telephone. In so doing, we will define quality and related concepts, explain how it should be measured, and discuss how the measurements should be used.

QUALITY DEFINED

Quality is a nebulous and elusive concept; it is often poorly defined and applied. The concept of *quality* is ubiquitous in business and management literature. Quality has been defined operationally by various theorists and quality gurus such as Deming, Juran, Kano, and Crosby. Quality definitions have also been suggested by ISO 9000 and Six Sigma. Those of us old enough to remember may feel as if we've experienced "The Quality Flavor of the Month" transitioning from terms such as "Audit" to "Total Quality Management" (TQM) to "Continuous Quality Improvement" (CQI), while visiting concepts like "Customer Satisfaction," "Benchmarking," and "Root Cause Analysis" along the way. And there continues to be confusion regarding the processes of "Quality Assurance," "Quality Improvement," and "Quality Management."

The American Society for Quality[1] specifies that *quality* is "A subjective term for which each person or sector has its own definition. In technical usage, quality can have two meanings: 1. the characteristics of a product or service that bear on its ability to satisfy stated or implied needs; 2. a product or service free of deficiencies." Merriam-Webster On-Line Dictionary[2] defines *quality* as "a degree of excellence" and *quality assurance* (QA) as "a program for the systematic monitoring and evaluation of the various aspects of a project, service, or facility to ensure that standards of quality are being met." This definition begs the question: "What standards are we using?"

THE INFLUENCE OF THE NON-MEDICAL CALL CENTER INDUSTRY AND ITS IMPACT ON CARE

In the early days of call center management, we looked to the non-medical call center industry for guidance and were provided with standards that we then tried to adapt to our telephone triage settings. The primary influences were measurements reflecting productivity and return on investment (ROI).

Although productivity has long been a concern of nursing, the idea of productivity measurements as quality indicators was new for our profession. For example, in addition to providing patient care, telephone triage nurses were required to focus on technical concepts such as average speed of answer, call handling time, dropped calls, blocked calls, and service level. Thus, emphasis was placed on productivity and efficiency rather than on the quality of nursing care. Some call centers even took this to the level of dictating desired call length rather than more realistic expectations of allowing nurses as much time as necessary to safely and effectively complete a telephone triage encounter.

Cost effectiveness (e.g., measurements reflecting ROI) has also long been a driving force in the non-medical call center industry. Following suit, medical call centers began measuring data that reflected ROI, and this was accompanied by emphasis on productivity. As one nurse put it, referring to her call center, "It's all about the money." This focus becomes a problem, particularly in telephone triage, when ROI takes precedence over quality through efforts to streamline the calls, potentially short-circuiting the nursing process as a result. Under these conditions, the quality of care delivered, the quality of the patient-nurse interaction, and nurses' work satisfaction suffer.[3,4]

It was (and still is) common for call center managers to rank nurses anonymously, posting for review their call times or other types of "scores" compared to those of their peers. In fact, in some organizations, the successful shortening of a nurse's call time is rewarded with a bonus or a raise, thereby incentivizing nurses to focus more on call length than on quality.[5] This type of reporting is potentially damaging, and can lead to nurses focusing on their score or their rank among their peers rather than on the quality of care they deliver to their patients.

One call center manager was using such a strategy to compare call dispositions. She posted, among other metrics, the percent of patients each nurse referred to the emergency department (ED). When advised to discontinue that practice for fear it might negatively impact performance, she replied, "They (the nurses) know I don't care." However, obviously she did care, or she wouldn't have posted the information on the wall. Indeed, when the nurse with the highest referral rate was questioned about whether it concerned her, she replied, "Oh yes! Every time I send a patient to the ED, I stop and consider what it will do to my statistics." When a nurse is talking to a patient who is sick enough to require evaluation in the ED, the last thing you want her thinking about is her performance scores or disposition statistics.

Fortunately, at present, the number of call centers attempting to track ROI is decreasing.[6] With the trend clearly moving away from a spotlight on cost and productivity measures toward a focus on the quality of care, can we assume that giving good care will be cost effective in the long run? According to Deming, "...when people and organizations focus primarily on *costs*, costs tend to rise and quality declines over time" (¶ 3).[7] And, conversely, "When people and organizations focus primarily on quality, quality tends to increase and costs fall over time" (¶ 3).[7] This makes sense because factors such as improved patient satisfaction and loyalty, appropriate utilization of resources, and improved overall health of our society are surely "cost effective."[8]

Despite this trend, some services still focus excessively on demonstrating their monetary value to the organization. This is usually an unnecessary effort because, over the years, the cost effectiveness of telephone triage has been well-established.[9,10,11,12] Although often difficult to measure directly, cost effectiveness can be reflected in cost avoidance. For example, money is saved when patients are appropriately redirected to a lower, less-expensive level of care, or directed to a level of care that avoids unnecessary expenditures. But also included in cost avoidance is getting the patient to the right care even if it is a higher, more expensive level of care, because this often prevents increased morbidity and costly associated medical interventions. While there is no doubt that all businesses must demonstrate their worth in a variety of ways, the value of providing safe and effective high-quality patient care over the telephone is immeasurable.

Eventually, after several years of metrics-driven "quality management," the non-medical call center industry arrived at the realization that productivity didn't necessarily equal quality. With this realization they shifted the emphasis from call handling time to customer satisfaction and one-call resolution.[13] Although their eye was never far from the clock or the bottom line, making the customer happy superseded handling calls quickly. Similarly, after several years of metrics-driven "quality management" in telephone triage, it is time to shift our primary focus from productivity measures to measures of actual quality.

THE VALUE OF PRODUCTIVITY MEASURES

To understand the value of volume and productivity, it is helpful to introduce the concepts of efficiency and effectiveness. Efficiency is a matter of resource utilization. *Efficiency* is the "ability to accomplish a job with a minimum expenditure of time and effort."[14] In telephone triage settings, this is often translated into completing a triage encounter with the least use of resources. *Effectiveness* can be a measure of quality. Effectiveness is being "adequate to accomplish a purpose; producing the intended or expected result."[15] In telephone triage settings, this is best translated into providing quality nursing care that meets the needs of the patient. Efficiency and effectiveness often go hand in hand, but efficiency is no guarantee of effectiveness.

Why We Still Need to Measure Volume and Productivity

Volume and productivity are not measures of quality, but they are important factors that can affect efficiency and effectiveness. Because they may impact the quality of care delivered, they are addressed in this chapter. Volume and productivity measurements provide managers with the information required to make changes necessary to improve quality. Managers need volume and productivity data to answer questions such as, "How many nurses do we need?" "Are our nurses being utilized appropriately?" "What time should they be scheduled?" and "How many phone lines do we need?" These metrics are necessary for program management because failure to attend to them (e.g., failure to provide adequate staffing) can have a negative impact on quality. Therefore, call volume must be measured and tracked so that predictions regarding future volume and staffing needs can be made and changes can be implemented based on those predictions.

If call volume is excessive, it has the potential to impact quality negatively. For example, nurses who have many calls to return or several callers in the queue are more likely to rush through a call, possibly omitting important aspects of care. Likewise, variables such as call length may impact quality.[3] For example, while conventional wisdom dictates that the quicker a nurse gets off the phone, the better (within reason), research shows that patient satisfaction is related in part to the nurse's ability to identify and meet the needs of the individual,[11,16,17] and this requires time.

The length of a call may be influenced by well-honed interviewing skills and efficient strategies such as use of a documentation template; however, regardless of the efficiency measures implemented, calls will still take as long as they take. Call length varies based on factors such as patient age, co-morbidities, educational level, and available resources, in addition to the nature and urgency of the patient's problem. For example, call length in the adult population increases significantly with age.[18] Thus, one can anticipate that triage calls with the geriatric population will be longer than the "average" call. While some nurses may take less or more time to handle calls than their peers, such call statistics should be viewed critically with an eye more on quality than time. Consistent variations from the averages may indicate opportunities for coaching and subsequent practice improvements, or they might represent best practices that should be emulated by their peers.

Common Cause and Special Cause Variation

Variability in volume and productivity can often be attributed to *common cause* or *special cause* variation. For example, call volume is observed in many settings to be higher on Monday morning than other days of the week; or in other settings, all mornings might consistently be busier than afternoons. These differences represent *common cause* variation, which is predictable, and thus staffing can be designed to handle the anticipated volume. However, *special cause* variation, such as would be seen with an outbreak of an infectious disease in the community, would not be anticipated and would thus cause unanticipated spikes in call volume, for which staffing might prove to be inadequate. Likewise, even in well-controlled situations, if one or more nurses calls in sick, the amount of time the caller will have to wait to speak to a nurse will probably be increased.

Common cause variability should be anticipated and addressed in advance. For example, more staff might be scheduled during peak call times such as Monday mornings. This additional staffing would prevent quality from suffering during times of high volume. However, special cause variation, such as an unanticipated drug recall or an epidemic cannot be predicted or controlled. Therefore, it is possible and even likely that the sudden unexpected surges in volume related to special cause variation may negatively impact quality. For example, nurses might rush through calls, skipping important steps, or patient satisfaction might suffer due to unusually high wait times. Because these events are outside the control of the organization, it is best to not hold the staff accountable for dips in quality performance during these periods. However, knowing that we can expect the unexpected will serve as a basis for crisis planning in the future. Let's apply the principles of common cause and special cause variation to call management and related quality assurance (see Table 1).

Application Exercise

As illustrated in Table 1, call volume will be higher during an epidemic (special cause variation). During that time, nurses are likely to reduce their call length, handle more calls, and therefore increase their efficiency and productivity. However, these apparent changes in productivity and efficiency may very well come at the expense of quality in clinical and administrative processes. In other words, nurses can be very efficient in the manner in which they handle a call and still fail to provide safe and effective (quality) care. This exercise illustrates the importance of deciding how to measure quality and under what circumstances. So while efficiency is desirable, effectiveness is an *imperative*.

QUALITY IN TELEPHONE TRIAGE

Quality in health care is "the degree to which health services for individuals and populations increase the likelihood of desired health outcomes and are consistent with current professional knowledge" (p. 21).[19] How then do we measure quality, or "doing it right" in telephone triage?

In saying, "choice of aim is clearly a matter of clarification of values," Deming[20] was aptly pointing out that we should measure what we value. Values are a basis for what a person thinks about, chooses,

Table 1.
Productivity, Efficiency, and Performance Measures Under Common Cause and Special Cause Circumstances

Conditions	Normal Common Cause		Epidemic Special Cause	
Nurses	**Janet**	**Julie**	**Janet**	**Julie**
PRODUCTIVITY & EFFICIENCY MEASURES				
Number of calls/shift	42	60	65	90
Average number of minutes/call	10	7	7	5
EFFICIENCY				
Number of calls/shift	Med	High	High	High
Number of minutes/call	Med	High	High	High
PRODUCTIVITY *				
Percent of productive time/shift	93%	93%	100%	100%
PERFORMANCE MEASURES				
Clinical process	High	Med	Med	Low
Patient satisfaction	High	Med	Med	Low
Administrative process (documentation)	High	Med	Med	Low
Patient safety	High	Acceptable	Acceptable	Compromised

*__Note:__ Possible productive minutes/8-hour shift, providing two 15-minute breaks = 450

- **Efficiency**
  Calls/Shift Julie was more efficient than Janet
  Minutes/Call Julie was more efficient than Janet

- **Productivity**
  Productive Time/Shift: Both nurses had equal productivity per shift

- **Performance Measures**
  All performance measures were negatively affected by the increased call volume.

Discussion

- Under normal circumstances, common cause variability related to different call management styles between Janet and Julie still yielded acceptable performance measurements in all categories, although with Julie, there was room for improvement in all performance measurements.
- However, during the epidemic that caused significantly increased call volume (special cause variability), all parameters suffered for both nurses. Because this was an unusual circumstance, remedial action was not taken for slips in performance with the exception that clinical process indicators had to be reviewed for Julie because her patient safety was unacceptable.
- So, although circumstances can force the efficiency and productivity to increase, it can be at the expense of quality.

feels for, and acts upon.[21] Therefore, telephone triage leadership must be very deliberate in what they decide to measure and report to the staff because the nurses will learn to value and thus emphasize the parameters upon which they are being evaluated. And, administrators will take the cue as well. In other words, if what we measure isn't already important to the team, it very soon will be.

Traditionally, the concept of quality management in health care has addressed structure, process, and outcome.[23] The structure and design of a program is critical to the delivery of safe and effective care. Without proper program elements in place, providing quality care is an uphill battle at best. Therefore Chapters 14 and 15 are devoted to program design and implementation.

"It's not enough to do your best; you must know what to do and then do your best" (p.1).[22]

First and foremost we want to facilitate optimum patient health outcomes. Thus, *effectiveness*, or providing safe care the right way in order to achieve the desired outcomes, is our primary goal in telephone triage. Right processes are what lead to desirable outcomes. This understanding carries a strong and clear message that we must measure *how* we do what we do from a patient care perspective.

While it is critical to monitor outcomes for a variety of important reasons, the primary focus in measuring quality in telephone triage must be on process.[24] This focus on *process* is based on sound theory.[25,26,27,28,29] In telephone triage, process is the most appropriate indicator of quality due in part to the difficulties encountered in measuring and controlling outcomes, which will be discussed later.

"We should work on our process, not the outcome of our processes" (p. 2).[22]

PROCESS AS A QUALITY INDICATOR

How the nurse conducts the call represents process. To measure process, however, we must first understand what we are measuring. Process indicators can be divided into administrative processes and clinical processes.

- *Administrative processes* include such factors as technical skills and knowledge of and adherence to organizational policies. Is the nurse able to type and use the computer and software proficiently? Did the nurse "fill in all the blanks" (or complete all fields) on the form? While measuring these performance indicators is an important managerial function, it is important to keep in mind that competency (using the software proficiently) and compliance (following policy), while important, don't necessarily ensure quality. However, they may impact quality because, for example, if the nurse fails to verify a telephone number and the one on file is wrong, that omission might result in impaired quality of care if the nurse needs to call the patient back.

"If you can't describe what you are doing as a process, you don't know what you're doing" (p. 1).[22]

- *Clinical processes* reflect elements of professional nursing. The key question here might be, "How are we providing care?" For example, are we asking the right questions? Are we using the right decision support tool? Is there evidence of critical thinking in the assessment, interaction with the caller, and decision making? In other words, is there evidence of professional nursing? The most basic, direct, and comprehensive measure of professional nursing is found in the nursing process.

Measuring Process

In measuring process as it relates to quality, management must be sensitive to what data are measured, how they are measured, and by whom. A tool should be developed for telephone triage nurses that will help determine whether established standards of care have been met. A key question in the measurement of quality is whether the nurse is following the defined processes for telephone triage, such as the nursing process[24], and more specifically, those described in the Greenberg Model of Telephone Nursing Practice.[27] In measuring the quality of the nursing process, it is important to look for the following evidence:

- *Assessment.* Is there adequate and descriptive subjective and objective data? Does the assessment documentation provide a complete clinical picture?
- *Diagnosis.* Has the nurse determined the nature and urgency of the patient's problem and associated nursing care needs as reflected in the assessment?
- *Planning.* Is the disposition consistent with the diagnosis and is there evidence of collaborative planning with which the patient is comfortable? Will it meet desired outcomes?
- *Intervention.* Has the nurse provided the necessary information to the patient, family, and/or other health care providers who will actually be carrying out the plan of care?
- *Evaluation.* Is there clear evidence of how the nurse will know if the patient's problem isn't resolved or doesn't follow the expected course? Is there a method for providing the nurse feedback regarding whether the particular problem was resolved, or not?

In reviewing calls, specific knowledge must be applied to assess the quality of each component of the process. For example, when evaluating nursing assessment and diagnosis, if the patient's chief complaint is headache, is it clear that the nurse began by anticipating worst possible, documenting the high-risk pertinent negatives? In the case of a patient who is vomiting, are likely associated problems such as dehydration considered and ruled out? Process in telephone triage is more than just filling in the blanks. There must be solid evidence of critical thinking and application of clinical judgment.

Peer Review and Self-Assessment in Evaluation of Process

In measuring the presence or absence of quality in telephone triage, with a mature group of nurses in a supportive culture, peer review can be a very effective strategy. Elements of the call that reflect quality in the process include collecting adequate data, documenting to paint a picture, accurately identifying the nature and urgency of the problem, identifying desired outcomes, developing a collaborative plan to meet those outcomes, assuring the patient's ability to implement the plan, and evaluating the effectiveness of the encounter. These activities can really only be evaluated by another nurse who understands the process well. The strategies described in the Greenberg Model (e.g., getting to know, verifying) are best recognized by monitoring a live or a recorded call, and their presence can be documented using a written evaluation tool. Care must be taken not to assign the task of doing quality audits to anyone other than an experienced telephone triage nurse. Quality reviews by a non-telephone triage nurse who is removed from or unfamiliar with the intricacies of the practice, increases the likelihood of misunderstanding the process and documentation, potentially yielding misleading QA findings.

Another effective strategy for quality analysis is self-assessment. Having nurses listen to their own calls or review their own records with a tool to measure the presence and quality of the nursing process and selected strategies identified in the Greenberg Model can be a real eye opener. In fact, listening to one's own calls or the calls of others, guided by the model of the telephone triage process, can be an excellent teaching tool for telephone triage nurses. It will provide a clear look at the process and focus on the nurse-patient interactions, driving home questions like, "Do I really listen?" and "Am I interpreting what I am hearing correctly and responding appropriately?"

When engaged in peer evaluation, we should be looking to see if the nurse is using a reasonable, professional thought process appropriate to each particular patient encounter. When using QA audit tools to collect data about performance, it is tempting to reduce our analysis to a numeric score, such as a percent or proportion. However, possibly because of experiences from our childhood, we often have a visceral reaction to the notion of receiving a "grade." Scores such as these are likely dissatisfiers rather than satisfiers. In other words, any score less than 100% is likely to elicit a negative reaction in many people, with the process focusing on what they did wrong instead of reinforcing what they did right. While coaching is an important part of mentoring and supervising a nurse, we believe that this should be done apart from reporting QA findings so that it can be regarded as an opportunity rather than as a punishment.

"We should be guided by theory, not by numbers" (p. 21).[30]

Perhaps a better approach would be to simply observe the nurses' calls and documentation, providing positive reinforcement to the nurse and making suggestions for improvement (when a trend is recognized) rather than assigning a score to each call. Nurses want timely feedback about whether they "made the right decision," or in other words, whether their process was right.[27,31,32] They also want timely feedback on outcomes and will seek it independently if it's not offered as a matter of routine.[27] Rather than one nurse (manager, QA coordinator, or peer) trying to objectively evaluate the quality of a particular interaction and assign a score, it would be more accurate and meaningful to observe the nurse's interactions and documentation over a period of time and reflect those observations back to the nurse in aggregate in a timely manner. Another meaningful exercise would be to review challenging calls with the staff as a group, providing constructive feedback in private to individual nurses when needed.

Constructive Use of Feedback

When framed in a manner that emphasizes the promotion of optimal practice, as opposed to a manner that emphasizes individual performance evaluation, the nurse is more likely to incorporate feedback into his or her practice. Constructive feedback obtained from self-evaluation, peer evaluation, and the designated QA coordinator or manager, plus timely feedback from our physician colleagues provide opportunities for professional growth and should be welcomed by the clinical nursing staff.

- Nurses should receive non-pejorative feedback on use of decision support tools, documentation, critical-thinking processes, and actual patient outcomes.
- Call review of self and peers, either as a record review or listening to a recorded call, can be instructional and informative if the nurse has a well-designed audit tool in hand.
- Educational offerings based on QA findings will help the entire staff grow. For example, widespread evidence of knowledge deficit should trigger an in-service offering relative to the specific problem. Individual mentoring should be offered if the knowledge deficit is limited to one nurse.
- Development of quality improvement teams to address process improvement is desirable and necessary when negative quality trends or inconsistencies are identified.

OUTCOME AS A QUALITY INDICATOR

Defining outcome measurements in telephone triage has proven challenging. While there are some outcome indicators that do measure quality indirectly, outcome continues to be an elusive measurement in telephone triage. Due to a variety of circumstances including the nature of the patient's problem, where and when the patient chooses to access care, and the quality of care the patient receives from others, telephone triage nurses are not generally able to control ultimate outcomes. In other words, whether the patient suffers increased morbidity or mortality is usually not within the control of the telephone triage nurse, nor is it always measurable, since in many cases, subsequent contact with the patient is not feasible. Thus, traditional outcome measures such as, "Did the patient get better?" or "Did the patient survive?" cannot be applied, given that telephone triage is often an initial component of the delivery of care rather than the entire basis of the care given to the patient. Once the patient goes to the ED, clinic, or other care delivery venue, the quality of the care provided and consequent outcomes are beyond the control of the telephone triage nurse. However, by assuring quality processes in telephone triage, we can facilitate appropriate care and thereby influence outcomes. Having established the importance of focusing on process to evaluate and improve quality, we will review and discuss outcome measures that have traditionally been used to assess telephone triage quality: customer satisfaction, cost effectiveness, and accuracy in decision making.

Customer Satisfaction as an Outcome Indicator

Patient satisfaction has long been used as a measure of quality. It is typically assessed by gathering individual or aggregated opinions regarding either a specific encounter or the service in general. Providing care that elicits a high degree of customer satisfaction is important because it impacts the financial viability and the reputation of the organization and positively influences patient compliance with the plan of care.[33] Satisfied customers are often repeat customers who talk to others about their satisfaction with your organization. Dissatisfied customers will also talk to others about their negative perception of your organization, potentially damaging your image in the community. And dissatisfied customers are more likely to sue if they experience a bad outcome. So in addition to being a good marketing tool, customer satisfaction is also a good risk-management strategy.

Studies measuring patient satisfaction as an outcome indicator have greatly supported the value of telephone triage to patients.[11,34,35]

This research has shown that patient satisfaction is influenced by aspects of the process of telephone triage as well as by telephone triage outcomes. Regarding the process, patients are most satisfied with care that is individualized, collaborative, and provides clear communication and problem resolution.[16,36,37] Regarding the outcomes, patients have been found to be satisfied with the value of the telephone triage service because of the access to care and convenience it provides.[11,37,38]

In a large survey of patients seeking care over the telephone in Quebec, researchers concluded that patients were very satisfied. Patients reported that after talking with the nurse, they understood their problem well, had clarity about the plan of care, understood the instructions, and believed their care was appropriate. They were also satisfied that the interaction provided the information needed for them to make the best decision, given their particular circumstances.

Of special interest was the patients' perception of the financial value of the encounter. The survey found that a significant number of patients believed they saved money because they were redirected to a less-expensive level of care. Other cost savings were noted as well. Eighty percent of the patients saved 5 hours of time, 60% avoided transportation costs, 33% saved an average of 3 hours in child care costs, and 25% avoided lost wages due to missing work.[11]

Clearly customer satisfaction is desirable. But it is not always achievable. For example, during times of unexpectedly high call volume, the quality of the interpersonal elements of care as well as access and convenience might suffer. Proper staffing strategies can help minimize such problems. The mother who wants only information on the "normal" temperature for her baby without first allowing the nurse to assess the child may be satisfied although she may not have received quality care. Therefore, while useful to measure and desirable to achieve, customer satisfaction should not be relied upon as the sole indicator of quality of a specific telephone triage encounter or of a telephone triage program in general.

Cost Savings as an Outcome Indicator

As discussed earlier in this chapter, cost effectiveness was one of the primary outcome measures in the early days of the medical call center. Tracking ROI was a key focus because many call centers were initially developed as community outreach and/or marketing strategies. If a program isn't regarded as being financially viable, and especially if it's viewed as being a financial drain on the organization, it won't be around long.

Cost saving has been used as an outcome measure for decades. How the cost savings are actually measured varies widely. The most common method to assess cost savings in telephone triage is by comparing what the caller would have done to the recommendation from the nurse and then calculating the cost difference.[9,10,39] This can give a good idea of how much money has potentially been saved. Beyond calculating these savings, there are underlying cost savings (and safety issues) that are often unseen or unrecognized and therefore difficult to measure. For example, telephone triage often results in the redirection of patients with emergent problems away from the office setting to the ED. Telephone triage also prevents unnecessary and inappropriate clinic walk-in visits which can translate into potentially significant savings in staff and provider resources.[10] Evidence of cost savings also supports the idea that telephone triage helps get the right patient to the right level of care, thereby saving money by reducing unnecessary use of resources.[40]

Although reduced cost as an outcome indicator helps to support the idea of the financial benefits associated with telephone triage, there are multiple limitations to this approach. Because the information is not usually readily available, it is often difficult to determine the actual outcome of the call or exactly what action the patient took after the telephone call. The outcome following the disposition given is dependent upon multiple variables, many of which are out of the nurse's control. Compliance with the disposition is one factor that must be considered when measuring cost as an outcome indicator and using the disposition to measure that cost. If patients are compliant with the disposition, substantial cost savings from telephone triage are possible.[39,41]

Decision-Making Accuracy as an Outcome Indicator

Although accurate decision making is essential to effective telephone triage, it is very difficult to evaluate. In the past, measures of accuracy of nurse decisions have often been based on appropriate choice of protocol and adherence to that protocol.[42,43] We have previously discussed at length why adherence to protocols is not an appropriate measure of quality in telephone triage. Also, organizations have occasionally compared the nurse's disposition with the patient's eventual medical diagnosis. But because triage assessment is based on symptoms, not diagnoses, the actual diagnosis often provides little meaningful information. Since nurses have been taught to err on the side of caution, a nurse can't be faulted for sending a patient with chest pain to the ED when the ultimate diagnosis is indigestion. Thus, accuracy in decision making can't be measured in the context of the medical diagnosis. Instead, the focus must be on the soundness of application of the principles of telephone triage nursing.

Researchers have also assessed decision-making accuracy by measuring the quality of the nurse assessment using simulated scenarios.[3,44,45] In such studies, the nurses' dispositions are compared to opinions of experts, usually physicians, regarding the appropriate disposition. However, the use of physicians is not appropriate to measure quality of telephone triage because their focus is most often on medical diagnoses and treatment whereas the telephone triage nurse focuses on symptoms, incorporating individual contextual factors and patient characteristics into his or her decision making. In other words, the goal of the physician contact is usually definitive care, while the goal of the telephone triage nurse is to facilitate care.

The basic problem with use of physician-intepreted scenarios as measures of accurate decision making is that: "Routine clinical practice can be so varied that even clinicians who work closely with each other do not necessarily agree about the information required to make safe decisions" (p. 556).[45] We maintain, and research suggests, that the appropriateness of the decision made is dependent on the individual characteristics of the call and the caller.[46]

Evaluation of the appropriateness of the nurse's decision making by someone other than a telephone triage nurse listening to a live or recorded call is not likely to yield an accurate assessment. Because each nurse is a professional, responsible for the consequences of his or her own actions, evaluation of decision making outside the context of the actual call itself and certainly by someone other than a peer is ill-advised and potentially misleading. Peer review, as described earlier, remains the recommended way to measure accuracy of decision making and advice given.

IMPROVING QUALITY: PRACTICAL IMPLICATIONS

Once the decision is made regarding *what* to measure in assessing quality (i.e., clinical process and evidence of professional nursing), the next question is *how*. In an effort to keep call length, compliance with policy, outcomes, and clinical processes in proper perspective, some organizations have tried developing QA forms that assign relative value to various call elements, with call length and form completion being noted but given less weight than professional nursing practices. However, we recommend that each of these parameters be tracked *separately* and reviewed in the context of each other so that both the efficiency and the effectiveness of the telephone triage program can be optimized. In other words, review of these metrics is an important management function even though not all of these parameters should be regarded as quality metrics.

Call Volume. Whether electronically or on paper, call volume should be tracked daily (and by shift if you have a 24-hour operation). This volume should be compared to performance data with an awareness that unusually high volume will impact quality indicators. During unexpected surges, the nursing staff will be under unusual pressure and multiple quality parameters may suffer (see Table 1). For example, nurses may take shortcuts that result in incomplete documentation. Customer service may suffer as well. However, patient safety must *never* be put in jeopardy. During these times it would be reasonable for quality assurance analysis to focus primarily on patient safety parameters, such as adequate assessment, accurate diagnosis of urgency, and evidence of collaborative planning that meets the needs of the patient.

Nurse Productivity. Although not necessary to track on a daily basis, periodic review of average call length for the department and by individual nurse will help the nurse manager determine if the service is adequately staffed. It is unrealistic to expect nurses to shorten their call time to fit a desired call length that is born of insufficient staffing, and it's not possible to "wish" the excess call volume away. However, tracking this information provides the manager with an opportunity to identify nurses who are outliers in terms of productive minutes or call length (i.e., they consistently have significantly shorter or longer call times than those of their peers). These RNs deserve a more focused assessment and should be provided with coaching if necessary. Although it is potentially counterproductive to share this information routinely with the staff, triage nurses should be able to access their own information as desired.

Administrative Processes/Compliance with Policy. In the distant and recent past, quality assurance activities have often resulted in "chart audits" largely directed at review of whether the medical record was completed in accordance with policy. The nurse manager or QA coordinator might select a few fields as indicators to assess the extent to which the prescribed documentation is completed. Compliance with documentation standards should be monitored periodically and staff held accountable both individually and in aggregate for compliance with policy. Additionally, other information, such as demographic data, might be spot-checked for completeness and accuracy. If a trend is noted in one area of documentation, before discussing it with staff, it would be wise to review the policy to be certain that it is both reasonable and achievable. While compliance with policy is important, it doesn't represent *quality*, although it, like call volume, can impact quality. The example was given previously of failure to confirm a telephone number. Other omissions can similarly have direct or "trickle-down" effects, but it is important to keep in mind that the type and amount of documentation for calls of a life-threatening nature should be less than for a patient who receives home care recommendations. It would be appropriate for the policy to indicate that only documentation the nurse considers necessary should be completed on patients with emergent dispositions. In other words, to "ding" a nurse for failure to document allergies on a patient experiencing respiratory distress would be unreasonable and might negatively influence the nurse's behavior in the future.

Outcome. Outcomes are defined by many factors. Good outcomes don't always reflect high-quality telephone triage and bad outcomes are not necessarily the result of poor telephone triage. However, bad outcomes such as sentinel events might spotlight an unsafe practice or policy that needs to be addressed. Undesirable outcomes, either in aggregate or singularly, provide opportunities to review the processes leading up to the event in an effort to prevent such occurrences in the future. In these cases, a root cause analysis and a team dedicated to process improvement might lead to improved care in the future.

Likewise, patient satisfaction should be monitored routinely through an ongoing customer service program. Telephone or written surveys provide valuable feedback if organizational factors are negatively impacting patient satisfaction. Nurses and providers should be surveyed periodically to assess satisfaction, and a qualitative review should be conducted of anecdotal concerns or complaints.

Evidence of accurate decision making should be measured by peer assessment. It should thus be conducted by another nurse familiar with the telephone triage process. It is best accomplished by reviewing records or listening to taped or live calls.

Clinical Processes. Evidence of professional nursing should receive the bulk of the department's attention in quality assurance activities and should be tracked on an ongoing basis, rotating the topic but routinely evaluating calls for evidence of the nursing process. When deficiencies are identified in this area, educational opportunities exist and should be addressed promptly.

It is a good idea to select charts of patients with high-volume complaints, as well as those with high-risk complaints. An initial review of frequency of chief complaints would establish a baseline to identify the most frequent complaints, while an expert panel might determine which high-risk complaints will be monitored. The clinical complaints should vary periodically (such as monthly or quarterly). In reviewing these chief complaints, key indicators should be used to determine completeness of the assessment. For example, verification of assessment of oral mucosa, urine output, and level of consciousness would provide more meaningful information about a patient with a chief complaint of vomiting than a simple description of the number of times the patient has vomited. Documentation of pertinent negatives should also be audited for high-risk complaints such as shortness of breath, nausea, and diaphoresis in any patient complaining of chest pain or indigestion. And finally, independent of the nature of the chief complaint, the record should be reviewed for evidence that all steps of the nursing process are present and complete, with emphasis on such elements as assessment, diagnosis of urgency, patient comfort with the plan of care, and discharge instructions.

MAINTAINING QUALITY

Peer review and ongoing timely feedback will help assure that quality is maintained. Keeping in mind that positive reinforcement works much better than criticism, a mechanism should be in place to provide regular positive reinforcement. Everyone will have an off day. Everyone will eventually mishandle a call. However, unless this is a pattern, as Deming says, "When a system is stable, telling the worker about mistakes is only tampering" (p. 4).[22] In other words, sometimes it's just best to leave well enough alone unless troublesome trends are emerging.

SUMMARY

The norm in telephone triage quality programs has long been to emphasize productivity metrics and customer satisfaction. However, measurement and analysis of professional nursing behaviors provide a more appropriate quality assurance mechanism for telephone triage nurses. Peer review of medical records or recorded calls is an effective strategy for identifying both best practices and opportunities for improvement. Emphasis should be placed on positive reinforcement with areas for improvement being presented in a nonpejorative manner, emphasizing good principles and practices rather than numerical scores or grades. Because we value what is measured, some joint values clarification involving both staff and management might be in order prior to development or redesign of a telephone triage quality review tool. RNs are professionals and want to do a good job. In the proper environment, given the proper support, most nurses will rise to the challenge.

When nurses aren't doing a good job, it's more likely to be because of system flaws such as inadequate or improper staffing, poor call flow, lacking appointments, insufficient training, lack of decision support tools, and lack of policies and procedures directing practice than because of an inherent flaw in the nurse.

Consistent with the findings of the IOM report[47], *To Err is Human,* we believe quality problems are more often caused by flaws in systems than problems with individual nurses. In the next two chapters, we will examine program elements that support quality care.

References

1. American Society for Quality (n.d.). *Glossary.* Retrieved from http://asq.org/glossary/q.html
2. Merriam Webster On-line Dictionary. (2011). *Quality.* Merriam-Webster, Inc. Retrieved from http://www.merriam-webster.com/dictionary/quality
3. Derkx, H.P., Rethans, J.J., Maiburg, B.H., Winkens, R.A., Muijtjens, A.M., van Rooij, H., & Knottnerus, J.A. (2009). Quality of communication during telephone triage at Dutch out-of-hours centres. *Patient Education & Counseling, 74*(2), 174-178.
4. Charles-Jones, H., May, C., Latimer, J., & Roland, M. (2003). Telephone triage by nurses in primary care: What is it for and what are the consequences likely to be? *Journal of Health Services Research & Policy, 8*(3), 154-159.
5. Larsen, A. (2005). In the public interest: Autonomy and resistance to methods of standardising nurses' advice and practices from a health call centre in Perth, Western Australia. *Nursing Inquiry, 12*(2), 135-143. doi:10.1111/j.1440-1800.2005.00265.x
6. Cohen, R. (2010, February). Calculating ROI is still important and expanding in scope. *Physician Referral & Telephone Triage Times,* p.1.
7. Clayton, M. (2011). *Deming's system of profound knowledge.* [Web log message] Retrieved from https://managementpocketbooks.wordpress.com/2011/08/30/demings-system-of-profound-knowledge/
8. Swan, B., Conway-Phillips, R., & Griffin, K.F. (2006). Demonstrating the value of the RN in ambulatory care. *Nursing Economic$, 24*(6), 315-322.
9. Cariello, F. (2003). Computerized telephone nurse triage: An evaluation of service quality and cost. *Journal of Ambulatory Care Management, 26*(2), 124-137.
10. Greenberg, M.E. (2000). Telephone nursing: Evidence of client and organizational benefits. *Nursing Economic$, 18*(3), 117-123.
11. Hagan, L., Morin, D., & Lepine, R. (2000). Evaluation of telenursing outcomes: Satisfaction, self-care practices, and cost savings. *Public Health Nursing, 17*(4), 305-313.
12. Marklund, B., Ström, M., Månsson, J., Borgquist, L., Baigi, A., & Fridlund, B. (2007). Computer-supported telephone nurse triage: An evaluation of medical quality and costs. *Journal of Nursing Management, 15*(2), 180-187. doi:10.1111/j.13652834.2007.00659.

13. Campbell, S. (2007). Customer satisfaction with call center largely relies on first call resolution and offshoring. *TMC news.* Retrieved from http://www.tmcnet.com/news/2007/06/12/2706248.htm
14. Efficiency. (n.d.). *Collins English dictionary - complete & unabridged* (10th ed.). Retrieved from http://dictionary.reference.com/browse/efficiency
15. Effective. (n.d.). *Online etymology dictionary.* Retrieved from http://dictionary.reference.com/browse/effective
16. Ström, M., Marklund, B., & Hildingh, C. (2009). Callers' perceptions of receiving advice via a medical care help line. *Scandinavian Journal of Caring Sciences, 23*(4), 682-690. doi:10.1111/j.1471-6712.2008.00661.x
17. Uden, C., Ament, A., Hobma, S.O., Zwietering, P.J., & Crebolder, H. (2005). Patient satisfaction with out-of-hours primary care in the Netherlands. *BMC Health Services Research, 5,* 6-10. doi:10.1186/1472-6963-5-6.
18. North, F., & Varkey, P. (2009). A retrospective study of adult telephone triage calls in a US call centre. *Journal of Telemedicine and Telecare, 15*(4), 165-170.
19. Institute of Medicine. (1991). *Improving information services for health services researchers: A report to the National Library of Medicine.* Washington, DC: National Academies Press.
20. WikiQuote. (2011). *W. Edwards Deming.* Retrieved from http://en.wikiquote.org/wiki/W._Edwards_Deming
21. Uustal, D. (1978). Values clarification in nursing: Application to practice. *The American Journal of Nursing, 78*(12), 2058-2063.
22. ThinkExist.com Quotations. (1999-2011). *W. Edwards Deming quotes.* Retrieved from http://thinkexist.com/quotes/w._edwards_deming/
23. Donabedian, A. (1966). Evaluating the quality of medical care. *Milbank Memorial Fund Quarterly, 44,* 166-206.
24. American Nurses Association. (2011). *The nursing process: A common thread amongst all nurses.* Washington, DC: Author. Retrieved from http://www.nursingworld.org/EspeciallyForYou/StudentNurses/Thenursingprocess.aspx
25. American Nurses Association. (1998). *Core principles on telehealth.* Washington, DC: Author.
26. American Academy of Ambulatory Care Nursing. (2011). *Scope and standards of practice for professional telehealth nurses* (5th ed.). Pitman, NJ: Author.
27. Greenberg, M.E. (2009). A comprehensive model of the process of telephone nursing. *Journal of Advanced Nursing, 65*(12), 2621-2629. doi:10.1111/j.13652648.2009.05132.x
28. Valanis, B., Tanner, C., Moscato, S. R., Shapiro, S., Izumi, S., David, M., & Mayo, A. (2003). A model for examining predictors of outcomes of telephone nursing advice. *Journal of Nursing Administration, 33*(2), 91-95.
29. Institute of Medicine. (2001). *Crossing the quality chasm: A new health system for the 21st century.* Washington, DC: National Academy Press.
30. The One Hundred Best Deming Quotations. (n.d.). Retrieved from http://www.deming.ch/E_quotations.html
31. Knowles, E., O'Cathain, A., Morrell, J., Munro, J.F., & Nicholl, J.P. (2002). NHS direct and nurses – opportunity or monotony? *International Journal of Nursing Studies, 39*(8), 857-866.

32. Valanis, B., Moscato, S., Tanner, C., Shapiro, S., Izumi, S., David, M., & Mayo, A. (2003). Making it work: Organization and processes of telephone nursing advice services. *Journal of Nursing Administration, 33*(4), 216-223.
33. Moore, J.D., Saywell, R.M., Thakker, N., & Jones, T.A. (2002). An analysis of patient compliance with nurse recommendations from an after-hours call center. *The American Journal of Managed Care, 8*(4), 343-351.
34. Kempe, A., Luberti, A., Hertz, A., Sherman, H., Amin, D., Dempsey, C., ... Hegarty, T. (2001). Delivery of pediatric after-hours care by call centers: A multicenter study of parental perception and compliance. *Pediatrics, 108*(6), e111.
35. O'Connell, J.M., Stanley, J.L., & Malakar, C.L. (2001). Satisfaction and patient outcomes of a telephone-based nurse triage service. *Managed Care, 10*(7), 55-65.
36. Moscato, S.R., Valanis, B., Gullion, C.M., Tanner, C., Shapiro, S.E., & Izumi, S. (2007). Predictors of patient satisfaction with telephone nursing services. *Clinical Nursing Research, 16*(2), 119-137.
37. Wahlberg, A.C., & Wredling, R. (2001). Telephone advice nursing – callers' experiences. *Journal of Telemedicine and Telecare, 7*(5), 272-276.
38. Greenberg, M.E., & Schultz, C. (2002). Telephone nursing: Client experiences and perceptions. *Nursing Economic$, 20*(4), 181-187.
39. Bunik, M., Glazner, J.E., Chandramouli, V., Emsermann, C.B., Hegarty, T., & Kempe, A. (2007). Pediatric telephone call centers: How do they affect health care use and costs? *Pediatrics, 119*(2), e305-313.
40. Hertz, A., & Schmitt, B. (2011). Decreasing ER utilization with nursing telephone triage and establishing a National Network of medical call centers. *Articles and Research in Schmitt-Thompson Clinical Content.* Retrieved from http://www.stcc-triage.com/research.htm
41. Bogdan, G.M., Green, J.L., Swanson, D., Gabow, P., & Dart, R.C. (2004). Evaluating patient compliance with nurse advice line recommendations and the impact on healthcare costs. *American Journal of Managed Care, 10*(8), 534-542.
42. Poole, S., Schmitt, B., Carruth, T., Peterson-Smith, A., & Slusarski, M. (1993). After-hours telephone coverage: The application of an area-wide telephone triage and advice system for pediatric practices. *Pediatrics, 92*(5), 670-679.
43. Wachter, D.A., Brillman, J.C., Lewis, J., & Sapien, R.E. (1999). Pediatric telephone triage protocols: Standardized decisionmaking or a false sense of security? *Annals of Emergency Medicine, 33*(4), 388-394.
44. Montalto, M., Dunt, D.R., Day, S.E., & Kelaher, M.A. (2010). Testing the safety of after-hours telephone triage: Patient simulations with validated scenarios. *Australasian Emergency Nursing Journal, 13*(1-2), 7-16. doi:10.1016/j.aenj.2009.11.003
45. Richards, D.A., Meakins, J., Tawfik, J., Godfrey, L., Dutton, E., & Heywood, P. (2004). Quality monitoring of nurse telephone triage: Pilot study. *Journal of Advanced Nursing, 47*(5), 551-560. doi:10.1111/j.1365-2648.2004.03132.x
46. Purc-Stephenson, R., & Thrasher, C. (2010). Nurses' experiences with telephone triage and advice: A meta-ethnography. *Journal of Advanced Nursing, 66*(3), 482-494. doi:10.1111/j.1365-2648.2010.05275.x
47. Kohn, L.T., Corrigan, J., & Donaldson, M.S. (2000). *To err is human: Building a safer health system.* Washington, DC: National Academies Press.

Chapter 14

Program Design and Implementation Part I: Organizational Culture and Staffing

A well-designed program is necessary for successful implementation of telephone triage in any setting. The content offered in this chapter and the following chapter provides a blueprint for optimum program design. Chapters 14 and 15 provide practical suggestions about how to create an infrastructure that supports safe, effective telephone triage and allows the nurse to succeed. The suggestions and recommendations in this chapter represent best practices which have been observed in a variety of settings, are consistent with theory and research, and are supported by logic and good common sense. If a program is lacking in structure or resources, efforts to give good care over the telephone can be jeopardized or even stymied.

Nurses are accustomed to working in settings that are occasionally lacking of staff and resources (and sometimes support). The telephone triage nurse who tries to provide care in a less-than-optimal situation may be set up to fail. It's possible that the suggestions contained in these two chapters may seem daunting or impossible to implement. You may believe that you have insufficient staff to support the recommendations provided. You might reflexively say, "I'm not the boss, so I'm not empowered to implement change," or "My doctor won't let me do that." If you believe you can't implement these recommendations in your organization, we challenge you to just stand by...

The vision of an ideal telephone triage program will begin to emerge but will not fully materialize until the end of these two chapters. It will all come together and reveal workable solutions in the end, providing guidance for excellence in patient care. The suggestions made in these chapters will not only enhance your telephone triage services, but they also have the potential to positively impact other elements of care and organizational operations in the ambulatory care setting.

The best practices described in this and the next chapter will work in essentially any setting. However, sometimes change requires one baby step at a time. These chapters will provide direction to those who are interested in designing and implementing telephone triage in their organization, or to those interested in revising or enhancing their existing program. We also hope that these chapters will provide validation of best practices for those who have well-designed telephone triage programs.

ORGANIZATIONAL NECESSITIES

To help identify resources and obstacles that may potentially affect program design, it is important to review your organizational goals, philosophy, and mission, and how they are applied within your organization. We have discussed how telephone triage, done right, can assure patient safety and quality of care, enhance patient and staff satisfaction, decrease organizational liability, and improve efficiency and cost effectiveness. However, these benefits don't just materialize; they must be created. For a telephone triage program to be successful, some overarching prerequisites must be in place. These are discussed in this chapter and offer a starting point for you to evaluate your current situation.

Patient-Centered Culture

Most health care organizations pride themselves on being patient-centered or customer-oriented. The sad fact is that many are not. Just take an honest look at your policies and assess with fresh eyes how patient-friendly they really are. For example, in many clinics, patients who arrive late are scolded and sent home. Even when the words are acceptable ("You're late. We've moved on with our schedule and therefore we're going to have to reschedule you"), the attitude may not be. The underlying message is, "You should have been here on time! Since you weren't, your 'punishment' is being sent home to return another day." Although many of us are uncomfortable with that approach, we sometimes use it because we've been taught it's the appropriate reaction to a late patient.

Be realistic! We've all been late. Using the Golden Rule, it becomes clear that we should make every effort to accommodate the late patient if possible, and if not, to at least speak to him or her in an empathetic, caring, and respectful fashion. Consider an alternative approach of, "Oh, I'm so glad you made it! We were afraid you weren't going to be able to come. Unfortunately, we had to go ahead and see other patients who were already here, but we'll get you worked in as soon as possible. Please make yourself comfortable and we'll try to keep you posted. Of course, if you don't have time to wait, we could certainly reschedule you for another day."

See the difference in the two approaches? And frankly, the primary difference in the two is probably in the heart of the individual dealing with the patient. If an individual is aggravated, it will show in her voice and actions. However, if she is empathetic, understanding that the patient wasn't late maliciously, that will also be apparent in the way she interacts with the patient. The kinder, softer approach is consistent with a patient-centered culture. Scolding the late patient or sending him or her home to return another day is definitely not patient-centered. Instead, it is designed to meet the needs of the staff.

But you might be thinking, "No! If we see the late patient, it's not fair to the other patients, and how are we going to teach them our expectations, and that actions come with consequences?" The truth is that if you're managing your patient flow properly, you didn't wait for that patient at all but rather went ahead and saw one of the many patients who came early. And why do we think it's our job to teach adults to differentiate right from wrong? If someone doesn't already know that being late is inconsiderate and essentially socially unacceptable, we're probably not going to teach him or her now. And, if the patient was unavoidably delayed, our understanding and support may be invaluable on multiple levels.

Other illustrations of a staff-centric policy can be seen in a pediatric office that is open 9-5 Monday through Friday, while parents are at work and the kids are in school. If the practice were really patient-focused, it would extend office hours on evenings and weekends. And another problem is represented by offices that turn their phones off during lunch. Many clinics evidently fail to recognize that a number of patients are unable to access the phone during work hours, making their lunch period the only time they can call the doctor's office. It would be more patient-friendly to have at least one employee man the phones while the office is closed for lunch.

One more example of our staff-focused culture is the policy regarding the desired lead time on prescription renewals. While those policies are created to give the staff a buffer and keep the patient from developing unrealistic expectations, there are times that, for one reason or another, patients call needing a refill that same day. Their reason may be legitimate in our opinion, or we may think the patient is irresponsible. In any case, it is good for us to remember that patients have many more responsibilities than keeping up with their prescription renewals, and sometimes, last-minute refill requests occur, whether we like them or not.

So what do you do when the patient calls the day she runs out of her pills? Do you renew her prescription, or do you "think about it?" If it's a beta blocker, you know you must renew it to prevent the patient from experiencing an unpleasant and potentially dangerous side effect. However, if the consequences to the patient are only a little discomfort or inconvenience, Herculean efforts might not be made to renew it today. It can be interesting when we honestly evaluate our motivates.

A nurse in a nephrology practice complained that their transplant patients, although aware of their office policy requiring a 3-day lead time for prescription renewals, often called requesting a refill after they had already run out of their immunosuppressive medications. She indignantly commented that, after telling a patient he wouldn't get his renewal for 3 days, he pointed out that if he suffered kidney rejection, it would be her fault! It's hard to believe that a nurse could be so committed to an organizational policy that she would actually jeopardize a patient's transplant by not renewing his critical medications promptly. Where is the greater good?

If you look carefully, you might be surprised to realize that many of your organizational policies are developed, not with patients and their needs in mind, but rather for the convenience of your staff. So as a springboard, take a look at your organizational culture and see whose needs are given primary attention: the patients or the staff?

Clarity of Purpose

As nurses, we believe we're doing telephone triage to facilitate care. Before moving forward with a new or reorganized telephone triage program, it is critical to be clear about the purpose of the program and to determine whether it is consistent with your organizational goals and mission. It is also critical to determine whether the goal for the telephone triage program is understood and shared by the organization at large. Evaluate how many of your colleagues believe telephone triage is supposed to be a barrier to care. We know our goal is to get the right patient to the right place at the right time, but is that understanding shared by all?

Staffing Model

Due to a variety of factors discussed in earlier chapters, it is important to be aware that the majority of professional nursing care delivered in the ambulatory care setting will likely be telephonic.[1] Especially in the setting of Medical Homes and Accountable Care Organizations, RNs will play a pivotal role in managing acute and chronic illness over the phone and facilitating appropriate care. Therefore, having a staffing model that supports telephone care delivery and *appropriate* utilization of all personnel is critical. Specifically, each person should function at his or her highest level of preparation and licensure. RNs must be reserved for patient management and other functions that require independent judgment and critical thinking as well as supervision of LPNs, LVNs, and UAP as appropriate and necessary. LPNs and LVNs should be responsible for all nursing that requires licensure but does not require the level of preparation or licensure of the RN. UAP should be utilized to perform functions that don't require a nursing license or specialized training beyond that which they have received. Differentiation of roles is necessary to support efficient and effective patient care delivery.[1,2,3]

Access (Availability of Appointments)

One frequent observation is that many offices lack access, or available appointments, for patients who are experiencing acute problems. Same-day appointment scheduling is often a problem, and triage nurses are unfortunately utilized as a "last ditch" mechanism to provide care to patients who should be seen but for whom access is not available. If the organization is committed to meeting patient needs, then options for the patient to receive care must be available. Evidence shows that in a variety of settings, patients are given inappropriate dispositions as a result of lack of access to appointments, and that in general, lack of resources affect the ability of the nurses to provide quality care.[4,5,6,7] This issue is discussed at length in Chapter 15.

Strong Leadership Support

The success of a telephone triage program is often directly related to the strength of leadership support for the program. The provision of safe and effective care over the telephone often requires some degree of operational reorganization. Health care delivered via telecommunications technology is swiftly becoming a way of life. Our rapidly changing health care environment has demonstrated increasing dependence on telecommunications technology and the skilled professionals that utilize this technology effectively. Recognition of the potential contribution of telephone triage will increase the viability and improve effectiveness of health care organizations in the future. Organizations with visionary leaders, who are knowledgeable about and committed to telephone triage as a strategy for care delivery, are ideally positioned to meet the challenges that the health care industry will face in the coming years.[8]

Organizational policies are often not patient centered; thus telephone triage is often regarded as a barrier to care. RNs continue to be under-valued and under-utilized in many settings, often viewed as a commodity that is interchangeable with and replaceable by LPNs, LVNs, and UAP. We give our best to determine the appropriate disposition for our patients only to discover that access is often not available for those who need it. Finally, when we look to leadership for support, we find inconsistent understanding of both our role and the challenges we face in providing excellent care over the telephone. If this sounds familiar, it is likely your organization lacks the necessities discussed and that there is an opportunity for change.

FORMALIZED TELEPHONE TRIAGE

When errors occur in the health care setting, or suboptimal care is delivered, it is often due to faulty system design rather than worker error. If attention is not given to program design elements, even the most competent RN can make significant practice errors due to lack of training, insufficient resources, or problems with work design. A formalized telephone triage program will go a long way toward preventing practice errors. Components of a formal telephone triage program include, at a minimum: dedicated staff with specialized training, decision support tools, access strategies, attention to call flow, a documentation template, and policies and procedures that support safe telephone practices in the organization.

As with other forms of clinical practice, there are some program design imperatives that hold steady, independent of the clinical setting. These imperatives start to become clear once an organization acknowledges that telephone triage is more than "just a phone call." This leads to the critical realization that rather than just managing calls in between other patient care activities, it is prudent to develop a formalized approach to delivery of patient care over the telephone. Call centers with nurses dedicated to the telephone have made significant inroads in establishing such a discreet service; other settings, most notably doctor's offices, have not.[9,10] However, patients must be able to expect the same level of competent care regardless of the source from which they seek advice.

All settings wishing to deliver care effectively over the phone must provide adequate resources, polices, and procedures that support safe care. In a formalized telephone triage program, attention must be given to proper staffing, access to appointments or other resources to provide appropriate care, and call flow that is designed to get calls promptly into the hands of the right person. Organizational structure and resources, including decision support tools, documentation templates, a policy manual, and a quality assurance program are also essential to program success. And finally, as discussed previously, clarity of purpose, a patient-driven culture, and strong leadership support provide the environment in which a telephone triage program can flourish. The integration of these elements is what creates a "telephone triage program," yielding a service that is identifiable and distinct from other organizational operations and forms of patient care.

The rest of this chapter will focus on appropriate staff utilization. The following chapter will address access, appropriate call flow, and formalized program policies, including protocols and documentation tools.

STAFFING

We have been very clear that telephone triage must be performed by RNs who are experienced and specially trained. But what are the specific traits that lend themselves to success, and how are those RNs best utilized? And what is the best utilization of other personnel who might be participating in management of patients over the telephone? Attention to development of a staffing model that addresses optimal utilization of all personnel is a key component to a successful telephone triage program.

The Telephone Triage Nurse

In addition to experience and specialized training, telephone triage nurses must have excellent assessment and communication skills and strong critical-thinking skills complemented by sound clinical judgment. These traits require a huge and diverse knowledge base, so the ideal professional experience would be in a variety of areas over a number of years. Although there is a perception that emergency department (ED) nurses, having experience with triage, would be ideally prepared for telephone triage, nurses from a number of clinical areas also bring special skills and strengths to the job. In addition to clinical competence, respect for the patient, a generous dose of empathy and compassion, and strong patient advocacy skills will serve the telephone triage nurse well. Telephone triage nurses must also have the ability to collaborate and a healthy respect for intuition (both their own and that of the patient's). The need to control is a personality trait of many ED nurses,[11] but experience and observation confirms that this need to control is not limited to ED nurses and is instead a trait of many nurses in general. To collaborate effectively, the telephone triage nurse must be willing to relinquish control and support the patient in decision making that is consistent with the patient's wishes and values.

A study investigating the characteristics of effective telephone triage nurses found four primary traits.[12] A description of these attributes follows.

1. *Telephone triage nurses are self-directed.* This trait is accompanied by a good work ethic and flexibility. Self-directed nurses realize the importance of their role, although their authority is often limited to the nurse/patient interaction.

2. *Effective telephone triage nurses are able to focus on short-term results.* This trait is supported by good time management skills. They enjoy measurable outcomes and use them to mark their own success, appreciating checklists and bite-sized tasks.

3. *Telephone triage nurses are strong patient advocates.* This quality requires empathy, which leads to patient trust and enhances the nurse's effectiveness.

4. *Telephone triage nurses have a good measure of practical intelligence.* This trait supports the fact that telephone triage nurses must be quick learners who enjoy learning and are able to relate new information to their existing knowledge base.

Experience

A question always in search of an answer is "How much experience does a nurse need in order to do telephone triage?" Various organizations have attempted to set criteria based on the number of years experience, but these criteria are based on opinion, not on hard data. A minimum of 3 to 5 years of experience is a common requirement for a telephone triage nurse. To perform at the Competent-to-Expert practice level often requires 3 to 5 years of experience (see Chapter 7). It is important to note that although Benner addresses experience in her book, *From Novice to Expert,* she also aptly points out that a nurse can be an expert in one area and revert to a lower level of competency when he or she changes to another clinical specialty.[13]

It is unlikely that a reliable or specific answer will emerge because of the multitude of variables that may impact clinical competence in telephone triage. Each individual nurse brings a unique background to the telephone. Due to the number of factors, both personal and professional, that might impact performance, it will likely never be possible (or advisable) to dictate a fixed number of years of experience necessary for the practice of telephone triage. Education, clinical experience, and personal exposure to health care as a patient or a caregiver are factors which might significantly impact clinical competence, regardless of total years of experience as a nurse. Also, each nurse has individual characteristics which might facilitate or hinder clinical competence in telephone triage. For example, nurses who are empathetic, strong patient advocates, good listeners with excellent communication, and strong critical-thinking skills are likely to function at a higher level than a colleague with essentially identical experience but lacking in these or other critical traits discussed previously.[12]

For example, a nurse could have a number of years of experience in a clinical area so far removed from telephone triage that his or her clinical experience is of limited value. Likewise, even new graduates can have an impressive level of competence if they have worked in a related ambulatory care setting in the past as an LVN or LPN. Individuals who enter nursing as a second career might have previous professional or job-related experience relevant to telephone triage. Likewise, life experience can be invaluable for a telephone triage nurse, especially if it corresponds with the needs of the patient population being served. For example, being a parent of several children might provide a relatively new graduate a measure of meaningful experience that would be helpful in a pediatric practice. A nurse who has cared for an aging parent and returned to nursing late in life might possess valuable clinical and life experience that would serve him or her well in a geriatric practice. A nurse who has personally experienced a chronic illness might have unique knowledge in that clinical area, even with minimal experience as an RN.

Thus, because of the wide variability in professional and personal experience and individual characteristics of each nurse, it is unlikely that a specific number of years experience will be the key; however, the importance of experience can't be overestimated. Further research is necessary to identify types of experience and traits of the ideal telephone triage nurse.

Basic Practice Model

Telephone triage conducted by RNs requires no direct clinical supervision since RNs function autonomously and telephone triage is within their scope of practice. Ideally, these telephone triage nurses are dedicated to the telephone rather than being multitasked. If a red flag is going up for you at this point and you are concerned that you will never have adequate staff to justify dedicating RNs to the telephone, consider the risk associated with not doing so (see Chapter 12). Telephone triage is risky business, even under the best of circumstances. Frequently, however, dedicating RNs to the phone doesn't require additional FTEs. If your organization presently utilizes RNs, LPNs, and UAP in nearly interchangeable roles, the opportunity exists to differentiate practice. Relieving RNs of responsibilities that don't require their specialized knowledge and skills will provide them with more time to perform more appropriate functions, such as telephone triage. Ideally, all telephone triage calls (symptom-based calls and requests for same-day appointments) should be managed by RNs because these calls are of an uncertain nature and require considerable assessment skills and clinical judgement.

The Role of Non-RNs in the Delivery of Care Over the Telephone

Although professional standards require RNs to manage calls requiring assessment (see Chapter 5), some state boards of nursing regard telephone triage as being within the scope of practice of LPNs or LVNs, providing they are supervised and using decision support tools. Further, the Captain of the Ship doctrine allows physicians to delegate tasks, including data collection, to medical assistants in many states. It is noteworthy, however, that at least one state, California, prohibits the practice of telephone triage by medical assistants.[14]

If the organization makes the questionable decision to utilize personnel other than RNs in managing patients over the telephone (even if it's only regarded as "collecting information"), basic policy decisions must be made and put in place to provide adequate supervision and support. These decisions require identifying who will supervise the non-RN and what that supervision will look like. For example, will the supervision consist of being on the telephone with the non-RN, sitting beside her as she takes calls, being available when she needs assistance, or simply co-signing her notes at the end of the day? Finally, is there documentation that the supervision is actually taking place? To illustrate the potential for disaster when staff are inadequately supervised, refer to the case involving the LPN who phoned in a prescription for hydrocodone for the patient who had a post-op septic joint (see Chapter 12).

This discussion notwithstanding, it is important to keep in mind that because telephone triage requires assessment, it is inappropriate for LPNs and LVNs to perform this task. Such practice would represent a deviation from current practice standards.[1,3] Use of LPNs and LVNs in this role also violates the scope of practice in most states in that it requires independent assessment.

In most states,[15] LPNs or LVNs may be utilized on the telephone to provide care that does not require independent assessment, providing that their telephone responsibilities are consistent with their defined scope of practice. For example, most states permit LPNs or LVNs to participate in the implementation of an existing plan of care. Thus, there are a variety of ways LPNs and LVNs can provide an educated conduit for two-way communication with patients. For example, they might take requests for prescription renewals, often being ideally prepared for this task because they usually know the names of the medications and, following policy, can take an adequate history for the physician to make a decision about renewing most drugs. Likewise, at the direction of an RN or provider, they could return results of selected ancillary tests, explaining basic findings of many tests to patients, especially if the results are normal. Of course, there are occasions in which the RN or even the provider must handle those calls. The point is that unless the call requires assessment, the knowledge base of LPNs and LVNs is often adequate to manage many of these calls and deemed appropriate by many state boards of nursing.[15]

Finally, medical assistants and clerical personnel may also be delegated telephone responsibilities, understanding that the final accountability for their actions rests with the delegator. While we will not create an exhaustive list of telephone tasks that may be performed by unlicensed personnel, the key is whether the action requires the knowledge, skill, judgment, or expertise of a licensed nurse. If not, and if the task fits the Five Rights of Delegation from the National Council of State Boards of Nursing,[16] delegate it! RNs should do *only* those things that require an RN license, LPNs or LVNs should do all other nursing that doesn't require an RN license, and everything else should be delegated to unlicensed personnel.

The Five Rights of Delegation[16]

- ***Right task***
- ***Right circumstances***
- ***Right person***
- ***Right direction/communication***
- ***Right supervision/evaluation***

Where Do We Get the Staff?

As mentioned previously, often organizations have enough RNs to manage all symptom-based calls without hiring additional FTEs. The problem usually isn't insufficient staff but rather misutilization of the organization's existing staff. RNs, LPNs, and LVNs should not be utilized to perform tasks such as rooming patients (taking a patient from the waiting room to the exam room), measuring vital signs, or scheduling a patient for a class, which can be performed by less-expensive personnel. Once RNs are relieved of those basic tasks, they have more time to devote to functions requiring their unique knowledge and judgment. In other words, you might have the staff but can't see them because they (or you) are too deeply immersed in the "weeds."

One organization, wishing to dedicate RNs to telephone triage, surveyed their existing staff, and performed a workload analysis to determine how each of their staff members were spending their time. Among many other surprises, they learned that both of their pediatric RNs, each assigned to work directly with a particular physician's panel of patients, were spending about 85% of their time on the phone, not all of which required the expertise of an RN. A little arithmetic revealed that of the two RNs in the clinic, 1.7 full-time equivalents (FTEs), were dedicated to the telephone. By performing a more in-depth data analysis, the chief nurse executive (CNE) determined that the nurses spent about half the time they were on the phone dealing with "nurse calls" (those requiring the expertise of an RN) while the other half of their phone time was devoted to activities that could appropriately be delegated to others. Thus, the CNE assigned one of the RNs to a dedicated, centralized telephone triage function, and the other to patient management in the clinic, delegating all other calls (not requiring an RN) to other, more appropriate personnel.

The preceding is an example of how one organization addressed improper utilization of its nursing staff, thereby recapturing RN time to appropiately manage telephone triage calls. In other words, this clinic had already devoted 1.7 FTEs to the telephone and realized that although they were handling the calls, they were often doing it in the most inefficient and potentially risky way possible. Multi-tasked nurses who are up and down, back and forth, into and back out of a critical-thinking mode, are nurses in a prime position to overlook an important element of care and thus mismanage a call.[17]

While it might have appeared that the clinic lost an RN FTE to the telephone triage program, in reality, the clinic functionally regained 70% of an RN. This nurse was then able to devote time to patients in the clinic rather than managing calls that could better be managed by the triage nurse or delegated to others. In this case, everybody won, especially the patients.

How Do We Train the Staff?

Extensive training of the telephone triage nursing staff is an essential element of program design and is necessary for the delivery of safe care. All too often, as referenced in Chapter 3, telephone triage is considered "just a phone call," something we've all done since childhood. But now there are standards, a minimum skill set, and often decision support and documentation software that the telephone triage nurse must use proficiently. Thus, a formalized education, training, and orientation program must be developed to include the following essential content.

- Initial Telephone Triage Education, Training, and Orientation to include
  - Purpose and standards (see Chapters 1-5),
  - Decision making and critical thinking (see Chapters 6-7)
  - Telephone triage as a specialized skill set, including but not limited to communication skills (see Chapters 8 and 9), assessment over the telephone (see Chapter 10), documation and use of decision support tools (see Chapter 11), and telephone triage pitfalls to avoid (see Chapter 12)
  - Training on the use of the computerized electronic health record and decision support software, if used
  - Orientation to the department and organization, including complete review and comprehension of the departmental policy manual, quality assurance program, and an introduction to resources available in the organization and within the community

- Practical Education and Experience
  - Listen to recorded calls if available, ideally with QA form in hand as a guide.
  - Monitor preceptor and other telephone triage nurses taking calls, analyzing and discussing together the particulars of the call such as decision making and application of the nursing process.
  - Review practice scenarios to demonstrate various practice principles.
  - Take live calls monitored by a preceptor with in-depth discussion and analysis of each call.
  - Participate in review and analysis of call documentation forms.
  - Receive timely feedback on their own clinical performance.
- Ongoing Continuing Education
  - Schedule routine in-service offerings regarding areas of clinical concern, especially as identified by QA activities or areas of interest for nursing staff.
  - Review and discuss examples of both good and bad calls as a group (listening to them if a recording is available) in order to encourage skills development.
  - Create a journal club, in which each nurse agrees to review a specific journal monthly and report to the group on any article of interest.
  - Attend continuing nursing education (CNE) offerings specific to areas of relevance; these offerings may be developed in your organization, provided by a nursing CNE company, or attended

"Training in active listening for telephone nurses should be compulsory, including regular listening to authentic calls by the individual nurse, but also discussing calls in a group" (p. 407).[18]

at professional meetings, such as the American Academy of Ambulatory Care Nursing's (AAACN) Annual Conference.

The nurse's participation in educational activities should be documented and a copy of any certificates retained in the nurse's personnel file. The nurse should, of course, retain any original documentation of CNE activities and certifications. Reading and researching new, unknown, or obscure topics is a good way for nurses to keep their knowledge up-to-date, and, fortunately, access to that type of information is readily available on the Internet. Finally, as listed earlier and discussed in Chapter 13, timely feedback regarding decision making on the nurse's own calls allows the nurse to incorporate information gleaned from management of actual telephone triage calls into his or her new knowledge base. It is critical that telephone triage nurses embrace lifelong learning and understand that this is a part of their responsibility as professionals.

The Multitasked Nurse

The concept of the multitasked nurse was mentioned previously in this chapter, but the risks associated with multitasking are so great that it deserves specific discussion. A good deal of research has been done regarding multitasking in various situations. For example, driving while talking on a cell phone has received a great deal of attention. In fact, legislation has been passed in some states prohibiting driving while talking on the phone unless using a hands-free device. However, it's interesting to consider that the act of holding the telephone in one's hand is not the dangerous part of talking on the phone while driving. If it were, driving while holding a cup of coffee should be prohibited as well. In other words, it is clearly not the psychomotor component of talking on the phone that leads to increased risk. It is the cognitive distraction associated with the need to be "present" while having a conversation over the phone that puts the driver and others in his or her vicinity in harm's way.[19]

Nurses in the ambulatory care setting are certainly engaging in activities that require even more cognitive processing than is necessary to carry on a simple social telephone conversation. Evidence specific to nursing shows that multitasked nurses are more apt to make medication errors than when not multitasked.[21] In a discussion of decision making and expertise, Facione and Facione,[22] state, "But experts also err due to problem misidentification, and they are more prone to being inattentive to those differences in the problem which make it the odd exception to the pattern..." (p. 3). This suggests that even well-prepared, expert telephone triage nurses need to focus on the nuances, the process, and the opportunities for decision making that are present in each call. It stands to reason that the risks associated with the provision of care over the telephone are significant in the office or clinic setting, where nurses are often performing or responsible for multiple cognitive activities simultaneously. While this poses a potential risk for any type of behavior,[23] the nurse responsible for telephone triage must face the additional challenge of not being able to see or touch the patient. Without the visual cues that are available in the face-to-face setting to help the nurse "keep his or her place," the result may be disorganized thinking. In addition to the challenges of keeping information organized, it is difficult to switch from one type of task to another, the end result being (at a minimum) loss of efficiency. And worse, critical thinking, essential to the telephone triage process, may be jeopardized when the nurse is multitasked.[24]

"Interruptions and multitasking are implicated as a major cause of clinical inefficiency and error" (p. 284).[20]

Nurses responsible for telephone triage should be doing *only* telephone triage. Unfortunately, it is not unusual for nurses who are dedicated to telephone triage to be required to be the "phone nurse," taking a variety of calls that don't require their level of expertise or critical-thinking skills. Likewise, it is not atypical for dedicated telephone triage nurses to be expected to do walk-in triage as well. These are just additional forms of multitasking that impede the telephone triage nurse's ability to do his or her job effectively.[26]

Interruptions in the nursing work environment can have significant, detrimental effects on patient safety.[25]

Thus, even dedicated telephone triage nurses should not themselves be multitasked with multiple "types" of calls.[26] This refers to the telephone triage nurse who has to report lab results, handle medication renewals, schedule classes, manage physician referrals, and juggle post-hospital discharge calls in the course of taking incoming telephone triage calls. The nurse must maintain focus without being disturbed by calls that do not require high-level critical thinking or the education and licensure of an RN. However, the flip side of that argument is that even calls as seemingly straightforward as a request for a name of a neurologist in the community must be screened to see if assessment is necessary. A patient requesting a neurologist for back and leg pain might instead need to see an orthopedist, a neurosurgeon, or even a rheumatologist. Or perhaps the patient needs to be refered to the ED or encouraged to see his or her primary care provider for evaluation and possible referral. Likewise, a simple request for a medication refill or test result might mask a concern regarding a symptom the patient is currently experiencing.

Nurses in both the clinic and call center settings who are multitasked and thus stepping into and out of a critical thinking mode throughout the day are at greater risk. Nurses required to move from critical thinking to the provision of health information, to critical thinking, and then to the provision of directions to the clinic, are likely to be asked a question such as, "What is the right dose of Tylenol® for my baby?" If not careful, that nurse might respond, "How much does he weigh?" rather than recognizing this as a possible triage call requiring patient assessment. The results could be devastating.

Staffing Model

Accepting the premise that the telephone triage nurse must be dedicated (not multitasked), the next step is to identify roles and responsibilities and determine how to best staff the triage program/service. The first consideration is whether it would be preferable in your organization to have permanent or rotating staff. The following is a discussion of the pros and cons of each of these staffing alternatives.

Rotating Staff. Often, in non-call center settings, the prevailing sentiment is that rotating telephone triage staff would be preferable. The rationale most often offered is that, not having enough staff in the first place, it is necessary to "rob Peter to pay Paul." The belief is that because there is no excess staff, each nurse should "take a turn" performing the telephone triage duties for the group. On the other hand, this often means that each nurse has one day they are unable to manage their routine responsibilities, resulting in double work the next day. Plus, it is likely that, because the nurse assigned to triage has ongoing patient care responsibilities, he or she may be interrupted repeatedly to manage pressing in-person patient care issues while trying to perform telephone triage.

Another reason cited in favor of rotating staff is that, if the responsibility were assigned to any one person, he or she might "quit." It isn't surprising that nurses who are responsible for telephone triage, but who are also multitasked, don't relish the idea of managing calls full time. This perspective is probably related in part to the way telephone responsibilities are handled in many settings. Unfortunately, the practice of telephone triage in such systems often involves multiple interruptions. Nurses also receive a variety of calls that don't require the knowledge and expertise of a nurse, diminishing the nurse's sense of satisfaction with the job. These calls, such as prescription refills, requests for test results, and directions to the clinic, are necessary, but most can be handled appropriately by others. Differentiation and proper routing of call types (discussed in Chapter 15) allows the nurse to focus on triage calls and remain in the critical-thinking mode, rather than being distracted by "other" calls. However, formalization of telephone triage with focus on the appropriate role of the telephone triage nurse will go a long way in promoting telephone triage as an enjoyable form of professional nursing.

The final reason often cited for rotating telephone triage nursing staff is that if dedicated full time to the telephone, the nurse will eventually lose his or her skills. There is actually some validity to this statement, especially for less-experienced RNs. Because their experience is already somewhat limited, taking them completely out of the face-to-face clinical setting might deprive them of valuable clinical experience. Until a nurse has had considerable exposure to a variety of clinical entities, has performed specific psychomotor skills repeatedly, and has generally gained robust and varied experience, the potential for losing some of his or her new skills may be a reality. However, many nurses who do telephone triage are already so experienced in the face-to-face setting that the risk of losing psychomotor skills is limited. And with good experience in telephone triage, the nurse's assessment skills will only improve by leaps and bounds. Keeping in mind that nursing is cognitive, not psychomotor, makes it less important for a nurse to "keep up" with new technology. If he or she decides to return to the bedside or other face-to-face patient care setting, the experienced nurse should have little difficulty getting up to speed on new technology, if necessary.

A primary concern with rotating staff is that telephone triage is not their "job," and thus they are less likely to feel ownership of the task. Instead of being regarded as their primary responsibility, telephone triage is the assignment that *interferes* with their ability to do their principal job. Needless to say, that attitude is unlikely to foster a commitment to quality care equal to that of the nurse assigned to do telephone triage full time. It is important to note, however, that exceptions have been observed, and rotating staff has worked well within individual organizations.

Permanent Staff. In our experience, dedicating specific staff to the telephone as their only or primary job is usually preferable. When a nurse works in telephone triage full time, he or she develops a professional identity as a telephone triage nurse. The nurse assigned to telephone triage full time will *value* the practice rather than regarding it as the pesky task that keeps him from doing his *real* job. The telephone triage nurse is more likely to seek continuing education opportunities relevant to the practice and, when reading literature, he will probably focus on articles that apply to managing patients over the telephone.

An additional advantage to telephone triage as a permanent assignment is reflected in the adage that "practice makes perfect." The nurse's skill set in telephone triage will grow with continuing experience. The ideal telephone triage nurse recognizes the value of the service being rendered, is effective at connecting with patients over the telephone, enjoys this type of patient interaction, and has the other skills and characteristics previously described in this chapter. Ownership of the specialized nature of the practice, ownership of the patient outcomes, ownership of the role of the telephone triage nurse, and even ownership of his or her own workspace enhances connectedness and thus effectiveness in the practice of telephone triage.

Strategies for Peak Call Times

Another challenge faced by telephone triage programs is how to manage peak call times. Much like EDs, patient volume fluctuates by time of day, day of week, and season, but the peaks and valleys will vary depending on the organization. For example, in the office or clinic setting, heavy call volume is often seen on Monday mornings, Friday afternoons and during the lunch hour. Call centers that answer after-hours calls for doctors' offices find their call volume to be high in the early evenings and on weekends; and in the military environment, heavy call volume is expected early every weekday morning.

Some organizations solve this dilemma by hiring part-time nurses to cover their peak call times. Retired nurses are often great candidates for this type of employment. Other telephone triage programs utilize a "virtual" call center setting in which nurses can take calls from home, thus helping out during periods of heavy call volume.[27]

A third way to plan coverage for peak call times is to utilize other RN staff in the clinic to "pitch in and help" when the volume exceeds the ability of the triage nurse(s) to keep up. This can be accomplished by providing other RNs with a telephone display indicating how many patients are waiting in queue to talk to a triage nurse and the maximum length of hold time for those in the queue. Then, when the queue reaches a pre-established threshold, the nurses would sign in as specified by policy (similar to the previously described "virtual" as-needed model), and take calls until the queue is once again manageable. The caveat with this approach is that the alternate RNs shouldn't schedule tasks that would need their undivided attention during the time they might be taking telephone triage calls. That practice would lead to multitasking, heightening the risk and decreasing efficiency. And, of course, all nurses would need to be trained and have the skill set necessary to function competently on the telephone.

Of course, last but not least, it is helpful to educate patients about the best time to call, advising them of the heavy call volume times and encouraging them to call outside of peak time if possible. Patients would undoubtedly be able to speak to a nurse more quickly if their calls were placed during a time of lower call volume.

One reason patients call early in the morning, thus making this peak call time, is their concern about not being able to get an appointment if they wait to call until later in the day. In many settings, this is a valid concern because same-day appointments are scheduled on a "first come, first served" basis by appointment clerks without benefit of an assessment to determine the appropriate disposition. This practice depletes the organization of appointments early in the day, often because patients are scheduled who would have been managed more appropriately elsewhere. In Chapter 15, we discuss access strategies which would help assure that appointments are available when needed.

Workload Analysis

Prior to any decisions about staff reallocation, it is helpful for the organization to conduct a comprehensive telephone workload analysis. The purpose of the analysis is to determine the number of calls received, the call type (or reason for the call), and the time of day each call is received. It might also be helpful to track acuity and dispositions. This doesn't have to be a long, drawn-out, or complicated process. Comprehensive data collection for a period of one (normal) week is generally sufficient to establish a baseline. If the study is then repeated quarterly, it would be possible to identify and compare seasonal trends, and annual comparisons would be possible as well.

While there are many different formats that can be used, it is generally desirable to determine what information you want to collect and then develop a form that suits your needs. We believe a form with a separate line for each call is ideal. Although this is the most labor-intensive way to collect data, if it's only for a week or two, it's usually worth it to go the extra mile. Consider the following example of a tally sheet illustrating basic data collection. A key is suggested to indicate possible call types, but this will vary from setting to setting. The first example might be a tally sheet used by an operator or receptionist who is answering incoming calls.

Example 1.

Time	Type	Specify	Transfer to	Comment
8:10	SDA		RN	
8:14	Rx		LPN	
8:15	HCP	Home Health	MD	
8:20	Sx		RN	

The following example is more suitable for the RN who manages calls, assuming no triage function currently exists.

Example 2.

Time	Call Type	Chief Complaint	Age	Triage Category	Disposition	Comment
8:10	SDA	Cold	42	R	HC	
8:20	Rx	NA	18	NA	NA	
8:40	O	NA	66	NA	NA	Report blood glucose levels
8:45	Sx	Shoulder pain	52	E	911	

Call Type
- SDA: Request for same-day appointment (record primary symptom)
- Sx: Symptom-based, no appointment requested
- R: Request for routine appointment (e.g., well-visit or routine followup; non-symptom based)
- Rx: Prescription refill
- T: Test results
- B: Billing/insurance question
- HCP: Health care professional (MD, home health nurse, hospital nurse, pharmacist, etc.)
- O: Other (specify)

Triage Category
- E: Emergent
- U: Urgent
- R: Routine/Non-urgent
- NA: Non-triage

Disposition
- 911: ED via 911
- ED: Emergency department
- UC: Urgent care
- Ofc T: Office today
- Ofc D: Office delayed care
- HC: Home care
- NA: Non-triage

If you would also like information such as how often someone other than the patient makes the call, how often a translator is necessary, which calls are transferred, etc., this information could be collected during the course of recording the call data. Additionally, recording the time the call begins and ends will facilitate determination of average call lengths for various call types.

Experience indicates that the following are important considerations when planning a workload analysis project.

- *Track all incoming calls during the study period.* These should include calls answered by both clerical and clinical personnel. If other personnel receive clinical calls, they should be included as well. Place a stack of paper tally sheets on the desk at each telephone and instruct the individual using the form about the important but short-term nature of the exercise.

- *Determine early how (or if) to track transfer calls.* If this nuance is overlooked, some calls will be tallied twice. It is best to uniformly have them tallied by the person who answers and then transfers the phone *or* by the person to whom the call is transferred. However, it might also be helpful to have a separate column on the form to record the number of calls transferred. These calls are important to include because they require the time of at least two staff and result in a "two-stop shopping" experience for the caller.

- *Collect data in a manner that will yield one solid week of data.* For example, this will be Monday through Friday in some settings and 24 hours/day for seven consecutive days in others. It is important to take measures to avoid periods with unusual call volume such as holidays, epidemics, unusual weather events, etc. Because of the traditionally heavy volume on Mondays, experience dictates that it may be best to begin data collection on a Tuesday. It might also be worthwhile to plan to discard the first day's sheets, since the learning curve on remembering to tally calls is fairly steep the first day or two. It is usually only necessary to collect data for a consecutive week for adequate analysis.

- *Enter data in a spreadsheet or data base program that will enable manipulation and analysis.* The more columns on the form, and thus the more data collected, the more information will be available pursuant to your short study.

- *Pilot the form prior to initiation of the data collection period.* Generally, a few hours will be sufficient to identify areas that might be problematic, such as ambiguity in how to code particular call types or an excessive number of calls that are coded as "other."

The information obtained from this workload analysis will be helpful in determining staffing needs, managing the appointment template to improve access, and developing a plan for call flow which gets the callers into the right hands. Additionally, this exercise will assist in identification of the most common chief complaints in your setting. This information has educational implications for your staff and may assist in selection, development, or customization of decision support tools for your practice.

Calculating Staffing Needs

The previously described workload analysis should provide sufficient information to begin development of a staffing plan. Besides call volume, two other variables must be considered.

First, the average length of a *triage* call in your setting should be measured. Characteristics of the patient population such as age, comorbidities, resources, educational level, and health literacy can impact call length significantly. Whether appointments are available can speed or lengthen the call. And the method of call intake and management can modify call length considerably. For example, the amount of time spent on an inbound call (one taken real-time when the patient calls) will usually be shorter all together than outbound calls (those that are returned by the nurse) for a variety of reasons which will be discussed later

The second variable is the number of productive minutes per nurse. This is a complex but often overlooked or miscalculated factor. It should be obvious that telephone triage nurses can not work 8.5 hours with a 30-minute lunch and two 15-minute breaks, and be productive the remaining 450 minutes of their shift. Some "down time" is necessary. Even nurses working in a hospital get a "break" of sorts when walking the length of the hall without someone talking to them. Telephone triage is an intense practice that requires time to stand up and walk around, time to collaborate with and support colleagues, and sometimes just a few minutes to defuse after a particularly taxing call.[28] This phenomenon has also been observed in ED settings when, after a major trauma, the staff retreats to the lounge or to the patio to refresh and refuel. Productivity will vary based on factors such as the clinical setting (e.g., pediatric vs. oncology), the geographical set up (e.g., secluded workspace vs. taking calls at a busy nurses' station), and the organizational culture (e.g., how much support and collaboration do your nurses engage in?). While data are not available that speak to productivity per shift per telephone triage nurse, it is possible to calculate it for your own setting through observation. A starting point for the sake of discussion might be 10 minutes of "nonproductive" time per hour, resulting in 375 productive minutes per 8-hour shift.

To illustrate how to calculate staffing needs, the following formula may prove helpful:

- Determine average number of triage calls received per 8-hour day
- Determine average length of telephone triage calls
- Determine productive minutes per FTE per 8-hour shift

$$\frac{\text{\# of calls x avg call length}}{\text{productive min per FTE}} = \text{\# of RNs}$$

The following example provides further clarification:

- Average calls 100/day
- Average call length 10 minutes
- Productive minutes per FTE 375 minutes/day

$$\frac{\text{100 calls x 10 min}}{\text{375 prod min per FTE}} = \text{2.6 RNs}$$

In the previous example, 1,000 minutes of calls per day divided by 375 productive minutes per nurse indicates a need for 2.6 RNs on duty during the course of that 8-hour day. Looking at call time statistics, it might be determined that the organization needs to start out the day with three nurses on the phone, perhaps with one of the three working 4.5 hours, staying to cover lunch and then leaving or returning to the clinic.

Of course, it will usually require more than 2.6 FTEs to cover 2.6 positions, especially in a 24-hour operation. The general rule of thumb is that it takes about 1.6 FTEs to cover one position because time must be built in for vacation, holidays, sick time, and continuing education as appropriate to your setting. While this staffing formula might not work exactly as illustrated in your particular setting, the preceding example provides direction in determining appropriate staffing.

Centralized or Decentralized Staffing Model

Another fundamental program design element to be addressed is whether to centralize or decentralize your triage function. There are advantages and disadvantages to each model, but please keep in mind that it is yet to be determined how the concepts of Medical Home, Accountable Care Organizations, and other changes on the health care horizon will impact the usefulness of each model.

A key distinguishing factor for a decentralized program is whether the nurse is co-located with or very near the provider(s). Decentralization can take two forms:

- *Multitasked, Decentralized:* A multitasked nurse (or nurses) handling all clinical nursing functions, including the telephone
- *Dedicated, Decentralized:* One or more nurses handling only telephone triage calls for one or more providers (probably no more than 3 or 4 providers per nurse in a primary care setting)

One major drawback to the decentralized model is that the telephone triage nurse is likely to be interrupted during the course of the day such as being "pulled" to work in the clinic, chaperone a pelvic exam, educate a diabetic, or triage a walk-in patient.

Centralized telephone triage consists of a group of co-located nurses providing services for a population of patients managed by a group of physicians or an organization and can take the form of:

- *Locally Centralized:* In a single clinic or satellite location for multiple providers
- *Globally Centralized:* Enterprise-wide telephone triage offered from a centralized (often off-site) location, serving the needs of the entire patient population

Advantages of Centralized Telephone Triage

Although the concept of centralized triage seems to present logistic challenges including staffing, the solution often relatively simple. Consider a multispecialty clinic which has several satellites. While many clinics fit the previously described profile in which the RNs spend a considerable amount of time on the telephone, some clinics have only one RN and others may have none. To staff a centralized triage function, FTEs would be dedicated to telephone triage from clinics in which the nurses were already spending a significant amount of time on the phone. For example, if family practice, internal medicine, pediatrics, and obstetrics and gynecology were co-located in a satellite of a large organization, perhaps each clinic could provide one FTE to the telephone triage center. This "trade" would be in exchange for having the nurses in that center manage their patient's requests for same-day appointments and other sick or symptom-based calls. While it might superficially seem that the clinic is losing staff, in reality, they are relinquishing more work than staff. This trade-off would assure telephone triage by dedicated staff and increase efficiency in the clinics.

Of course, this concept could be enlarged to function enterprise-wide, serving the needs of all satellites and all clinics. Although some clinics wouldn't be able to contribute FTEs to the call center (because they have only one or zero RNs), their call volume would likely be low enough that the centralized nurses would be able to absorb their calls without much difficulty.

The advantages of centralization are many. First, centralization is more cost effective, reducing duplication and improving efficiency throughout the organization. Second, the quality of telephone triage is likely to improve since the calls would be handled by specially trained, dedicated staff who are focused on telephone triage. Third, the opportunity for collaboration among the nurses would be considerable. This collaborative environment would facilitate growth in their knowledge base and formation of a tight-knit support group for each other.[6,29,30] Fourth, they would be able to cover each other for breaks and lunch. If one of them called in sick, telephone triage service might be a little slower, but not "out of business" as it would be if a single nurse responsible for telephone triage failed to come to work. Finally, there would be insulation, or protection, for the telephone triage nurses in that they would not likely be "pulled" into other areas to work when a clinic was short-staffed. The nurses would be more or less "out of sight" and thus "out of mind," making them less-handy targets to assist with a procedure or fill in during lunch breaks.

A frequent argument against centralization, especially in a large clinic or medical center setting, is the fear that quality will suffer if the patient doesn't get to interact with their "own" nurse over the telephone. Consider this dilemma from the perspectives of patients, providers, primary nurses, and specialty nurses.

Ambulatory care nurses who have close relationships with their patients might say, "I want to provide care to my own patients." However, in a well-designed telephone triage program, communication between the telephone triage nurse and the patient's primary nurse is intact. The primary nurse, or care manager, would remain involved in the care of the patient, but without the pressure of having to drop everything else to be sure the patient waiting for a call back doesn't have a time-sensitive, high-risk need.

Patients might resist a triage center, wishing to speak to "their" nurse. Once patients have established a relationship with a particular nurse who knows their medical history and perhaps a bit of their social history, the bond can be tight. However, with good communication and careful planning, the primary nurse can prepare the patient by explaining how the telephone triage nurse(s) and primary nurse will communicate about the patient's issues. It's helpful to point out to patients that they're not losing a nurse; they're gaining one (or several).

Providers might insist that they want their patients triaged by "their" nurse(s) because they know the patients better. However, evidence indicates that a clinician can know a patient *too* well. The decisions nurses make about patient care are often influenced by how well they know their patients. And not necessarily in a good way. Nurses may stereotype patients or develop prejudices about them, impairing the nurse's objectivity.[31,32] For example, it is not unheard of for a patient to suffer a cardiac arrest just weeks or months after a negative stress test. And, the risk of a nurse inadvertently minimizing the credibility of the frequent caller was explored in Chapter 3.

Specialty nurses may believe that telephone triage nurses, as generalists, can not provide safe and effective care for their specialty patients. Overcoming this prejudice requires recognition that there are at least two general types of telephone encounters requiring a nurse. One is triage and the other is care management.

Consider, for example, the patient who is seen in several clinics and/or by several specialists. If telephone triage is decentralized, and the patient develops a headache, the patient must determine which clinic to contact. For example, is this headache related to an ENT problem, a neurologic problem, or an endocrine problem? The patient must essentially self-diagnose in order to place the call for help. This problem is potentially compounded when the patient chooses a specific clinic which might not have been his or her best choice. In this case, the nurse who is oriented primarily to that specialty is likely to consider the patient's headache in the context of his or her own specialty, potentially overlooking other possibilities. Of course, if the patient selects the wrong clinic and the nurse doesn't look beyond his or her own specialty, the actual cause of the headache might be overlooked, and thus the patient might receive an inappropriate disposition. This is especially a problem for children who are seen in the pediatric medical center environment and are often followed by several specialties. The fact is that triage of a patient with a headache is the same, regardless of which specialty it's related to or the etiology of the headache. Centralized telephone triage would solve this problem for the patient and the specialty nurse, with the triage nurse first determining the nature and urgency of the call, and then if clinic nurse or physician involvement is necessary, referring the patient to the appropriate clinic. Centralized telephone triage removes the potential for specialty bias by the nurse, eliminates pressure on the patient to decide which clinic to call, and decreases the potential for misuse of organizational resources (see Figure 1).

Figure 1.
Patient with Headache
(Patient doesn't know which clinic to call.)

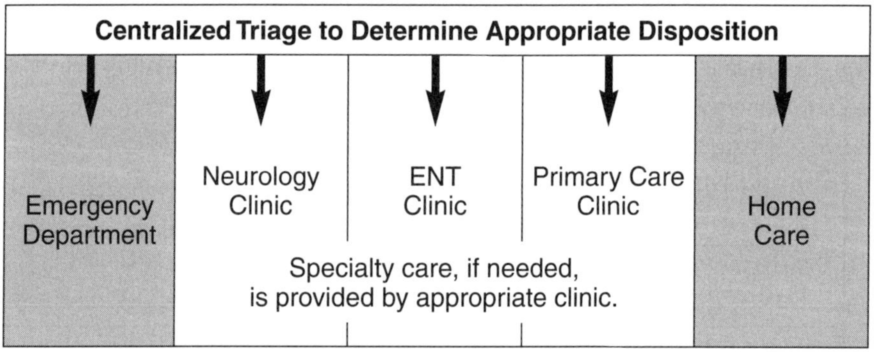

Consistent with the description of telehealth nursing in Chapter 1 is the understanding that while all calls require an unbiased assessment because they have the *potential* to be telephone triage calls, not all calls *are* telephone triage calls. As mentioned previously, there are a variety of types of interactions that occur over the telephone between the nurse and the patient. Following triage, involvement of the primary nurse is often required, resulting in a "patient management" call. Consider the following two examples.

The patient calls the triage nurse with a complaint of constipation, inquiring about the appropriate OTC laxative. The triage nurse rules out impaction and obstruction and determines the patient's appropriate disposition to be home care. The triage nurse, following a medically approved treatment protocol, recommends MiraLAX® and then sends a note to the patient's nurse, requesting a followup call to develop a more sustained plan of care, since this is the patient's third call for "constipation" this month. The primary nurse, at his or her convenience, then contacts the patient to inquire about diet, fluid intake, exercise, and medications to get to the root of the constipation and develop a plan of care which will better prevent it in the future.

A second example would be a patient with type 1 diabetes who has a repeatedly elevated blood sugar. The triage nurse would promptly evaluate the patient to rule out emergent or urgent problems associated with an elevated blood glucose. If the patient has symptoms of diabetic ketoacidosis, she needs to be sent to the ED now for evaluation. If the patient has symptoms of infection, she needs to be scheduled promptly for an appointment with her primary care provider. And if she's in the latter half of her pregnancy, she needs to be evaluated for possible preeclampsia. However, once all of those potentially life-threatening problems associated with diabetes are ruled out, the patient may be referred to his or her primary care nurse who, at the nurse's convenience, will call to discuss diet, exercise, stress, and medication regimen to help determine and address the cause of the blood sugar elevations.

The final concern about centralized triage is impairment of continuity of care. Trust in the nurse's understanding of the importance of collaboration, coupled with policies that support involvement of the provider, will facilitate continuity of care. To assure collaboration and proper involvement of the provider, a policy should require review of all telephone triage records by the end of the day by the patient's provider. While this might pose some unique challenges for nurses in a call center setting, it can be accomplished successfully.

One suggestion is to include a clause in the contract with client physicians specifying that all notes will be sent electronically or by fax to each physician's office for review by the close of business each day. Nurses working in medical centers with resident-staffed clinics should have their records reviewed by the appropriate house staff. However, if they aren't available to review the patient's record by the end of the day, an attending physician should assume that responsibility. Finally, when nurses in community-based call centers are taking calls from patients at large, independent of their relationship with a provider, other arrangements should be made for medical review if possible.

Telephone Triage in Home Health

We have discussed telephone triage in the office and call center settings. However, as mentioned early in the book, telephone triage is performed in essentially every setting in which a patient can access a nurse by telephone. One of those settings, home health, is unique enough that it deserves special mention.

Telephone triage in home health has taken on growing significance in recent years. Home health agencies have been charged with the responsibility of preventing acute care rehospitalizations. This is especially important in this time of early discharges and limited personal, financial, and health care resources. Telephone triage, performed properly, is a tool to assist the home health nurse in assessing the patient and his or her family to make a decision regarding the necessity of a home visit or a referral to the ED.

Home health nurses provide home visits and are also responsible for telephone consultation as necessary for their own casesload, and then they often take calls for the agency at night. This practice poses a multitude of potential risks including:

- Being multitasked while talking on the phone, possibly in transit between homes.

- Potentially knowing the patient "too well."
- Possible confidentiality issues arising from speaking with one patient in the home of another.
- Fatigue and foggy thinking related to being awakened at night to triage a call.
- Potential (usually unrecognized) conflict of interest for nurses taking calls at night and having to make the home visit themselves if one is indicated. Although difficult for any nurse to acknowledge, if making a decision that a patient needs a home visit at 3 a.m. during a snowstorm, and it's a close call, the nurse's judgment might be swayed by the warm bed, without him or her being aware of it.

Knowing there is a nurse "awake all night" to help them is comforting and reassuring to patients. Without a dedicated telephone triage program, there is a concern that the patient or family might not call the nurse, fearing that the call would awaken him or her. A final concern associated with telephone triage in home health is the possibility of perceived pressure to keep the patient out of the hospital due to the imperative to reduce acute care rehospitalizations.

It is essential that nurses who are making decisions about the health care needs of this high-risk population have the special training, resources, and other tools necessary for good decision making. In recent years, having dedicated nurses in somewhat formalized telephone triage roles for home health agencies has been a growing trend. This trend, also noted with hospice programs, is evidence of the growing role telephone triage is playing in providing care to patients in the home.

SUMMARY

In this chapter, we have outlined broad organizational necessities that provide a solid foundation for development of a telephone triage program in your organization. We have also explained the necessity of formalizing telephone triage. And we have discussed staffing considerations from the micro perspective of hiring the right person to the macro considerations associated with developing a centralized telephone triage program within an organization. In the following chapter, access, call flow, and policies necessary to support a safe and effective telephone triage program will be explored.

References

1. American Academy of Ambulatory Care Nursing. (2011). *Scope and standards of practice for professional telehealth nurses* (5th ed.). Pitman, NJ: Author.
2. Aita, V., Dodendorf, D.M., Lebsack, J.A., Tallia, A.F., & Crabtree, B.F. (2001). Patient care staffing patterns and roles in community-based family practices. *Journal of Family Practice, 50*(10), 889.
3. American Academy of Ambulatory Care Nursing. (2011). Position statement: The role of the registered nurse in ambulatory care. *Nursing Economic$, 29*(2), 96-66.
4. Custer, M., O'Rourke, K., King, R., Sprinkle, L., & Horne, E. (2003). The impact of a nursing triage line on the use of emergency department services in a military hospital. *Military Medicine, 168*(12), 981-985.
5. Ernesäter, A., Engström, M., Holmström, I., & Winblad, U. (2010). Incident reporting in nurse-led national telephone triage in Sweden: The reported errors reveal a pattern that needs to be broken. *Journal of Telemedicine and Telecare, 16*(5), 243-247.
6. Purc-Stephenson, R., & Thrasher, C. (2010). Nurses' experiences with telephone triage and advice: A meta-ethnography. *Journal of Advanced Nursing, 66*(3), 482-494. doi:10.1111/j.1365-2648.2010.05275.x
7. Wahlberg, A.C., Cedersund, E., & Wredling, R. (2003). Telephone nurses' experience of problems with telephone advice in Sweden. *Journal of Clinical Nursing, 12*(1), 37-45.
8. Haas, S.A. (2011). Health reform act: New models of care and delivery systems. *AAACN Viewpoint, 33*(2), 11-12.
9. Flannery, M., Phillips, S.M., & Lyons, C.A. (2009). Examining telephone calls in ambulatory oncology. *Journal of Oncology Practice, 5*(2), 57-60. doi:10.1200/JOP.0922002
10. Rupp, R.E., Ramsey, K.P., & Foley, J.D. (1994). Telephone triage: Results of adolescent clinic responses to a mock patient with pelvic pain. *Journal of Adolescent Health, 15*(3), 249-253.
11. Dare, C. (1994). *Control as a personality trait of emergency nurses.* Unpublished manuscript, College of Nursing, University of Arkansas Medical Science, Little Rock, AR.
12. Wells, S. (2009). *Due diligence: Assuring hiring the best candidate for your telehealth position.* Podium presentation. American Academy of Ambulatory Care Nursing 34th Annual Conference, Philadelphia, PA.
13. Benner, P. (1984). *From novice to expert: Excellence and power in clinical nursing practice.* Menlo Park, CA: Addison-Wesley.
14. Medical Board of California, (2010). *Medical Assistants - Frequently Asked Questions, Are medical assistants allowed to perform telephone triage?* State of California. Retrieved from http://www.mbc.ca.gov/allied/medical_assistants_questions.html#14
15. Rutenberg, C. (2012). [Surveys of Boards of Nursing]. Unpublished raw data.
16. National Council of State Boards of Nursing. (1997). *The five rights of delegation.* Retrieved from https://www.ncsbn.org/fiverights.pdf

17. Anderson, P. (August 2001). *Study: Multitasking is counterproductive.* Retrieved from http://archives.cnn.com/2001/CAREER/trends/08/05/multitasking.focus/index.html
18. Wahlberg, A.C., Cedersund, E., & Wredling, R. (2005). Bases for assessments made by telephone advice nurses. *Journal of Telemedicine & Telecare, 11*(8), 403-407.
19. Ophir, E., Nass, C., & Wagner, A. (2009). Cognitive control in media multitaskers. *Proceedings of the natural academy of sciences of the United States, 106*(37), 15563-15587.
20. Westbrook, J.I., Coiera, E., Dunsmuir, W.T.M., Brown, B.M., Kelk, N., Paoloni, R., & Tran, C. (2010). The impact of interruptions on clinical task completion. *Quality and Safety in Health Care, 19*, 284-289.
21. Greengold N.L., Shane R., Schneider P., Flynn E., Elashoff, J., Hoying C.L., Barker K. & Bolton, L.B. (2003). The impact of dedicated medication nurses on the medication administration error rate: A randomized controlled trial. *Archives of Internal Medicine, 163*, 2359-2367.
22. Facione, N.C., & Facione, P. A. (2008). Critical thinking and clinical judgment. In N.C. Facione & P.A. Facione (Eds.), *Critical thinking and clinical reasoning in the health sciences: An international and multidisciplinary teaching anthology* (pp. 1-13). Millbrae, CA: The California Academic Press, LLC.
23. Hedberg, B., & Larsson, U.S. (2004). Environmental elements affecting the decision-making process in nursing practice. *Journal of Clinical Nursing, 13*, 316-324.
24. Lin, L. (2009). Breadth-biased versus focused cognitive control in media multitasking behaviors. *Proceedings of the natural academy of sciences of the United States, 106*(37), 15521-15522.
25. Hall, L.M., Pedersen, C., & Fairley, L. (2010). Losing the moment: Understanding interruptions to nurses' work. *JONA 40*(4), 169-176.
26. D'Ausilio, R. (2009). The pitfalls of call center multitasking. *Medical Call Center News, 3*. Peter DeHaan Publishing, Inc. Mattawan MI. Retrieved from http://www.medicalcallcenternews.com/issue/2009/september.pdf
27. Hansen, B., Whelan, S.M., Barton, S.J., Hirokawa, C., White, P.A. & Chen-Lin, M.L. (2011). Pediatric telephone triage: There's no place like home. *AAACN Viewpoint, 33*(6), 1, 10-12.
28. Koehne, K. (2007). Nurse – care for thyself! Ergonomics in the nursing workplace. *AAACN Viewpoint, 29*(4), 1, 10-11.
29. O'Cathain, A., Sampson, F.C., Munro, J.F., Thomas, K.J., & Nicholl, J.P. (2004). Nurses' views of using computerized decision support software in NHS direct. *Journal of Advanced Nursing, 45*(3), 280-286.
30. Knowles, E., O'Cathain, A., Morrell, J., Munro, J.F., & Nicholl, J.P. (2002). NHS direct and nurses – opportunity or monotony? *International Journal of Nursing Studies, 39*(8), 857-866.
31. Casad, B. (2007). Confirmation bias. In R.F. Baumeister & K.D. Vohs (Eds.), *Encyclopedia of social psychology* (pp. 162-163). Los Angeles, CA: Sage Publications.
32. Lee, J., Chan, A., & Phillips, D. (2006). Diagnostic practise in nursing: A critical review of the literature. *Nursing & Health Sciences, 8*(1), 57-65.

Chapter 15

Program Design and Implementation Part II: Access, Call Flow, and Policy Development

In Chapter 14 we first described organizational necessities for successful program design and implementation and then focused at length on how to achieve optimal staffing. In this chapter we will look in-depth at how to optimize three additional components of successful telephone triage programs: access to services, call intake and routing, and program policies. Last we will take a look at change implementation and review risk management principles discussed throughout the book.

ACCESS TO HEALTH CARE SERVICES

Access is usually synonymous with getting an appointment in the doctor's office, but it is actually more than that. "Access" refers to the availability of health care resources and the ability of a patient to access those resources when needed. The health care resources might be accessed in a doctor's office, an urgent care center, an emergency department, over the telephone, or via a number of other methods and technologies. Specifically, in the context of this chapter, "access" is used to describe the patient's ability to get an appointment with his or her provider or another suitable resource for medical care.

Not having sufficient access to meet patient demand is a common problem faced by many health care organizations. It is not unusual for doctors' offices and clinics to have a paucity of appointments, especially for same-day access (for the patient to be scheduled and seen on the day of his or her call). This is frustrating and poses a challenge for telephone triage nurses who assess their patients and determine that they need to be seen that day by their health care provider but are unable to get them an appointment. Nurses in some settings find themselves spending a significant amount of their day trying to secure access for their patients. Without an organizational policy directing the telephone triage nurses on how to handle patients who need to be seen after all available appointments have been depleted, their day is often largely devoted to calling doctor after doctor asking for permission to work-in a patient between other appointments. To complicate matters further, some providers are more willing than others to see extra patients, with the outcome being that some providers are over-utilized while others don't see a comparable volume of patients. This inequity is frustrating for almost all involved, including the patient, who often can't get an appointment with his or her regular doctor. Nurses learn quickly which providers will see extra patients and which providers will resist if asked to increase their workload. The net result, unfortunately, is that nurses wind up abusing the "nice guys" and protecting those who resist extra work.

When this dysfunctional process was pointed out during a consultation, one CEO of a large organization (himself a physician) summed it up perfectly. He said, "With our current system, the nurses are frustrated because they're wasting their time trying to find someone to see the patient, the patients are frustrated because they don't get to see their doctor, and the compliant providers are frustrated because they are having to do more than their share of work. All of this is in an effort to accommodate those providers who refuse to see additional patients. If they're that unhappy seeing patients, we probably won't be able to make them happy regardless of what we do." He then asked the medical staff to develop an organizational policy instructing and empowering the nurses to schedule patients as they needed to, equitably, and without regard for individual physician personalities and preferences. Interestingly, the medical staff was all too happy to develop and enforce this policy because predictably, there were more overworked "nice guys" than recalcitrant "fit-pitchers."

Strategies to Improve Access

The solution to this conundrum is to have an organizational policy that details how patients should be scheduled or referred if they need to be seen today but no same-day appointments are available. The obvious solution is to utilize data from the previously mentioned workload analysis (see Chapter 14) to determine an average number of requested same-day appointments by day of the week and revise the clinic's appointment template (schedule) to include a sufficient number of slots for patients who need to be seen that day. For example, one large primary care organization needed about six same-day slots per day, representing 25% of daily appointments. Control of those slots should be given to the telephone triage nurse(s).

Another strategy might be a policy that allows the triage nurses to "work in" (overbook) a specified number of appointments each morning and each afternoon for every provider. This policy could also include rotation instructions for these appointment slots such as (a) first to the patient's primary care provider (PCP), and then (b) when the patient's PCP has met threshold, booking patients to the hall-mate, pod-mate, or partner. When both of those close associates have met threshold, patients could be booked to any other provider in the practice who still has openings or hasn't yet been overbooked. Of course, a cut-off time should also be established, after which no additional same-day appointments may be scheduled and all patients still needing to be seen are referred as appropriate to an UCC or the ED. Generally speaking, no patient should be sent to UCC unless all providers' work-in thresholds have been met, the cut-off time has arrived, or the patient's condition *requires* evaluation at the UCC. In other words, in organizations in which the question of work aversion exists among the medical staff, whether or not a provider is at liberty to decline to see extra patients should be a matter of policy, not personality.

Additional strategies to improve access might include having a team huddle in the morning prior to clinic in order to identify opportunities for schedule adjustments. For example, if an appointment clerk has given an appointment to a patient who could probably be managed over the telephone, the physician or RN could call this patient, conduct an assessment, and determine whether phone treatment might be indicated. Likewise, patients who are scheduled for follow-up of a previous acute illness (such as bronchitis), who could be appropriately assessed over the phone, might receive a call from an RN or provider. As a final example, patients who are known to frequently be late or are quick "in and outs" may be put in double-booked time slots.

Some practices have designed a role of "Dr. Acute" for the day, which might be assigned on a rotational basis. This involves having one provider a day (or per half day) who sees only patients in need of same-day appointments. To make this work, however, two criteria must be established. First, the provider must keep his or her schedule open in order to see patients needing an acute appointment. Second, all providers must accept the fact that, although seeing a provider other than the patient's own PCP does potentially impact continuity of care, it is not nearly as disruptive as sending patients to an UCC due to lack of appointment space.

Another solution might involve hiring mid-level providers to see acute patients for the practice. If the patient's own physician is unavailable, advanced practice nurses or physician's assistants can handle these patients and will benefit from access to the patient's electronic health record and his or her primary provider if necessary.

Finally, RN-run clinics could be added as the role of the RN in the ambulatory care setting continues to grow and develop. Although nurse-run clinics already exist in many settings, they usually take the form of wound care clinics, immunization clinics, or diabetic education classes. However, RNs should also be able to conduct follow-up visits on stable patients with chronic illnesses such as diabetes, hypertension, congestive heart failure, asthma, chronic bronchitis, and the like. Here, the key is that the patient be *stable,* with the provider seeing the patient every-other-visit and the RN seeing the patient in between. Reviewing a patient's labs, evaluating a patient's blood sugar or blood pressure diary, taking a history, and conducting an appropriate physical assessment are all well within the role of an RN. As long as the RN is following a plan of care put forth by a licensed provider and isn't making a medical diagnosis or prescribing, nurse-run clinics are within the RN's scope of practice. It should be considered the ambulatory care equivalent of caring for a patient on an inpatient unit. For example, patients who are in the hospital are occasionally on sliding-scale insulin based on a physician's order with criteria evaluated by the RN. In fact, the sickest patients with pulmonary edema, hypertensive crisis, respiratory failure, diabetic ketoacidosis, and other extreme problems are managed in intensive care units every day, by RNs who are following the orders of a physician while exercising judgment that is well within their own scope of practice. It only makes sense that RNs should be able to perform similar functions in the ambulatory care setting. Of course, this might raise the question of billing, but there should be no loss of revenue since the practice can bill for a "nurse visit" and will have freed up the provider's schedule to see another, presumably higher-acuity patient, instead.

While appointment or scheduling template design is not generally within the purview of the telephone triage nurse, without organizational support to assure access, telephone triage can be futile and frustrating. Collaboration and cooperation among all members of the team are necessary to design a program that provides adequate access options for patients who need to be seen.

Collaboration Between the Telephone Triage Nurse and the Provider

In addition to having sufficient available appointments, the telephone triage nurse must be empowered to access and utilize the appointments at their discretion (thus the policy outlining a prescribed course of action if a patient needs an appointment and none is available). However, nursing empowerment goes far beyond the ability to implement an existing policy. There must be a recognition that the nurse, who has talked with the patient and assessed the situation directly, is making a recommendation based on clinical judgment which incorporates clinical knowledge, the patient's specific circumstances, the patient's preference, professional standards, and organizational policy. Regardless of whether the recommendation is to dial 911, schedule an appointment, or provide home care advice, an experienced telephone triage nurse has considered all options, confirmed his or her decision making against the decision support tools, and developed a plan of care that is acceptable to the patient.

This is in no way intended to imply that nurses shouldn't collaborate with their physician colleagues if the RN is uncertain about the best course of action to take or reccommend. Collaboration and teamwork are keystones of professional nursing.[1] As discussed earlier, the provider should review each triage note by the end of the day to stay apprised of what is going on with his or her patients, and to provide collaborative expertise when indicated. If the provider is comfortable with the nurse's decision, it should be honored. If the provider or another member of the team wishes to supersede the triage nurse's decision, it should be based on his or her own direct assessment of the patient unless representing an upgrade (a change to a higher level of care). Superseding the triage nurse's recommended course of action (to a lower level of care) would, at a minimum, necessitate another phone call, potentially damage the credibility of the triage nurse, and possibly confuse the patient. But of potentially far greater significance is the possibility that the individual making the ultimate decision has not spoken directly with the patient and therefore may not have all the information necessary to make a fully informed decision. Thus, this option should be used judiciously. The triage process requires the nurse to utilize clinical judgment based on what the patient says and doesn't say, how she says it, and relevant contextual factors. If the provider is making a determination based on the documentation, regardless of its quality or completeness, it is possible that elements of the patient's tone of voice or other subtle cues would not be apparent. Remember, the triage nurse doesn't have a crystal ball and has been trained to err on the side of caution. While decision making by the physician or primary nurse may be based on intimate knowledge of the patient and can be helpful, it can also lead to loss of objectivity and thus oversight of an unexpected problem. Finally, having established that the patient gets 51% of the vote on whether or not she is seen, it is possible that the nurse has already offered home care, which the patient has declined. The staff working with the triage nurse should respect the process and follow the recommendation of the triage nurse unless there is a compelling reason to defer to the assessment of another team member.

In some settings, policy dictates that the nurse (often in a misguided effort to avoid liability), talk with the patient, only "taking a message," and then passing the patient's information on to the provider for final decision making. The notion of an RN being restricted to taking a message for the doctor instead of making a decision utilizing professional knowledge and judgment flies in the face of reason. Nursing accountability, critical thinking, clinical judgment, and the ability to individualize care for his or her patient is the role of the telephone triage nurse. The inappropriateness of a process that reduces an RN to the role of message taker may be difficult to recognize but impossible to side step. The serious flaws in this type of reasoning are illustrated below.

- This approach is based on an implicit assumption that the physician can make a better decision than the telephone triage nurse. Unless the nurse has a knowledge deficit, he or she, by virtue of having talked to the patient directly, currently knows more about this particular situation than the physician does, regardless of the physician's knowledge of the patient or the thoroughness and quality of the nurse's documentation. Therefore, deferring to the physician because of their medical knowledge base, devalues the unique contribution that can be made by the nurse. This principle will be discussed further in the *Policy* section of this chapter.
- When the nurse *takes a message* and delivers it to the doctor, the

nurse has already made an assessment, obviously concluding that the patient's situation is not life threatening. Otherwise, the nurse would have directed the patient to seek care immediately rather than forwarding the note to the physician. Because interpretation (assessment and diagnosis of urgency) is inherent in the practice of telephone triage, the belief that by not dispensing advice, the nurse is not "practicing nursing," is erroneous. RNs are accountable for their practice, as based on their interaction with the patient and their scope of practice, which requires use of the nursing process.

Second-Level Triage and Chain of Command

"RNs...maintain ultimate accountability for their actions, even if those actions are in response to a direct order from a physician. Having a physician's order does not relieve the nurse of the responsibility to act in the patient's best interest, within the constraints of the nurse's knowledge base (and their scope of practice, organizational policy, and the standard of care). It is therefore important to note that nurses may NOT carry out an order that they believe is contraindicated and would result in an adverse or potentially life-threatening outcome" (pp. 11-12).[2]

Second-level triage represents an organizational policy that requires the telephone triage nurse to consult with a provider for final determination regarding "the necessity of an after hours visit" (p. 226).[3] It has been advocated as a method to either improve quality or contain cost. However, if one is to evaluate it critically, it becomes apparent that at its root, there is a not-so-obvious implication that a physician, without talking to the patient, can make a better judgment than the nurse who has assessed the patient and his or her situation directly.

Reasons cited in support of second-level triage include promoting cost savings and increasing patient convenience by giving a physician an opportunity to see the patient in the office instead of referring him or her to a higher level of care, thereby eliminating an unnecessary ED visit. However, again, such policies consistently, if covertly, call into question the judgment of the RN.

We suggest that if the problem is that the decision support tool directs the patient to a higher level of care than is necessary, the nurses should be supported by policy in downgrading the disposition. If the problem is that the physician's "permission" is necessary to schedule a patient for an appointment, policies should be developed giving the triage nurse access to the schedule and empowerment to make the appointment without first involving the physician. If the problem is that the nurse is accessing the physician to encourage patient cooperation, there are other, less-costly strategies to motivate a non-compliant patient. And finally, if there are indeed errors in the nurse's judgment, they should be dealt with through education and other avenues. In other words, the physician's involvement should not routinely be necessary for an RN to provide appropriate care to his or her patient.

There may be other apparent advantages to second-level triage, but at the base of each of them is a question about the ability of the RN to make the right decision. Rather than muddying the water with a policy that *requires* the nurse to talk to the provider before making a decision, why not put the decision where it belongs: in the hands of the telephone triage nurse? Rather than *compelling* the nurse to seek the provider's input, the provider should be available as a resource for collaboration in those cases in which the RN is unsure of what action to take. One additional concern about second-level triage is that taking the time to contact the provider could result in a delay in care for patients who are in need of prompt evaluation as described in the next vignette.

Gladys, an experienced pediatric nurse of 30 years, received a call at 10 p.m. from a mother of a 6-year-old child who had a temperature of 100.2 orally, a "cold and a cough," and was "breathing funny at times." Mother denied nasal flaring, retractions, cyanosis, or other symptoms of concern and said that her child was "acting

normal." She just didn't know what to think of this "funny breathing." When the nurse asked to listen to the patient breathe, she was concerned about the character of the respirations and told the mother that she would need to take her child to the ED. The nurse said she would talk to the doctor and then call the mother back.

Because her organization required second-level triage for all ED referrals, the nurse discussed the patient with the doctor, suggesting an ED referral, but the RN was unable produce a term that would correctly describe the child's respiratory efforts. She told the physician it wasn't a wheeze, stridor, or even noisy breathing; there was just a "raspy" quality she hadn't heard before. Being unable to "name that tune," the nurse was unable to impress upon the patient's PCP the extent of her concern. The physician felt the child would benefit from croup measures and told the nurse to instruct the mother on home care recommendations for croup and to advise her to call back if her child didn't respond promptly to warm or cool mist and increased hydration.

Unfortunately, the child's condition did continue to deteriorate, resulting in a 911 call at about 5 a.m. He was later diagnosed with pneumonia for which he was hospitalized, thankfully followed by a full recovery.

Fortunately, the child did not suffer an adverse outcome other than a potentially preventable hospitalization. But had the nurse not been required to seek second-level triage, based on the independent judgment of the RN, the patient would have been evaluated and treated earlier, perhaps avoiding the subsequent hospitalization. In summary, the notion that a physician who has not spoken with the patient can make a better decision about disposition than the triage nurse has the potential to result in an inappropriate disposition, delay in care, and call into question the capabilities of the nurse to exercise proper clinical judgment. However, as mentioned previously, it is important to recognize that physicians have an extensive knowledge base regarding medical conditions and should be consulted freely if the nurse is in doubt about the appropriate action to take.

This discussion is in no way intended to discourage nurses from consulting with physicians when in doubt about what action to recommend. However, collaboration when the nurse feels that it is indicated does not represent second-level triage because the contact is made at the professional discretion of the nurse, not because it is required by policy. Regardless of the ostensible reason for second-level triage, with careful analysis, it almost always becomes apparent that the term is a euphemism for "the doctor knows best."

Of greatest concern is the fact that a larger professional issue can potentially surface with this policy requirement for second-level triage. Suppose the nurse feels strongly that the patient should be seen immediately, but the provider consulted for second-level triage disagrees and declines to "authorize" the ED visit. The nurse now finds him or herself in a predicament. A basic tenant of nursing is that a nurse may not follow an order he or she feels is inappropriate. However, the nurse may not ignore a direct order either. The difference of opinion needs to be resolved. Ideally, the relationship between the nurse and physician is mutually respectful enough for the nurse to express discomfort with the order and discuss it with the physician. However, if resolution through negotiation is not possible, the question must be elevated promptly through the chain of command, as outlined in policy. This, of course, further increases the potential for delay in care to the patient. For the safety of the patient and in order to maintain the quality of the professional relationship between the nurse and the physician, the chain of command policy should be discussed in advance, dispassionately, when a patient is not hanging in the balance.

"This chain of command should be established, discussed, and understood by all in your organization. In the event of unresolved disagreement about care of the patient, the provider should talk directly with the patient, shifting the final responsibility to the provider. If this is not possible, the chain of command should be utilized for ultimate resolution of the dispute" (pp. 11-12).[2]

A positive way to initiate a conversation about chain of command with the physician might be to say, "It is possible that eventually we are going to disagree about the management of a patient. When and if that happens, we should be able to negotiate an agreement. However, in the unlikely event that we are not able to do so, there must be a chain of command policy that gives us a route for arbitration because your order cannot supersede my judgment. I am equally as responsible to the patient, the board of nursing, and the standards of nursing practice as you are to the patient, the board of medicine, and the standards of medical practice." Unfortunately, this is a conversation that probably doesn't often take place, which is a mistake. Many physicians, having been taught that they are the "Captain of the Ship" (as discussed in Chapter 5), mistakenly believe that as long as the nurse has an order, the accountability for the RN's actions rests with the physician.

The Role of the Telephone Triage Nurse in Open Access

Open Access, also referred to as Advanced Access or Same-Day Scheduling, a method of giving patients appointments the same day they request them, gained popularity around 2000. The Open Access model allows the patient to bypass the "gatekeeper," permitting secretaries or appointment clerks to give patients appointments upon request.[4]

However patient-oriented this may seem, the fundamental problem this presents is that patients may request an appointment when it is not appropriate. And the error can go either way. Some patients will request an appointment when they would actually prefer and benefit from home care but don't realize the potential for care over the telephone exists. Of greater concern, however, is the patient who requests and is given an appointment and presents to the office in critical condition.

In an Open Access model in a large clinic, a patient called one morning requesting an appointment for a "cold." She was given an appointment, and when she presented to the clinic 45 minutes later, she was hypertensive, morbidly obese, and in respiratory failure. This patient had to be intubated in the clinic but due to the configuration of the doorway into the exam room, and the patient's size, it was extremely difficult for the EMTs to get the patient out of the exam room. Despite Herculean efforts on the part of the staff, the patient did not have a favorable outcome.

The preceding example demonstrates the importance of triaging every request for a same-day appointment, whether in an Open Access model or not. Assuring that patients access the right level of care in the right place at the right time is the enduring goal of telephone triage.

The Role of the Telephone Triage Nurse in Appointment Scheduling

Often, concern exists about the use of telephone triage nurses to triage and schedule requests for same-day appointments. As discussed previously, the purpose of telephone triage is not to decide whether the patient gets an appointment or not. If, after triage, it is determined that the patient needs or wants an appointment, the RN should go ahead and schedule it. Remember, if the patient wants an appointment, he or she should be given an appointment (or referred elsewhere).

Initially, the notion of having an RN schedule the appointment may seem like misuse of the nurse's time. However, it is indeed appropriate for the nurse to schedule the appointment because even if almost unconsciously, critical thinking goes into the process. Is the problem so urgent that the patient needs to see the first available provider, or is continuity of care so important that it's appropriate and desirable for the patient to wait until later in the afternoon to see her own PCP? If the nurse offers a patient a 10:00 a.m. appointment that the patient can't make because her husband won't be home with the car until 3:30 p.m., is it acceptable for the patient to be seen later that afternoon, or should the nurse help the patient explore options to get to the office sooner? Scheduling an appointment often requires some negotiation, which might involve additional patient education. Recognizing appointment scheduling as an important part of implementation of the care plan, utilization of triage nurses in this role is appropriate. In fact, in a large study of telephone advice services in the United States, researchers concluded that the professional skills of the nurse are consistently utilized even when making an appointment.[5]

CALL INTAKE AND ROUTING

How calls are received and routed can make the difference between a successful and unsuccessful triage program. Standards dictate that all calls requiring assessment must be taken by RNs; however, thought must be given to the method and implications of how the call is routed to the nurse. There are four identified methods of call intake. Each one will be discussed separately. They are call intake by clerical personnel, message taking by answering services, voice mail, and call intake by telephone triage nurses.

Call Intake by Clerical Personnel

In many offices and call centers, the call is answered initially by a clerical person, sometimes referred to as a customer service representative, patient service representative, contact center agent, or referral specialist. Use of these titles, while appropriate in a job description, may be misleading to the public. Terms that are well understood by the public such as *appointment clerk* or *secretary* are more straightforward and decrease the likelihood that patients will believe they are talking to a nurse.

In some organizations, these clerical personnel simply route calls according to the patient's request or perceived need. In others, the clerks take messages for the RN for the purpose of a call back. Still others utilize sometimes fairly sophisticated decision trees or algorithms that direct the clerk in decision making.

In each of these cases, it should be recognized that to a greater or lesser extent, the clerical personnel are being asked to perform triage. This is easiest to recognize in situations in which the clerks have been provided decision support tools. In fact, in one organization, the nurse manager said, "We're trying to get the nurses to a higher and higher level of functioning," meaning she only wanted the nurses to provide triage services to the highest acuity patients. The inference was that the nurse manager believed the clerks should be able to identify and handle the low-acuity calls. In the same organization, a nurse expressed frustration that "The clerks keep sending me non-cardiac chest pains!" The obvious implication was that she expected the front-end clerk to recognize cardiac chest pains, referring them immediately for triage by the nurse and to likewise recognize low-acuity chest pains, routing them through routine channels. Although probably unintentional, both examples illustrate expectations by the nurse manager and by the nurse that the clerk should be able to perform first-level triage.

In clinics in which clerks take messages and refer them to the nurse, the clerks are being expected to do triage, although just as in the more formal situation, it usually isn't recognized as such. In some settings, the clerks are provided with "hot lists," "red flags lists," or "cheat sheets" (lists of symptoms or situations) that should be brought to the immediate attention of the RN. Upon close inspection of these documents, it is apparent that their use requires some level of assessment. While these lists might be helpful to RNs who don't have protocols, in the hands of the clerks, they become triage tools that may or may not prove to be helpful, depending on how the patient describes his or her problem and the knowledge base of the clerk. For example, while chief complaints of "chest pain" or "shortness of breath" or "hemorrhage" or "dehydration" are meant to be referred immediately to the RN for evaluation, complaints of "toothache" (referred chest pain), "not sleeping well" (related to shortness of breath),"I want to talk about my period" (because I'm saturating two pads per hour), or "my child has been vomiting" (and is thus dehydrated), might not be. Just to be clear, there's nothing wrong with a clerk referring a patient with chest pain or shortness of breath to an RN. The problem arises when the "toothache" and other apparently low-acuity complaints, which could be life-threatening problems in disguise, receive delayed attention because the patient didn't say one of the "magic words." Similarly some red flag lists are so complicated that an assessment is necessary to identify them. For example, "Second degree burns on the hands, feet, or perineum;" do we really want our clerks taking that kind of history and making those kinds of judgments? Even identification of a fever of 100.4° F in an infant often requires patient education by a nurse. If the criteria for immediate transfer of an infant with a fever are (a) under 3 months of age and (b) temperature of 100.4° F or greater, a call from a mother who announces, "My 2-month old has a fever of 101," is clear cut. But again, our concern should be the mother with the febrile infant who has misinterpreted the problem and says, "My baby is teething and is crying when I offer her a bottle." Reliance on the red flag process to identify high-acuity patients is risky business and in fact represents telephone triage by unqualified personnel.

A 36-year-old female professor contacted her college health center with a complaint of, "I'm having some pain in my chest." The clerk inquired whether it was radiating into her arm, and the patient said, "Yes." The clerk's next question was, "Which arm?"

Fortunately, the patient responded that it was her left arm, and she was transferred immediately to an RN. That example, of course, begs the question of what the clerk would have done had the patient denied arm pain or stated that it was radiating into her right arm. Sometimes a little learning can be a dangerous thing.

In a study comparing the chief complaint as identified by clerks to their problem as identified by the RN, in 12% of the calls the problem (chief complaint) reported by the clerk was different than the problem identified by the nurse.[6] In almost one-third of those calls (3.8%), the discrepancies were considered to be potentially problematic, typically with the nurse advising the patient to seek immediate health care. Although in this particularly study most of the calls were returned within the organizational standard of 20 minutes, in many programs that is not the case. Delays in nurse call-back time would make these cases of problem misidentification especially troublesome. Even when calls are returned promptly, if the patient ultimately experiences a bad outcome, a delay in care, even if minimal, takes on huge significance, especially if it can be shown that the outcome was related to the delay. Furthermore, although only 3.8% potentially problematic calls may seem like acceptable odds, in an organization taking 100 triage calls per day, 5 days per week, that amounts to approximately 3.8 patients/day, 19 patients/week, 76 patients/month, and 912 patients/year who are potentially put at risk.

We realize that with any system there will inevitably be some bad outcomes, but is it acceptable to implement a program with a known design flaw that will put a significant number of patients at risk, even on a good day? Although this was one small study, it is consistent with our own experience and observations. And remember that our calculations were based on a small organization that takes only 100 triage calls per day. Imagine the volume in a large organization. The bottom line is that although these may represent just phone calls to many, the person on the other end of the phone is somebody's Somebody, and they are counting on us to get it right every time.

As disconcerting as those numbers might be, there is a another fundamental problem with clerks front-ending calls. Patients often think they are talking to a nurse. The nurse knows there is a problem when he or she calls the patient back, begins the interview, and the patient asks, "Why am I having to tell you all this? I already told it to the *other* nurse." This is much more than an annoying case of mistaken identity. It is likely that the patient, having told his story to someone presumed to be the nurse, is waiting for a return call after the nurse has "talked to the doctor." When the patient receives a call requiring him to retell his story, he may be cooking, driving, napping, or otherwise multitasked and distracted, and thus provide an incomplete history. In other words, once the patient has told his story, the chances of him telling it again in full detail are diminished. The end result is that the nurse may be making decisions based on potentially incomplete information.

The approach in the United States is mixed, with some call centers and doctors' offices utilizing clerical personnel in the initial intake role, and others recognizing the value of using only RNs to front-end and manage calls. In the previously cited study,[6] the impetus was to find a more cost-effective way to manage patients over the telephone. While cost effectiveness is a worthy goal, we must safeguard our patients, assuring that cost-containment measures do not impair patient safety. In summary, programs that utilize clerical personnel to front-end calls potentially put the patient, the organization, and the nurse at risk.

Message Taking by Answering Services

Many after-hours call centers and some doctors' offices utilize answering services to take messages and relay them to the telephone triage nurse or the physician. Although one might anticipate the same problems with an answering service that we have discussed with clerical front-end staff, the complaints about inaccuracy in this process are less frequent. Perhaps it's because the patient is aware he is talking to an answering service rather than to the doctor's "nurse." However, at least one study demonstrated problems with the answering service that resulted in bad outcomes. In this particular study, when parents placed calls to the pediatrician through the answering service, the service personnel asked the parents if they thought their problem was bad enough that it needed immediate contact with the doctor.[7] Of note, when asked, a significant number of callers opted out. When reviewed by physicians, 50% of all calls not referred to the doctor represented a potential emergency. In another study where calls were handled by answering service personnel, "one fourth of patients whose after-hours phone call was not forwarded to the on-call physician suffered ongoing pain and discomfort" (p. 440).[8] Obviously, if a telephone triage program uses an answering service, there must be proper training of personnel and control over what is said to the patient. Additionally, these studies point out that callers are not always able to accurately identify the severity of their problem, thus supporting the value of telephone triage by RNs.

Voice Mail

In the health care setting, we must be very careful with our use of voice mail. Not only are there patient confidentiality issues at stake, but there are patient safety issues as well. While most of us have voice mail, it becomes a problem when a patient can call and leave a symptom-based message in the nurse's mailbox. This might occur if someone transfers a patient call to your phone when you are out of the office. Or if you take calls live, and two calls come in at once, one of them could be routed to voice mail. And nurses may be inviting this potential disaster by providing patients with their direct telephone numbers. The potential danger associated with voice mail is compounded when patients leave messages after hours or over the weekend, when the phone is not monitored for extended periods of time.

Many of us have experienced firsthand the "red light terror" of knowing something is waiting for us on voice mail but not knowing what it is. Many nurses spend a good deal of time transcribing messages from their voice mail and then have very little time to return those calls. Calls are best handled promptly, ideally by a live person. However, if patients are allowed to leave voice mail messages, the following script is recommended:

- Do not leave an urgent message on this line as it is only checked periodically.
- We will call you back (provide realistic expectations when patient may expect return call).
- If you don't hear from us by then, please call us back.
- If your call can't wait, you may speak to someone now by (pressing or dialing a number).

Patients should be encouraged to call again if they do not receive a return call by the time expected. Numbers do get transposed, cell phone transmission can be interrupted, and many of us have gotten calls from a patient who requests a return call but does not leave a name or phone number. Finally, we must be tolerant and realize that not every call a patient considers urgent would represent a medical emergency to us. Patients have legitimate social reasons why their calls can't wait such as they can only access their phone at work during their break, or they're on a layover at an airport. This topic was addressed in Chapter 3. We are not walking in our patient's moccasins, so patience and the Golden Rule are key.

Call Intake by Telephone Triage Nurses

In making a policy decision regarding whether to have the nurses return calls so that patients don't have to wait on "hold" to talk to a nurse, or for nurses to take them "live," it is helpful to consider the advantages and disadvantages of each. Many organizations use a call-back policy so the patient doesn't have to remain on "hold." There are multiple variations of this arrangement, including clerks taking messages as described previously, having the patient use the touch-tone pad to place themselves in an electronic queue for a call back, or allowing the patient to leave a message on voice mail. Our motives are good in trying to provide a patient-friendly service that doesn't necessitate the patient holding for an extended period of time. However, with such a system, the minuses outweigh the plusses. The overall inefficiency of the processes described often results in an unnecessary waste of time and potentially decreases quality of care.

Consider the following examples, and the inefficient use of time associated with patient call backs.

- A frequent complaint of telephone triage nurses is that their "front-end personnel" fail to confirm or obtain the proper number for the nurse to return the call and a good deal of time is wasted in trying to identify a valid contact number.
- Another frustration is that patients often can't be reached at the number provided. And, even if they can be reached, it occasionally takes multiple calls to contact them.
- Then, once we finally get the patient on the phone, there is often additional time spent in allowing the patient time to collect his or her thoughts. As pointed out previously, this call-back process may interfere with the patient's ability to give a thorough history because of distractions at the time the call is received from the nurse.
- Additionally, we are asking patients to be tethered to their telephone until we call back at our convenience rather than theirs. They can't hop in the shower, walk to the mailbox, or even vacuum the floor for fear of not hearing the phone ring. Returning

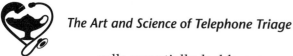

calls essentially holds many patients "hostage" until the call is returned and their problem is resolved.

Two final points are worth mentioning regarding the amount of time wasted in returning calls. First, the very process of determining whom to call first is a time-consuming process, usually requiring the nurse to review each message to determine the highest priority call. And then upon conclusion of that call, the nurse must go through the entire process again to identify the next highest priority. And so on and so on, with the nurse often having to review each note several times.

The second time-consuming activity is that the nurse often feels compelled to review the patient's record, at least as it relates to the chief complaint, prior to calling the patient back, so the nurse will feel somewhat informed when speaking with the patient. However, given that we're discussing a *triage* function and not patient management at this point, many problems can be triaged without review of the patient's record. If review of the record turns out to be necessary, the nurse can take time to review it with the patient on the telephone.

Consider the following example.

A triage nurse in a university clinic was scrolling through her messages and ran across one that said "chest pain." She reviewed the patient's record, noting that he had recently had a full cardiac work-up including a stress test, an echocardiogram, and a cardiac catheterization. All studies had been normal. After a rather lengthy chart review, the nurse called the patient only to learn that instead of "chest pain," the patient was experiencing musculoskeletal pain in his thorax, which he had referred to as his "chest."

Two problems are evident in this story. First, if a patient is experiencing "chest pain," the RN should return that call promptly, evaluating the urgency of the situation before reviewing the patient's record. Second, in this particular case, the RN spent a good deal of time reviewing elements of the record unrelated to the patient's chief complaint.

All things considered, it is better if telephone triage nurses take calls live, allowing the patient to remain on hold until the nurse answers. This is usually the safest and most efficient approach with the added benefit of using the hold time, if any, for relevant patient education announcements instead of music. It is important to recognize that often, in our efforts to be "patient friendly," we may be negatively impacting efficiency, and perhaps even patient safety.

To Have (the Nurse Now) or to Hold? Using logic and observation, we can identify many advantages to having nurses front-end their own calls, taking them live. We believe strongly that this is the best approach for a variety of reasons previously described. However, the question of whether patients prefer to hold or leave a message for a call return has not been studied. This probably varies from population to population. If the patient's history with your practice is that you call him or her back promptly, the patient might feel comfortable leaving a message. If call return is inconsistent or otherwise a problem in your practice, it is likely that the patient would rather devote a few minutes to being on hold than to wait all day by the phone for a return call that may or may not come. If the decision in your organization is to require patients to leave messages, two policies should be developed.

First, when the patient starts sharing information, the message taker should interrupt the patient, saying, "I'm not a nurse, and the nurse will want to hear all of this from you. So rather than having to tell your story twice, please save it for the nurse."

Second, the organization should develop a policy for how

quickly calls are returned, tempering the desired goal with reality. In other words, it is important to designate a time frame that is both achievable and safe. For example, don't tell or otherwise give the patient the impression that the nurse will call "right back." That is usually not achievable and thus sets up unreasonable expectations and may lead to frustration and disappointment. On the other hand, your policy must also be safe. For example, at a minimum, all symptom-based calls must be returned (or at least attempted) prior to the end of the day. It is risky and thus poor practice to delay evaluation of symptom-based calls until the next day. One exception to this rule might be a policy specifying that calls taken close to closing time will not be returned until the following day, but even this approach is fraught with potential risk.

Once this call-back policy is developed, it should be communicated to the patient. However, to make this approach acceptable, there is one other caveat. In communicating the call-back expectation to the patient, whether advising a return call later today under normal circumstances, or tomorrow for calls received late in the day, the message taker must ask, "Can it wait that long?" If the patient says "no," that call should be put directly through to a nurse or returned as soon as possible.

This is actually a more reasonable and safer approach than the previously described "red flag" lists in the hands of a non-RN. The clerk is usually a lay person; the patient is usually a lay person. Who is in a better position to know how long the patient can wait to talk to a nurse? The patient! While the clerk has some medical knowledge from experience in the health care arena, the patient has specific information about her concerns, how she feels, and what her needs are. Refer back to the call about the child with tonsillitis whose mother was concerned about his breathing (see Chapter 12). That call came at 4:00 p.m. and wasn't returned until almost 5:00 p.m. If the mother had been told, "The nurse will call you back around 5:00. Can it wait that long?" the mother would surely have said "No." The purpose of her call was to see if she should bring him back in for evaluation. Had that child been seen that afternoon, it is more than likely he would still be alive.

At this point, many readers probably believe that asking callers if they could wait 2 hours (or as specified by policy) for a call return would be unrealistic, with every patient saying "No, it can't wait that long." However, experience has shown that most patients are generally respectful of the nurse's time and will be willing to wait a specified length of time, providing the nurse is reliable in meeting that expectation.

Finally, it is important to realize that sometimes it can't "wait that long" because, for example, the patient is calling during a lunch break and can't receive calls during work. The "Can it wait that long?" rule will increase the safety of care delivered and improve patient satisfaction, but as discussed previously, the nurse must realize and tolerate the fact that patients will occasionally say it can't wait because of social, not health issues.

Suzanne, a single mother of three, underwent surgery for a congenital mitral valve prolapse when she was 8 years old. Because of an atrial-septal defect, she also had a pacemaker and was under the care of cardiologist. Now, at 45, she had developed an unexpected cough, which she attributed to allergies or exposure to chemicals at work. Over the next few days she developed progressive fatigue, insomnia (probably due to orthnopnea and/or nocturia), and dyspnea on exertion, leaving her too tired at the end of the day to do her shopping and cook dinner. It occurred to her that she should call her doctor's office, but by then, they were closed, so she resolved to call the next day. Working in a factory, she wasn't able to access the telephone at work outside of her lunch hour and two 15-minute breaks. She called during her morning break, requesting a call back during lunch.

She waited through her lunch but received no call. That night, still sick and having talked to no one, she decided to call again tomorrow. When she called the next morning, she was told, "The nurse got your note and she called you back yesterday, but you weren't home." Suzanne patiently explained that she was at work and was only able to accept calls from 12:00-1:00. She once again gave them the number of her cell phone and waited for the return call during lunch. By 12:50, fearing she was going to miss the nurse's call again, she called the office, only to reach the answering service, and left a message including the time of her afternoon break. Again, she didn't get a call at work, but that night, on her answering machine at home, there was a message from the nurse that she had called Suzanne twice; once at home and once on her cell phone and there was no answer. The nurse instructed her to call the office again tomorrow if she still needed to talk to them.

This went on for several days; Suzanne trying to reach her doctor's office the only time and way she could and the office returning her calls at inopportune times or to the wrong number. It was a case of phone tag in the worst degree. Eventually, having never talked with her doctor's office, Suzanne, in congestive heart failure (CHF), decompensated and presented to the ED in pulmonary edema. Eight diuresed liters of fluid later, she was discharged home with instructions to call if she gained more than 2 pounds overnight or 5 pounds in a week. Ten days later, she noted a 2 pound weight gain and called her doctor's office, staying home from work until her call was returned. She missed a half day of work waiting for a return call, but by talking to the nurse, she was able to double her Lasix® and remain at home in compensated CHF.

The lesson in this story is clear. We need to develop ways for patients to access a nurse if they, like Suzanne, face challenges in being available on *our* schedule. Perhaps we should make efforts to be available on *theirs*.

We have discussed various methods for patients to access a triage nurse, concluding that having nurses taking the calls directly, without clerical personnel or voice mail interceding, is the preferable mode, being safe, efficient, and generally patient friendly. Assuming we're all on the same page with that conclusion, let's now turn our attention to how an organization can get those calls into the hands of the nurse as expeditiously and safely as possible.

Call Routing: Getting the Calls into the Right Hands

Experience shows that a call routing system developed to complement the call types your organization receives can improve efficiency and patient safety. This can be accomplished by developing a menu, which is either electronic and accessed directly by the caller or utilized verbally by a switchboard operator. The objective of such a system is to allow the caller to route his or her own call based on a menu developed to meet the needs of patients and staff.

As a precursor to developing this menu, it is important to identify call types (through your workload analysis) and determine who in your organization is best equipped to handle each type. For example, calls for routine appointments (e.g., physicals and scheduled follow-ups), billing questions, and follow-up on referral paperwork should be handled by non-clinical personnel. Conversely, clinical calls should be delivered into the hands of the most appropriate and least-expensive person who can safely and legally handle the job. For example, in some organizations, pharmacists manage prescription renewals, so these types of calls might be forwarded to the pharmacy. Alternatively, clerical personnel, unlicensed assistive personnel, or LPNs or LVNs might best handle these calls. Requests for test results could be routed directly to designated personnel, with results being shared with the patient as previously authorized, based on review by a physician or

RN. If this review has not yet taken place, the request could be conveyed to the provider or RN who would review the results and make a determination of who is best equipped to call the patient with those results. For example, some test results could be reported by medical assistants, under the direction of a physician; others should be reported by LPNs or LVNs because the patient might have questions the nurse would be able to answer; or perhaps, because complex teaching or assessment is anticipated, the call might best be returned by an RN. And, of course, there are some results that should be disclosed only by the provider. Finally, calls requiring assessment, such as requests for same-day appointments or "sick calls," should be handled by the telephone triage nurse. There will be occasions when the patient's primary or team nurse (the nurse in the clinic) should also get involved in patient calls, but ideally, those will primarily be outbound calls, initiated by the RN, at his or her convenience.

During a telephone triage consultation at a large teaching facility, calls were placed to various clinics during the noon hour for the purpose of evaluating the organization's methods of call intake. In one instance, an RN answered the phone frantically, "This is Darlene. How can I help you?" The consultant explained who she was and why she was calling, to which the nurse replied, "Oh gosh! I can't talk to you now. I'm on a tight deadline, and I have to get a report to the CEO by 1:00."

While it was perfectly acceptable for the nurse to not talk with the consultant, what if the caller had been a patient who required a few minutes of the nurse's undivided attention? Both the nurse and the patient would have been in trouble. This is just one example of why attention must be given to call routing. Figure 1 illustrates the conceptual model for the previously described method of call routing. Please notice that while the primary nurse is in the loop on all clinical calls, he or she is not responsible for fielding any patient calls on demand. The primary nurse either gets notes for his or her information only, or if an action is necessary, it can be done at his or her convenience, knowing that any urgent problems have already been addressed by the triage nurse.

Figure 1.
Care Delivery Model (Call Flow)

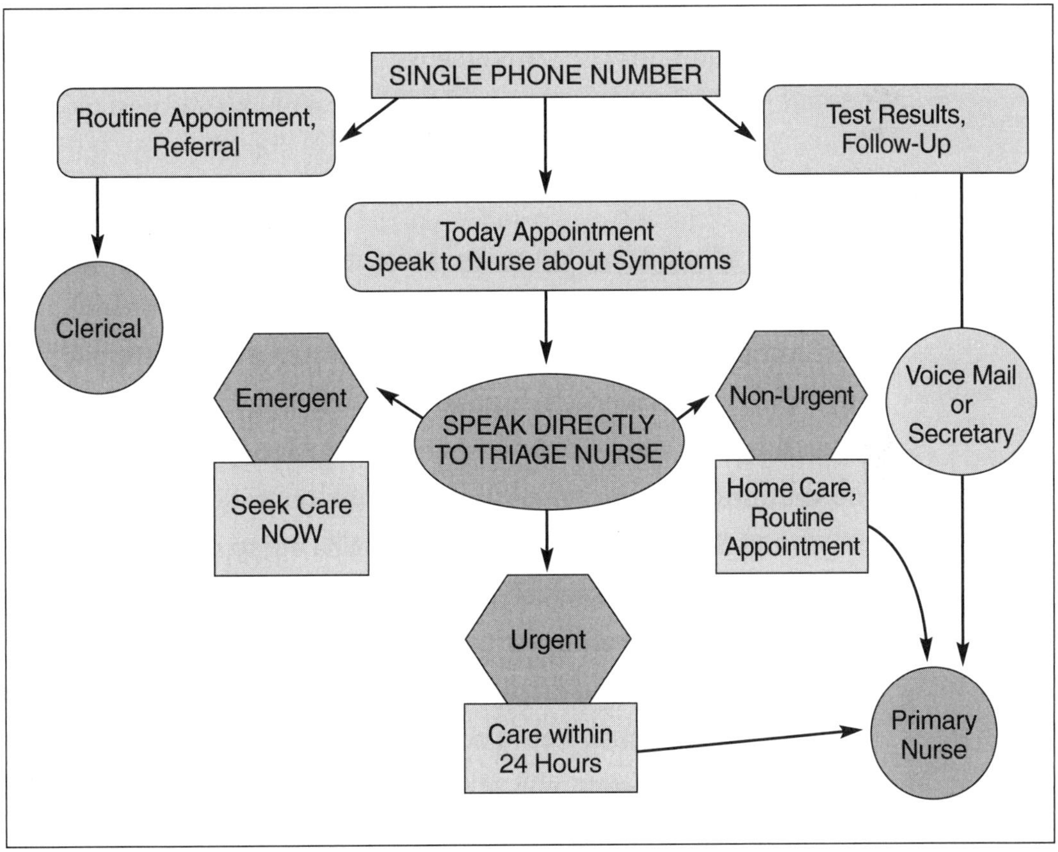

Menu Development

In the context of the preceding discussion, let's turn our attention to development of a telephone menu or tree that would support ideal call routing. As mentioned previously, design of this menu should be based on the findings of your workload analysis. The following menu and discussion are offered as a starting point for consideration of the benefits of such a system. While in many settings it is ideal to design this menu electronically (so that patients self-route their calls), the same menu could be utilized by an operator or clerk specially trained in its application. If using a person to route the calls instead of an electronic menu, it is important to note that instead of answering the phone with "How may I help you," a more effective opening for the person answering the call would be, "How may I direct your call?" At that point, the menu would be used by the operator to match the caller's request with the best option to meet his or her needs.

Organizations often shy away from electronic menus because the prevailing belief is that patients dislike automation and would resent the use of an electronic routing system. Often, when patients express displeasure about an electronic menu, it's not the electronic menu per se that poses the problem. Rather their concerns have more to do with how the menu is designed or utilized. Three types of menu problems often lead to dissatisfaction.

- *Many menus are too long or too "deep."* First, the menu should be as short as possible. One fatal flaw with many doctor's office greetings is that they provide hours of operation, fax number, and directions to the clinic *before* the patient is allowed to hear the routing options. The patient who has to listen to that information every time he or she calls will understandably get aggravated. That type of general information should be a menu option rather than a precursor to the menu. Additionally, the trite comment, "Please listen carefully, as our menu options have recently changed," is of little use and only adds to the length of the greeting. In fact, because this is clearly a machine rather than a human responder, it would be appropriate to take the "pleases" out of the instructions to further shorten the greeting. The menu should be not only short, but also not very deep. Options requiring the patient to drill down endlessly further increase the caller's frustration.

- *Second, most, if not all, options should route the call directly to a live person.* Perhaps one primary reason patients dislike electronic menus is that instead of being a call *routing* mechanism, they become a call *blocking* strategy. Menu options that end in voice mail should be used sparingly.

One organization identified a significant problem with their menu and call routing. In reviewing their existing system, it was noted that every single option went to someone's voice mail with greetings as uninformative as "Hi. This is Susan. Leave a message and I'll get back with you as soon as possible." There was no indication of who Susan was or when "as soon as possible" might be. Had she just stepped away from her desk, was she only a part-time worker, or was she on vacation? And if callers pressed "0," anticipating that it would take them to an operator, the system would hang up on them! This system was anything but customer friendly and was probably rarely helpful, only adding to the caller's frustration.

This is an example of a menu that was being used as a repository for messages left by callers but only if they followed the "rules." The message delivered by this system was one of lack of concern for the patient. Woe to those who actually needed to speak with someone promptly.

- *The third design flaw that will hopefully improve over time is the interactive voice response (IVR) type menu.* Clearly, some are better than others. But when a machine doesn't understand the word "no," imagine the caller's frustration! Also, many of the IVR systems are sensitive to background noises such as overhead pages and coughing, so in some settings, for some individuals, IVR poses an unnecessary and possibly insurmountable challenge.

We will continue with our discussion of call routing, based on the belief that callers will cope with and perhaps even appreciate a well-designed menu. The following outline illustrates a menu that can be used as a starting point for an organization wishing to streamline its call routing and handling and to "get the right mail into the right hands." The recommended menu is listed below followed by a discussion of each option.

You have reached Your Family Health Care Clinic.
If this is an emergency, hang up and dial 911.

- If you are a health care professional or a patient returning our call, press 1.
- If you wish to make, cancel, or change a routine appointment, press 2.
- If you are seeking test results or a prescription refill, press 3.
  - For test results, press 1*.
  - For prescription refills, press 2*.
- If you have a billing or referral issue, press 4.
  - For billing, press 1*.
  - For referrals, press 2*.
- If you would like to make a today appointment or speak with a nurse about symptoms, press 5.
- For fax number, hours of operation, or directions to the clinic, press 6.
- All other callers, or to speak to an operator, press 0.

*(Sub-menus are optional.)

Let's start with a few general comments about the menu. First, it is short. An effort should be made to limit the number of primary and secondary options so the caller doesn't feel like he or she is on the phone, endlessly pressing numbers.

If a specific clerk is responsible for two or more functions (such as test results, refills, and billing questions), make them one option. There is no benefit in listing several options that all go to the same individual, unless your system is sophisticated enough to alert the agent to the reason for the call.

Although an option to speak to the nurse is provided, it is at the bottom of the list, not the top, allowing the patient to select a different option, prior to getting to #5. Placing the "nurse" option too high in the menu will entice callers to access the nurse prematurely when other options might be more appropriate.

Give deliberate thought to who the appropriate level of personnel is to handle each call type. It is important to match the skill of the employee with the complexity of the function. Be certain that all personnel are familiar with the menu, its intent, and how to screen and reroute calls if necessary.

Now we will describe and discuss each previously suggested menu option.

☐ ***"If this is an emergency, hang up and dial 911."***

While this statement is certainly a standard in the industry, it might be of little benefit to most patients because they often don't know whether their problem is an emergency or not; that's why they are calling the clinic or call center. Some organizations have chosen instead to provide the caller with an option (such as # or *) to speak to a nurse now *(e.g., "If this is an emergency or you need to speak to a nurse immediately, press #")*. Some staff shudder at the thought of this option, concerned about excessive or inappropriate use. However, experience has shown that patients are usually respectful of the nurse's time and won't use that option unless, in their opinion, they do have an immediate need.

☐ ***"If you are a health care professional or a patient returning our call, press 1."***

This choice is offered as the first option because these are two categories of callers with whom we definitely don't want to play "telephone tag." Please note the term "health care professional" is used instead of the more traditional "doctor or doctor's representative." This is because there are myriad health care professionals who have reason to call a health care organization including home health nurses, hospital nurses, pharmacists, various types of therapists, and other health care providers or institutions. These calls should be routed to a secretary who is able to interview the caller, find out who he is, what he wants, and get him into the hands of someone who can handle the call promptly, even if it necessitates getting up out of her chair and finding someone to take the call.

☐ ***"If you wish to make, cancel, or change a routine appointment, press 2."***

These callers should be routed to an appointment clerk who has been trained to screen the caller and recognize the difference between a "routine" appointment (such as a wellness check or a routine follow-up) and a symptom-based call, which should be transferred to the triage nurse for assessment and disposition. Also, if a patient is canceling or changing an appointment, the clerk should find out why. If it's because the patient is "too sick to come in," he or she should be triaged.

☐ ***"If you are seeking test results or a prescription refill, press 3."***

This option might have a short sub-menu, separating requests for test results from prescription refill calls, but this is only necessary if these call types are managed by different personnel. For example, requests for test results could be routed to a voice mail, while as previously suggested, requests for prescription refills might be routed to the pharmacy. However, if a clerk or LPN is handling both of these, all calls in this category should go directly to that individual. And this category of patient must always be screened to identify the presence of any symptoms that would require transfer to the triage nurse. For example, if a patient is requesting the results of her Pap smear, it is appropriate to pose the question, "Are you having any symptoms?" If the patient responds to the affirmative, such as, "Yes, I'm having a vaginal discharge," the patient should be redirected to the triage nurse. Likewise, patients requesting prescription refills should also be screened for acute symptoms. Perhaps the patient is requesting a refill to treat a symptom-based problem, such as a refill on nitroglycerine for a patient who has run out because he's "taken them all and they're not working." Another example might be a patient who, instead of calling in advance, has run out of his clonidine, and abrupt discontinuation has resulted in undesirable effects. A final example might be a request for a refill on a PRN antihistamine by a patient who has self-diagnosed his sinus infection as "allergies." These calls must be screened, and if symptoms exist, the caller should be redirected to the triage nurse. Thus, this is an ideal role for an LPN or LVN who can recognize high-risk situations and calls requiring triage that should be redirected to the triage RN.

☐ ***"If you have a billing or referral issue, press 4."***

This category of calls might best be directed to a staff member who can deal with or properly route non-clinical questions. Because of the huge variety of non-clinical issues for which patients might need to contact the office, it is usually difficult to combine these calls into a general category. For example "referral" questions might be of three different types.

- First, with some health plans, if a patient visits an ED or UCC, she needs what is commonly referred to as a "retro-referral," which authorizes the visit after the fact, assuring insurance coverage. In some settings, because of the clinical judgment necessary in this process, these requests might need to be handled by a nurse but are generally non-urgent, thus not requiring the involvement of the triage nurse.

- A second type of referral might be "you told me you were processing the paperwork for my MRI, but they say they haven't received it yet." These types of referrals can usually be handled by a referral specialist who is not an RN.

- Finally, there is the potential for a referral request "because my son has an ear infection *again,* and I want to take him to an ENT doctor." Of course, this type of "referral" request should be triaged.

☐ ***"If you would like to make a today appointment or speak with a nurse about symptoms, press 5."***

This category is for patients who are presumably sick or in need of health education and thus must be assessed by an RN. Again, both the patient and the staff must understand that the purpose of speaking with a triage nurse prior to receiving an appointment isn't because the nurse is trying to keep the gate closed. Quite the contrary; the gate is wide open, but the triage nurse will help the patient decide when and how to access the appropriate level of care.

☐ ***For fax number, hours of operation or directions to the clinic, press 6.***

This information can be helpful and appreciated if it is an option and not the preface of every greeting as previously described.

☐ ***For all other callers, or to speak to an operator, press 0.***

As discussed previously, "0" should be the universal sign for "I want to talk to somebody now." Having the option to speak with a live person is essential for callers who might be hearing impaired, elderly, or otherwise unwilling or unable to deal with the electronic menu.

Strategic call routing allows the primary or team nurse to remain informed of what is going on with the patient, but relieves the nurse of the arduous task of being a slave to the telephone.

POLICY DEVELOPMENT

Policy development is an essential element of formalized telephone triage (see Chapter 14). Policies necessary to support your telephone triage practice have been discussed throughout this book, and an outline for a policy manual is offered in Appendix B. Formalized policies encourage clear communication, standardization within the organization, consistency among personnel, and compliance with accreditation and regulatory standards.

Decision support tools and documation templates are two critical areas of telephone triage program design that fall under the heading of "policies," but both are clinical tools. In other words, they represent much more than a policy and thus deserve special discussion.

Selecting Decision Support Tools

Use of protocols has been discussed at length throughout this book. However, here, we will focus on the necessary selection and approval process.

Types of Decision Support Tools. Decision support tools are available as software programs, Web-based programs, and as paper manuals. It is also possible for organizations to develop their own resources. Each type of format has advantages and disadvantages. Although most protocols follow the same "top-down" approach (most serious to least serious), the actual layout varies considerably. Furthermore, the thought process encouraged by the format of each set also varies somewhat, based on the orientation of the author; some protocols are authored by nurses, and others are written by physicians. Computerized programs have tracking and reporting capabilities that are incorporated into the software. Most electronic (computerized) protocols require the nurse to engage in sequential history taking and decision making, progressing through the decision support tool step by step. In using decision support software, nurses must be cautious of going into "rote" mode, following the protocol without enlisting critical thinking and clinical judgment. Paper protocols, on the other hand, provide lists of signs and symptoms to consider and recommend dispositions but rely more fully on the nurse to apply critical thinking to the situation and administer the protocol as indicated for each patient. However, regardless of the format used, the nurse must consistently perform an adequate assessment, utilize critical thinking, and individualize care as appropriate for each patient.

Triage Criteria vs. Treatment Recommendations. It is important to distinguish between triage criteria, which provide the basis for developing decision support tools, and treatment recommendations, which suggest or direct specific medications or other interventions that might otherwise require a physician's order. Treatment criteria (such as OTC medications) might be an integral part of the commercial protocols, or they might be added to the decision support tools as a customized, practice-specific enhancement according to the preferences and practices of the physicians. These treatment criteria may vary from clinic to clinic and provider to provider. It is important to keep in mind, however, that excessive variation in the treatment protocols presents potential conflicts for the telephone triage nurses and must be minimized. For example, if Dr. A treats fever with acetaminophen and Dr. B prefers to use ibuprofen, which drug does the nurse use when Dr. A is covering for Dr. B? It is desirable, to the fullest extent possible, for the organization to standardize basic treatment options for the sake of clarity and consistency.

Medical Approval. Protocol selection should be a committee effort with approval of content by both the medical and nursing staff. However, the format and layout should be the decision of the nurses who will be using them. Although medical direction and approval of triage protocols is desirable (and required by some boards of nursing), the triage criteria utilized should be mutually acceptable to both the medical staff and nursing staff. To facilitate adoption and use, they must be in a format that the nurse finds both practical and helpful. In gaining medical approval of decision support tools, requesting review of perhaps the five most common protocols first, followed by subsequent review of other small quantities, is less overwhelming for the medical staff than requesting approval of an entire set all at once. Although it is generally impossible to get unanimous agreement in organizations with several physicians, consensus can usually be achieved, with approval granted by the medical director and the chief nurse executive.

Routine Review and Approval. Once approved, the protocols should be reviewed and re-approved at regular intervals, usually defined by various standards as being annual or biannual. Maintenance of a "decision support tool approval task force" is a good idea, with one-twelfth of the protocols being reviewed each month, keeping the workload at a manageable level. Finally, once a set has been selected, the protocols chosen should be used consistently across the organization, regardless of the specialty or the provider. For example, the approved headache protocol should be available and used in each of the clinics in a multi-specialty practice. Careful attention to selection and approval of universally applicable decision support tools, with or without customization, is an important element of any formalized telephone triage program.

In selecting protocols, here are the elements you might want to look for.

- They should be perceived as user-friendly by your nurses and manageable in size, whether paper or electronic. Using them should not be a chore, or the nurses won't use them.

- Consider the orientation of the author(s). Are they written by nurses or physicians? Who were the reviewers? Keep in mind that the thought processes of physicians and nurses are (and should be) somewhat different. However, because telephone triage necessitates the diagnostic thinking referenced previously, perhaps the perspective of a physician or nurse practitioner would be helpful, given that diagnostic reasoning is not a skill formally taught in basic nursing education. At a minimum, however, they should utilize the nursing process and encourage a systematic assessment.

- Do the decision support tools have a proven track record? Are they flexible? Can they be customized for your organization and your community whether by reprogramming the software or making changes in the manual?

- They should be symptom-based and comprehensive, covering adult, OB/GYN, and pediatrics (if applicable), even if yours is a specialty clinic.

- If computerized, do they allow narrative documentation and support documentation of pertinent negatives?

- It's ideal if they are available both on paper and electronically. Some nurses prefer one format or the other, but even if you use electronic protocols, you will need a "hard copy" to use if your computer system goes down.

- You might find it helpful if they include additional topic information on each protocol, supplementing knowledge for the nurse.

- Flexibility in dispositions is best. "Today" or "within 24 hours" may prove to be more useful than those that give specific time frames and specify where to be seen. The nurse needs "wiggle room" to exercise nursing judgment, considering specific circumstances, such as patient and organizational resources, as well as patient preference, in making a disposition that's right for each individual patient.

- Protocols should promote (rather than discourage) critical thinking. Although they should be symptom based (rather than based on a medical diagnosis), it's helpful if they mention disease processes that should be considered or ruled out, rather than relying exclusively on symptoms to direct the disposition.

Development of a Documentation Tool

The documentation tool should include both administrative and clinical components. Ideally, the documentation tool should be designed in such a manner that it serves as a memory guide and provides structure to nurses during the encounter. The medical record should include such elements as:

- Demographic and identifying information
- General patient information such as history, including a history of diabetes or immunosuppression; medications and allergies; reproductive status and last menstrual period; and habits such as tobacco, alcohol, and drug use
- Patient assessment data (such as POSHPATE and TICOSMO described in Chapter 10)
- The triage diagnosis should express the level of urgency (emergent, urgent, or non-urgent), identify the primary problem (ideally expressed as a symptom or symptoms), and include additional confounding factors (such as lack of transportation or patient motivation). For example, a complete triage diagnosis might be: non-urgent fever, knowledge deficit, patient requesting antibiotics.
- A plan, which includes the disposition specifying where, when, and how, the patient will seek treatment (e.g., if the patient is being transported by ambulance or if another adult will drive); or if home care is provided, specifically what is advised
- Any interventions such as patient education, advice, or calling report to the referral facility, with special attention to continuity of care
- A method for evaluating the effectiveness of the plan and anticipated interventions including patient call-back instructions and nurse follow-up if indicated

Additionally, specific closing statements are customarily documented, such as "patient verbalizes understanding," "patient expresses intent to comply," "patient verbalizes comfort with the plan of care," and "patient denies other questions or concerns." As discussed previously, documentation should be thorough, including all pertinent positives and negatives, so adequate space to record clinical information should be provided. In other words, narrative fields should be available for elaboration by the nurse to provide adequate documentation to paint a complete picture.

A final word of caution is given to organizations that rely on decision support tools to supplement documentation. A specific concern is the assumption that protocol elements not selected represent indirect documentation of pertinent negatives. In other words, some organizations have policies that encourage the nurse to select the "first positive response" on the list and then document (or infer) that "all previous protocol questions negative." The problem with this approach is two-fold. Primarily, in addition to being a legal document, the medical record is first and foremost a communication tool. Comments such as these leave the reader wondering about the content of "all previous protocol questions." Additionally, the medical record is where the nurse indicates critical thinking, often reflected by documentation of pertinent positives and negatives. If a nurse documents "chest pain" but doesn't comment on nausea, shortness of breath, and diaphoresis, how does the reader, whether colleague or attorney, know whether or not the nurse ever considered the significance of those pertinent findings? Direct documentation of both pertinent positives and negatives is an important element of any triage note.

CHANGE IMPLEMENTATION

While this section is not intended to be an exhaustive discussion regarding change implementation, it is hoped that these practical suggestions will help the reader who is interested in implementing some of the suggestions in this book within his or her organization. By now, hopefully, the reader feels validated and positive about his or her practice. However, it would certainly be possible at this point to feel a little overwhelmed, especially if you are interested in implementing change. So, here are some words of encouragement and suggestions for how to proceed.

- First, every suggestion in this chapter has been successfully implemented in an actual telephone triage setting. If the suggestions seem insurmountable, it may be because you are presently in a broken system and some policy and practice adjustments might need to be made before you can effectively make significant changes. For example, if you're working in a setting where RNs and unlicensed personnel are utilized interchangeably, perhaps role differentiation is a good place to start. If you're in a good system, but your nurses haven't been adequately trained, that might be your starting point. In other words, the ground will need to be fertile before the seeds will grow, but often a bit of tilling must come first.

- Sometimes, timing is everything. But if change is going to occur, *someone* has to start the ball rolling. Maybe that someone is *you*. And often, there's no time like the present.

- Instead of approaching the project with the attitude that "we're doing everything wrong," the change ahead of you will go more smoothly and be better accepted if you regard the things you've learned in this book as opportunities for improvement. You are more likely to be successful if you are positive; you should be able to identify multiple strategies to improve the care you deliver. And who can argue that they aren't interested in "opportunities" or "improvement?"

- If you are not in a formal management position, you can still be a change agent. In fact, sometimes change works best when it begins as a grassroots effort. And a word to the RNs reading this book. You are a leader. Nursing must be defined by nurses, not others. You have a professional responsibility to design, implement, and administer nursing services delivered under your direction. If you are the only nurse in your practice, you are the chief nurse executive, and if change is needed in the way nursing services are managed and delivered in your setting, it is your responsibility to get it done.

- Change will usually go more smoothly if the recommended changes are consistent with the organization's goals and objectives. A well-designed telephone triage program can accomplish many things that may be in line with organizational initiatives. For example, to secure leadership buy-in, perhaps you need to focus on the cost-effectiveness of telephone triage. Perhaps your primary selling point will be patient satisfaction or improved quality of care. Well-designed telephone triage programs will accomplish these goals.[9,10] Or perhaps your best strategy will be to approach desired change as a risk management strategy. But keep in mind that while "risk" may get management's attention, some administrators and physicians are risk-tolerant and may take the stance, "We haven't had a bad outcome yet. If it's not broken, let's not try to fix it." If that is your situation, rather than becoming discouraged, realize that's what risk management is all about. Do you have a $200 deductible on your car insurance or $1,000? If your deductible is $200, you're essentially betting you're going to have a wreck. However, if you have a $1,000 deductible, evidently you're betting you won't. We all engage in risk management to a certain extent. And we realize that, working in the health care industry, all of our outcomes are not going to be good ones. If we hadn't been able to come to grips with that reality, we would have left nursing or health care a long time ago. However, even though we know intellectually that we will have some bad outcomes, the approach we hope to engender is "Not on my watch!" We must always remember that the patient on the other end of the phone is somebody's Somebody. We must value, assist, and respect callers as patients, customers, and our fellows. Always be guided by the Golden Rule.

- Remember, even with good leadership support, change takes time. This process might be a little bit of three steps forward and two steps back. But even if you're only making baby steps, if you're persistent, you'll eventually get to where you're going. We're all familiar with the riddle, "How do you eat an elephant?" Of course, the answer is "One bite at a time." And many reading this book have a plate full of elephant, but if you keep plodding, you'll surely reach your goal.

Telephone Triage Steering Committee

It is helpful for organizations planning to implement change in their telephone triage services to form a telephone triage steering committee. "Having an organization-wide steering committee will enhance buy-in; facilitate multilevel, interdepartmental problem solving; and provide a vehicle for exploration of standardization and possibly eventually centralization of telephone triage services within the organization" (p. 4).[2] The following is a suggested list of committee members, based on previous experience with various organizations, both large and small.

- *Chief nurse executive (CNE).* The CNE should be involved from the outset and be actively involved throughout the process. The CNE will understand and have a good grasp on important professional issues. The CNE will also understand the "big picture" and be in a position to influence organizational change as appropriate and necessary.

- *Telephone triage nurse manager.* If your organization intends to develop a formal program, it is a good idea to hire a nurse manager to oversee this process. Policies will need to be developed, decision support tools selected, training and quality assurance programs designed, and staff hiring processes initiated. Additionally, logistic concerns such as physical space, furnishings, computers, and telephones will need to be addressed and coordinated. In some organizations, especially in the past, non-nurses have been appointed as call center or telephone triage managers. When the focus was on call center efficiencies or marketing, it seemed to make sense to hire managers with non-medical call center experience or with marketing backgrounds. However, recognition that telephone triage is professional nursing practice punctuates the advantages if the policymaker and manager is an RN.

- *Telephone triage nurses.* If you plan to implement telephone triage formally in your organization, it is a good idea to provide education to personnel at all levels about the practice of telephone triage. Often, after nurses understand the value and challenge associated with this form of nursing, they are anxious to practice as telephone triage nurses. These positions are often highly coveted, and in many organizations, little turnover is experienced. Posting telephone triage positions and allowing nurses to apply for them from within is a good strategy to support staff growth, reward excellence in practice, and staff your department with nurses who have internal knowledge of your organization. In military facilities, it is recommended that at least 75% of the telephone triage staff be civilian nurses who will not move from base to base, thereby providing stability to the department. Once the staff is selected, the telephone triage nurses should be included in the planning for the department.

- *Non-telephone triage nurses.* Because telephone triage will impact the operations of essentially every nursing department in your organization, it is helpful to have non-telephone triage nurses (both RNs and LPNs or LVNs) on the task force. These individuals can help the other members of the task force "look downstream" to predict how the telephone triage process will integrate with and affect the rest of the organization.

- *Practice administrator, group practice manager, department director.* While the title of this position will vary from organization to organization, the individual you are looking for is probably a middle manager, and sometimes not a nurse. This is the person responsible in the office setting for managing clerical personnel and operational issues such as organizational budgeting, schedule template management, communications, information technology and similar support functions. In the call center setting, this middle manager might be responsible for overall departmental operations, program development, and integrating the call center into the organization.

- *Clerical personnel.* Inclusion of clerical personnel and/or the person who manages them is critical because formalized telephone triage will often precipitate significant changes in the functions of clerical personnel. Additionally, these personnel will generally have a good handle on call volume and other information helpful to program design.

- *Physician champion.* Because of the collaborative nature of nursing and the collegial relationship between the telephone triage nurse and the provider staff, having a physician champion on the task force is extremely helpful. This individual should have respect for nursing and grassroots support from his or her colleagues. This provider would participate in protocol approval and modification as necessary for your setting. He or she would also represent the medical staff to the task force and the telephone triage function to his or her colleagues, enhancing interdisciplinary understanding. This provider should participate in telephone triage quality assurance and be the medical resource for the telephone triage program. Note: Depending upon your organizational structure and culture, it is sometimes helpful for this individual to be a nurse practitioner who can more clearly understand both the nursing and medical perspectives.

- *Patient focus group.* To ensure that any changes will be viewed as positive for your patient population, it is a good idea to include input from a representative patient panel or focus group. Ideally, at least one member of this focus group should be a nurse who receives care from your practice or call center, since nurses who are patients often view care through a lens of nursing values and are less intimidated by the process than lay patients. Examples of appropriate use of this group would be to get feedback on menu design, development of strategies for information dissemination about your new or improved program (such as newsletters, etc.), and general feedback on their telephone triage experiences as patients of your organization.

Blueprint for Program Design

Additionally, if your organization is interested in moving forward in developing or improving your existing services, the following approach is offered to your task force as a blueprint for program design.

- Begin with a risk assessment, based on the information included in this book. Give special attention to staff utilization, protocol use, documentation, and professional practice.

- Develop a vision for your telephone triage service. Here, we don't mean the concise, two-sentence "Vision" that organizations use as a guiding document. We're referring to an actual vision or picture. What does it look like? Do you have a group of RNs sitting in a room together (hopefully with windows), wearing headsets, sitting in their ergonomic chairs, each with a set of decision support tools open on the desk or computer monitor in front of them? Does the quality assurance program utilize peer review and is there routine in-service education such as a journal club brown bag lunch? Are the positions so highly conveted that other nurses in the organization want to transfer into the telephone triage department? Do the physicians respect the judgment of the nurses, capture "teachable moments," and provide regular feedback on interesting cases? Do patients look forward to speaking with their triage nurse when they have a health care concern?

- Identify what changes are needed to make your vision a reality. What are your goals and objectives? Do you need to purchase or upgrade your telephones and computers? Do you need to find physical space? Do you need to select decision support tools? Do you need to educate your staff about telephone triage? Occasionally, education is needed to help the staff identify problems with the status quo so that employees will be motivated to change. However, caution should be exercised to avoid creating dissatisfaction with the current situation too far in advance of the program implementation.

- Develop a list of tasks that must be accomplished, such as development of a quality assurance program, design of a medical record template, selection of protocols, hiring and training of staff, and development of a policy book. You should also give some consideration to internal and external marketing, and provide appropriate education for various groups of stakeholders when the time is right.

- Develop a work group to address each task, naming a group chair and defining the goal of each group. Identify the proper individuals to work on each task.

- Develop a sequence of events. What do you need to do first? Is it to provide education for the key stakeholders? Is it to hire a telephone triage manager? What will you do next and in what order?

- Once the program begins to take shape, it is time to develop a budget and a timeline.

While this is a very basic and rough outline of the steps that might be taken in program design, there are much more exhaustive works on the subject.[10,11] The ideas provided here constitute a set of principles and strategies that have worked in numerous types of settings, both small and large, office and call center, military and civilian. Any efforts at change in your organization must be in line with overall organizational objectives, approved by senior leadership, and planned and implemented in a manner consistent with your organizational culture. The reason this information is provided is to help the reader recognize that change of any scope, small or large, can, and usually must be, approached one bite at a time. Keep the faith! Your goal is worthy, with the payoff being improved patient care and increased staff satisfaction.

RISK MANAGEMENT

In any well-designed program, attention to risk management is essential. Although probably a basic review for most readers, the following information is offered, outlining the elements an attorney must prove in order to establish negligence.

- *Duty.* The nurse has a duty to provide patient care consistent with the standard of care. When a nurse begins talking to a patient on the telephone, that duty has been established.
- *Breach.* The nurse breaches that duty by not meeting the standard of care. The standard of care is defined in legal terms as what any reasonable, prudent nurse would do under the same or similar circumstances.
- *Damages.* Any injury or harm to the patient could be construed as damages.
- *Causation.* The attorney must establish that the nurse's action or failure to act was the cause of the harm to the patient.

Risk Management Principles

Strategies to reduce risk have been interwoven throughout the content of this book. The compilation listed here is not exhaustive, but it provides an inventory of practices that should be considered when developing telephone triage program policies. Futhermore, if used with careful and consistent attention, these measures will significantly decrease the potential for a bad outcome. The best way to control risk is to ensure that high-quality, safe care is delivered. If your focus is on the patient (rather than on "being covered" legally), you will give the best care possible, which is the best risk management strategy of all.

Rules of Thumb

- Consider every call life threatening until proven otherwise.

- If in doubt, err on the side of caution.
- Patients who call more than once for the same problem should be re-evaluated with an open mind and should probably be seen.
- If you don't see it often, you often don't see it – look for zebras.
- Always speak to the patient (or at least listen to him or her breathe, regardless of age or condition) unless he or she is physically absent.

High-Risk Patients

- Extremes of age (the very young and the very old)
- Those with co-morbidities, such as diabetes, immunosuppression, asthma, and other chronic illnesses
- Patients who have recently undergone surgery or other invasive procedures
- Frequent callers, especially those well known to the staff
- Patients with multiple complaints
- Poor historians
- Those who are not present when you talk to the family/caregiver

Red Flags

- Repeat callers (more than once for the same problem)
- Pathognomonic symptoms (e.g., "Worst headache of my life," "Elephant sitting on my chest," "Shades coming over my eyes")
- High-risk symptoms such as lethargy, altered level of consciousness, nuchal rigidity, shortness of breath
- Worse, or different, than usual

- New, unexpected symptoms
- Symptoms inconsistent with the presumed diagnosis
- Symptoms that follow an unexpected course

Remember if they don't need an appointment, they need something.

- Getting better then worse (a "relapse")
- Extremely sick (toxic) patients
- Concerned patients or callers
- When you are concerned, whether for obvious reasons or intuitively

Organizational Safeguards (Critical Policies Impacting Patient Care)

- Symptom management calls require assessment and should be handled by an RN.
- Develop a system for rapid identification of high-risk callers.
- Avoid triage or clinical decision making by unlicensed personnel.
- Avoid having multitasked telephone triage nurses.
- Telephone triage nurses must have experience and specialized training.
- Telephone triage nurse competency must be assured.
- Maintain a chain of command for clinical disputes.
- Consider clinical implications of all policies, even those that don't seem "clinical" (such as call routing).
- Standardize practice among nurses and locations.

- Protocols should be available but must never supersede nursing judgment.
- Telephone triage RNs should be empowered to act in the patient's best interest.
- Documentation tool must facilitate systematic assessment and thorough documentation.

Nursing Behaviors to Decrease Risk

- Use the nursing process on every call.
- Use critical thinking and exercise clinical judgment.
- Don't over-rely on the decision support tools.
- Remember, you're being paid for your knowledge and clinical expertise. Think!
- Follow policy and protocol unless it doesn't fit and then deviate and document why.
- Document both pertinent positives and negatives.
- Document to paint a picture.
- Know and function within your scope of practice.
- Communicate with your team and collaborate when indicated.
- Remember, you maintain accountability for your decisions and (usually) patient outcomes.
- Use extreme caution when multitasked or rushed.
- Avoid pitfalls such as accepting patient diagnosis and jumping to a conclusion.
- If the caller is concerned or you are concerned, the patient should be seen promptly.

- Think continuity. What's next? Who's next? Is follow-up indicated?
- You can never be *wrong* if you bring them in...you can only be wrong if you *don't*.
- Remember, patients, while just another call to us, are somebody's Somebody.

The Patient's Role (They can't do their part unless we help them)

- Confirm their comfort with the plan of care.
- Confirm their understanding of the plan.
- Confirm their intent to comply.
- Confirm their ability to carry out the plan of care.

Telephone triage nurses don't have to be right. We just can't afford to be wrong.

- Confirm that they know the likely consequences of their actions if non-compliant.
- Know what they need to do if they don't get better.
- Know what "worse" looks like.
- The patient gets 51% of the vote if he or she insists on being seen.

SUMMARY

The information contained in the last two chapters provide a blueprint for program design that incorporates risk management principles and focuses on quality care delivery. While not an exhaustive list of risk management principles, these suggestions will help you evaluate the safety of the care you are delivering. Remember that putting the patient first is usually the best risk management strategy available to us.

In the next chapter, we will explore some real-life situations in which nurses have implemented the principles discussed in this book.

References

1. Institute of Medicine. (2011). *The future of nursing: Leading change, advancing health.* Washington, DC: The National Academies Press.
2. Rutenberg, C. (2009). *Customizable telephone triage policy book/how-to manual on CD.* Little Rock, AK: Telephone Triage Consulting, Inc.
3. Kempe, A., Dempsey, C., Hegarty, T., Frei, N., Chandramouli, V., & Poole, S.R. (2000). Reducing after-hours referrals by an after-hours call center with second-level physician triage. *Pediatrics, 106*(1), 226-230.
4. U.S. Department of Health and Human Services, Agency for Healthcare Research and Quality. (2011). *Open access scheduling for routine and urgent appointments.* Retrieved from https://www.cahps.ahrq.gov/Quality-Improvement/Improvement- Guide/Browse-Interventions/Access/Open-Access.aspx
5. Shapiro, S.E., Izumi, S., Tanner, C.A., Moscato, S.R., Valanis, B.G., David, M.R., & Gullion, C.M. (2004). Telephone advice nursing services in a US health maintenance organization. *Journal of Telemedicine & Telecare, 10*(1), 50-54.
6. Klasner, A.E., King, W.D., Crews, T.B., & Monroe, K.W. (2006). Accuracy and response time when clerks are used for telephone triage. *Clinical Pediatrics, 45*(3), 267-269.
7. Hildebrandt, D.E., Westfall, J.M., & Smith, P.C. (2003). After-hours telephone triage affects patient safety. *Journal of Family Practice, 52*(3), 222-227.
8. Hildebrandt, D.E., Westfall, J.M., Fernald, D.H., & Pace, W.D. (2006). Harm resulting from inappropriate telephone triage in primary care. *Journal of the American Board of Family Medicine: JABFM, 19*(5), 437-442.
9. Edington, L.A. (2011). Improving access, patient flow, and nurse triage in a college health setting. *AAACN Viewpoint, 33*(4), 1.
10. Vinson, M.H., McCallum, R., Thornlow, D.K., & Chanpagne, M.T. (2011). Design, implementation, and evaluation of population-specific telehealth nursing services. *Nursing Economic$, 29*(5), 265-272, 277.
11. American Academy of Pediatrics. (1998, November). Strategies for practice management. Provisional section of pediatric telephone care and committee on practice and ambulatory medicine. *Pediatric call centers and the practice of telephone triage and advice: Critical success factors.* Chicago, IL: Author.

Chapter 16

Best Practices

The information presented in this book may resonate with the reader. Many nurses, when exposed to this information, are given validation that the course they are following is the right one. Others may feel overwhelmed, believing that the principles described in this book are "nice in theory," but unachievable in real life. While we acknowledge that practice as we have described it may seem lofty, we contend that it represents nothing more or less than the duty we owe our patients, our organizations, and our profession.

We have had experience with a great many organizations that offer telephone triage services, representing a full range of program types including clinics and call centers of all sizes in both formal and informal settings. These services have been associated with medical practices ranging from small groups to large health care systems to gigantic health maintenance organizations. In this book, we have also represented both the private and public sectors including county health departments; state and private university settings including college health services; Air Force, Navy, and Army medical treatment facilities; Indian Health Services; the Veterans Affairs; home health agencies; agencies serving persons with developmental disabilities; and a wide variety of call centers.

In an effort to illustrate the feasibility of the practices recommended in our book, we have identified "best practices" which we believe provide real-life examples of various facets of telephone triage "done right." It is our hope that the examples provided will both reassure and inspire readers to reach for the stars in their own setting.

- **"Making Your Call Center Indispensable to Your Organization"** by Pat Reynaga, RN, and Charlene Albertson, RN
- **"Care for the Caregiver"** by Kathryn Koehne, BSN, RNC-TNP
- **"Promoting Nurse Triage in a College Health Center Setting"** by Lyn Edington, RNC-TNP
- **"Call Center Innovations in Reward, Recognition, and Selective Recruitment"** by Suzanne Wells, MSN, RN
- **"Nurse-Developed Algorithms and Protocols in Electronic Decision Support Tools for Telephone Triage Practice"** by Debra Cox, MS, RN
- **"Telephone Triage Education and Program Development in an Urban Teaching Environment"** by Wanda Mayo, BSN, RN
- **"Process Improvement for Telephone Triage and Same-Day Appointment Management in an Air Force Family Health Clinic"** by Holli McDonald, MHL, BSN, RN; Allison Plunk, RN, USAF NC Col (Ret); and Maureen Koch, RN, USAF NC Lt Col (Ret)
- **"One Military Treatment Facility's Journey in Setting Up Nurse-Led Telephone Triage"** by Capt Elizabeth Anne Hoettels, NC, USAF
- **"Considerations for Development and Management of a Work-at-Home Telehealth Program"** by Kathryn Scheidt, MSN, MS, RN

The following best practice is an outstanding example of a nurse manager making her call center indispensable to her organization. This call center provides services for nurse advice, follow-up calls for "left the emergency department without being seen by a provider," scheduling for Joint Camp, after-hours employee exposure, after-hours complaint line, care line for families, instruction review for discharged patients, discharge follow-up calls, and inpatient tobacco cessation. During a recent survey by The Joint Commission (formerly known as JCAHO), multiple departments referenced the call center's services as being an integral part of the care delivery system. As a matter of fact, what appeared to the Joint Commission to be departments numbering in double digits was actually the call center discussed below.

MAKING YOUR CALL CENTER INDISPENSABLE TO YOUR ORGANIZATION

Pat Reynaga, RN
Charlene Albertson, RN

Telephone triage services can fill a niche on several levels both inside and outside an organization. What specific niche this service fills is often dependent upon the type of organization with which it is affiliated. Whether a stand-alone call center or a department in a large organization, the call center is a dynamic business which should promote and support growth.

Telephone triage as a business model inside your organization should be built on some basic tenants that when followed will provide a strong foundation for visibility and viability. These tenants, or building blocks, will enable your call center business to expand and adjust while making it indispensable to your organization. The building blocks identified by experience are:

1. Be specific in your plan.
2. Know your market.
3. Position for growth.

4. Always say "YES."
5. Maintain financial viability.
6. Focus on customer service.
7. Assure organizational visibility.

Be Specific in Your Plan

Every business, in order to survive and thrive, must have a plan of action. There are as many plan models to choose from in the business world as ideas under the sun, any number of which may initially seem daunting. Your plan must be specific. This means declaring your vision for the call center. Plan what percentage of growth you wish to achieve over what period of time, what type of personnel you will hire, how often you plan to add a program or client, and where the funding for your center will come from. This plan needs to align with the mission and objectives of the parent organization, be flexible enough to transform as the business model adjusts overall, and to benefit both the patient and the organization as well. Be prepared to demonstrate and document your call center's contribution and how your business supports the organization's strategic plan and objectives. To do this, you must know your audience and the key initiatives supported by the top executives. Assuring your administration's understanding of the value your service provides to the organization is imperative for their financial support and commitment to your program.

Know Your Market

To know your market you must work with marketing and business development departments to identify and analyze current trends. Seek their assistance in assessing the types of products and services your call center will offer by identifying your customers and determining whether your service will meet their needs. Be ready to adjust your service plan as trends change both internally and externally according to market conditions. Be aware of the competition and develop a strategy to compete. Have a plan in place that serves current needs and is able to respond to changes in your organization's strategic plan or market forces. This will enable you to provide beneficial customer services and continue to be competitive both internally and externally.

Position for Growth

Initially each call center opens with a client base made up of contracted physicians/clinics, hospital-based cold calls, or any combination thereof, which connects callers to your call center. Your specific plan from this point, in encouraging growth for the telehealth center, may be adding or realigning services as necessary. Specifically, it would not be unusual to adjust one internal program every 1-2 quarters or contract with new outside clinics or organizations. For example, you might be charged with the responsibility of developing an internal program for patients to contact the center's "triage nurse" for clarification of discharge instructions. Or you might be asked to resume or revitalize a stalled operation like contacting patients who left the emergency department (ED) before they could be evaluated. Another example of growth, over this same time frame, would be adding an external client through contracting with another hospital that transfers all its ED calls to the call center nurse for triage. What you add and when you add it should be consistent with your personal vision and direction. *Do not* be afraid to tentacle into every area of your health care organization by advertising your willingness *to do.*

Always Say "YES"

Be the YES person. In the arena of ideas there is never a vacuum, and when your organization wants to try something new be ready to say YES! This will facilitate growth for your department while making your services visible and viable within your organization and community. You can always figure out later how to make these new ideas functional in the call center. Remember, you are never alone; you are supported by talented professionals who are often full of ideas. Rely on them to help work out how to do this new thing. It's their job, it's what they do, and they know how to do it!

But you must also know when to say "no." Never be afraid to admit something failed. Take your ego out of the equation. For instance, if you do a trial for a new program, the trial should last 2-3 days, at the most, before you evaluate the program. It either is working well or it's not. If it is not working well, evaluate whether it can be fixed or if the program should be eliminated. The same is true for any contract where the client or you decide to stop service for good cause such as when a service no longer supports the organization's mission. Or, if based on statistical analysis, your revenue per volume of calls indicates that a contract is no longer economically viable, just stop, unless you can see opportunities to rectify the situation, but do not take it *personally.* Nothing lasts forever. Learn from the experience and then move forward, adjusting your vision as you go. Market and client needs will change and your ability to adjust makes you invaluable as a customer service oriented entity.

Maintain Financial Viability

Keeping the call center viable and financially sound and running a large budget in current economic times is very challenging. Be aware of cost per call, cost per minute, speed to answer, and length of call, then translate those numbers into revenue which keeps the books in the black. Be creative in obtaining funding by seeking outside sources like contracts or grants that may apply to the type of calls your call center provides. There may also be funding sources from your local community, such as a university, municipality, or not-for-profit organization, where funding for a specific type of call would augment the budget for your call center. A grant from a local municipality to field calls about "flu" for a finite period of time is an example of outside funding. And if all goes well, this grant might be renewable or recurring. Regardless of where you obtain funding, be creative in your source-finding efforts, step out of your comfort zone, and be the visible spokesperson for your call center to create interest from those outside sources. Also, court sources inside and outside of your organization by reminding them that your call center is available and ready to serve. This will pay off because when a need arises, you will be the "squeaky wheel" they remember.

Focus on Customer Service

Customer service satisfaction is not just a cliché. It is an important and integral part of any call center. Your customers are the individual patient, physician, clinic, hospital, or payer who utilize your call center. And remember, the secretary, nurse, physician, or other employee working the call center is your customer as well. Creating a practice environment that meets the needs of both external and internal customers is essential. The call center manager must lead with vision in order to keep employees motivated. Begin developing this environment by hiring the right staff members. Look for individuals with experience and a knowledge base in medicine or nursing who are motivated and able to think independently. The ideal nurse is one who is not afraid to make a decision or exception in the best interest of the patient as long as it is within the parameters of organizational policy, national practice standards, and the laws governing his or her licensure.

Trust the staff to conduct themselves professionally. Encourage them to collaborate with each other, assume authority in making decisions about a call or their work schedule, continue their education, and participate in organizational or community committees. Lead by example and imbue a sense of belonging by allowing them to choose their destiny within the call center through open, respectful interaction with each person. Make opportunities for those who are motivated to participate in the growth and development of the call center by identifying their talents and putting those talents to use. For example, individuals may have strengths in writing educational materials for the call center or developing contracts, proposals, or surveys. Reward them for their participation. These measures will assist with staff development and retention. The only boss is the customer, and the staff is the first customer whose needs must be met. If you take care of your staff, they will take care of their patients.

Create an environment where there is open communication between the staff and call center director/manager. Be honest and upfront in your presentation of information to your staff and let them know you value their ideas. Discuss budget realities on a regular basis, ensuring understanding regarding the purchase of required equipment and its impact on salaries and staffing. When this kind of open communication is offered consistently, it translates into a cohesive, contented staff.

A satisfied staff is more able to interact with the call center patient/caller compassionately and professionally. When callers perceive compassion for their situation over the phone, they feel their needs are being met by the triage nurse or other medical personnel. Many opportunities arise during the triage call to meet the needs of the client caller, whether during the initial interview process or the eventual disposition. Meeting the needs of the contracted physician/clinic/hospital client is also critical and possible when the agreed-upon contacting process is consistently followed by the staff. Smooth, efficient delivery of services makes for loyal, committed contract clients both within and external to your organization.

Measuring patient satisfaction is important for your call center when potential clients (external or internal) are looking to make a decision about where to obtain care for their beneficiaries. Routine patient satisfaction monitoring can help identify and subsequently resolve potential problems before they affect the marketability of your call center. You can develop your own surveys for both patients and contracted customers, or you can purchase these services from an outside source that will conduct the survey and collate the collected information. Regardless of who develops and conducts the survey, the information gleaned from surveys of patients, physicians, payers, and employees is important. This information will help your call center identify strengths and areas for growth, measure successful ventures, benchmark standards and goals for your services and programs, and help justify your call center's existence.

Assure Organizational Visibility

Every opportunity to make your call center visible inside your organization should be seized and made a priority. Become involved with employee activities, such as committees or intramural contests, attend other department staff meetings to introduce or reintroduce your department to your organization, and make yourself known to leaders. These types of activities give you the opportunity to advertise internally, answer questions, and plant seeds for future projects with other departments. Attend new physician orientations where you can provide information advertising your services, thus creating an occasion to possibly obtain new contracts. Involve yourself with health fairs, give presentations to high schools, and publish a column about your call center in physician publications outside your organization. Attend an unlimited number of meetings and demonstrate willingness to step in on short notice. When you make your call center more visible by trumpeting your vision at every opportunity, your call center will become more viable and eventually indispensable to the overall organization.

Conclusion

Making your call center essential to your organization will not look exactly the same for each manager or director who is working hard to make this happen. However, it should contain the seven ingredients discussed and thus provide a basis for a flexible working template. These building blocks provide the basis upon which you can build and rebuild your business platform. Start by writing a specific plan of action that reflects your dream for the call center, is consistent with your organization's strategic plan, and supports its mission. Know your market, and position your call center for growth within your external and internal communities. Be assertive and bold by becoming the YES person while giving constant attention to maintaining financial viability. Support your staff and encourage them to acknowledge and use their strengths and gifts. This recognition and encouragement from you will assure their satisfaction and support in developing a "how to" plan of action for the next project. Demonstrate professionalism salted with compassion and peppered with knowledge of your call center's functionality to all of your customers. Lastly, "crow!" Make your voice heard by being visible within your organization and your community so others will come to you when they have an idea or need that your call center could support. Jump in there! Use these building blocks to structure your ideas and actions and watch your call center transform.

A good deal of attention has been given recently to the topic of care for the caregiver. Telephone triage is regarded by many as being a low-stress environment, but in reality it can be exactly the opposite. The following paper, written by an experienced telephone triage nurse, addresses critical elements of caring for the caregiver.

CARE FOR THE CAREGIVER

Kathryn Koehne, BSN, RNC-TNP

Currently, there is debate whether the nursing shortage is fact or fiction. Don't be deceived! A looming historical shortage is presently masked as baby boomers are still working and economic uncertainty is encouraging nurses to hang on to their employment. According to the Bureau of Labor Statistics' Employment Projections 2010-2020, "employment for registered nurses is expected to increase 26 percent...faster than the average for all occupations" (¶ 1).[1] Policy-makers, nursing organizations, universities, and the media are partnering to strategize a plan to increase nursing supply to meet the future demand. However, stabilizing a nursing workforce is not only about recruiting; it is also about retaining your own nursing team.

Nursing is a demanding profession. Nurse vacancy rates are low in environments that are positive. So, even if the work is hard, nurses will endure if they describe their work atmosphere as enriching. This type of setting increases engagement; nurses will stay and even thrive. If you are a manager, you can create this environment for your nursing staff. If you are a staff nurse, you can incorporate healthy behaviors that will increase your sense of personal and professional wellness. Caring for the caregiver is a shared responsibility between manager and nurse.

The practice of telephone triage impacts nurses physically, professionally, and personally. It is important that the individuals who manage nurses who provide this type of care realize that these nurses have needs that differ from other nurses who work in other settings. In addition, telephone triage nurses themselves need to actively participate in healthy career and lifestyle behaviors. I will share best practices that can ensure contentment and longevity for years to come.

Providing nursing care in a clinic or call center environment, involves spending a considerable amount of time on the telephone. Even though patients relay different issues, the repetitive nature of the work can lead to physical and mental exhaustion that other types of nursing roles do not. Many nurses report that they experience increased dissatisfaction as time passes due to the stationary and isolating nature of telephone triage. However, in my conversations with nurses who "love" telephone triage and cannot imagine working in any other area of nursing, I have discovered some common themes. A common reason why nurses find this area of nursing so enriching is the presence of a beloved manager who validates their contribution to the team and the patients they serve.

In research examining the reasons why nurses leave nursing, it was discovered that nurses abandon the profession because their desire to be validated at work is not being met.[2] Nurses express a need to be recognized and respected and when this need is not consistently met, they eventually exit their position or even the profession! There is significant value when managers take an opportunity to validate their nursing staff. Even a small gesture has great impact. Nursing staff will be happier and their positive emotions will contribute to a more dynamic environment. As a result, the manager may also experience an increase in job satisfaction. Nurses will be more satisfied and less restless; the turnover rate will be lower. The nursing team will be dedicated and stable.

MANAGERS

Managers provide the foundation for their department. It is the manager who is recognized as the core of the workplace community and it is often he or she who impacts the health of the community. To be successful, managers need to really know their team members as individuals. If you are a manager, you should be able to identify those who welcome change and those who resist it; those who are positive and those who are quick to complain; and those who rise to the occasion and those who lose confidence quickly. Yet, wherever your staff members are along the attitude spectrum, you can manage them effectively. As you identify their areas of strengths and fields that present opportunities for growth, you have the power to facilitate individualized professional development. This guidance demonstrates to your staff that you care about them as individuals. And when they realize how much you care, they are more positive and content.

Managing your staff is only one of your responsibilities. The complexity of an ever-changing health care environment demands that you need to manage so much more than people. You have to deal with regulatory requirements, organizational initiatives, and quality measures, and yet ensure that you are accessible to build relationships with your staff. Telephone nurses require some specialized "care" that, if effective, will increase their engagement. Managers can be instrumental in retaining staff when the physical, professional, and personal needs required of this work are addressed.

Physical Care

To provide your staff with physical care, you need to have an understanding of the physiological impact that telephone nursing care can have on nurses. Whether you manage a clinic department or call center, when nurses spend long hours on the phone, their movement is limited. They will eventually suffer metabolic and/or musculoskeletal consequences from this type of work if physical care is not provided.

As a first step, acknowledge that actions must be taken to decrease the physical "wear and tear" of this work. You have already made a difference when you don't assume that "sitting and taking calls" is easy. Your next step is creating an action plan that eliminates or reduces the potential problems related to immobility.

Ergonomics is the science of designing a workspace to meet an individual's capabilities and limitations. When you are able to provide an ergonomically correct workstation, employees experience an increase in comfort, health, safety, and productivity. An ergonomic assessment and provision of ergonomic accessories such as headsets, adjustable chairs, armrests, and footrests are expensive. Initially, you will incur expenses, but you will have a return on your investment. When preventative measures are put into place, absenteeism due to injury and cost of therapy may be eliminated. When I was working as a telephone nurse advisor at Gundersen Lutheran, an integrated health system located in southwestern Wisconsin, I was fortunate to have an ergonomic evaluation. Employees were able to receive this assessment as a response to physical complaints or proactively as a preventative measure. After I implemented the recommended changes, my back, neck, and arm discomfort were eliminated.

If you cannot provide an ergonomic assessment and accessories, you still can promote physical well-being among your staff. You can do this simply by ensuring that your staff takes breaks. Investing in inexpensive exercise equipment is a simple act that shows your employees you care. A group of telephone triage nurses shared that their manager provided their department with a set of hand weights, latex-free exercise bands, and a yoga mat so staff could do some simple exercises during break. The manager also invited a physical therapist to attend a staff meeting to demonstrate workstation exercises that could be done to relieve the nurses of common aches experienced from repetitive movements. Then she made copies of the exercise sheet and hung one in every cubicle as a visual reminder to staff to exercise periodically.

Professional Care

It also is important for managers to provide professional "care" for their telephone triage nurses. You can assist your nurses to grow professionally by taking time to explore areas of interest. A prime opportunity for this discussion to take place is during your employees' annual review. Once there is an identified area of focus, assist them in developing goals and an action plan to meet these targets and then periodically follow-up on their progress. This type of individualized planning increases staff optimism and commitment.

While in my role as a triage nurse at Gundersen Lutheran, I was having a conversation with other nurses. Prior to telephone triage, we had all been working in various specialty areas for a length of time and were considered experts. When we transferred into the telephone triage department, we became generalists. We agreed that we were content, but were experiencing a shared sense of loss. There were new developments —medications, protocols, and technologies — and sometimes we were hearing about them for the first time from our *patients!*

After that conversation, I had a talk with my manager. I relayed the concerns that we all had expressed. I proposed a solution: a specialty liaison responsibility. We could ask the nursing staff if they wanted to be a liaison to a specialty area. The responsibilities of this role included:

- Acting as a resource for current information related to that specialty.
- Serving as a link between the telephone triage department and the specialty area.
- Participating as a reviewer for the newest triage protocols related to that specialty.

My manager welcomed the idea and encouraged me to develop it. She energized me and did so to the rest of our staff. The nurse who had worked in inpatient psychiatry became the behavioral health liaison. The former labor and delivery nurse became the perinatal liaison. The former operating room nurse became the surgical liaison. The rest of the nurses quickly volunteered for other liaison roles. We became specialty experts again! This professional development tactic had more than one benefit. Nurses were excited, but our manager reaped benefits, too. She no longer had to single-handedly seek information and respond to questions from departments all over the organization. She was able to share her workload with her staff; there was a partnership. It was a win-win situation.

This type of innovative staff development strategy is only one of many things managers can do to keep their staff growing professionally. Managers also can encourage staff to attend telephone triage or other specialty conferences. If nurses are interested in continuing education, managers should facilitate appropriate continuing education, including specialty certification and/or additional education.

Personal Care

Managers need to facilitate physical and professional care for their staff. However, it is the individualized, special considerations that nurses identify as meaningful. The following are some "Simple Acts of Caring."

- Compliment your staff's strengths.
- Communicate clearly.
- Recognize exemplary care.
- Share success stories.
- Support the team through difficulty.
- Advocate for fairness.
- Strengthen departmental areas of weakness.
- Provide enriching opportunities for your team.
- Help your staff when they are busy.
- Say hello at the beginning of the day.

- Say good-bye at the end of the day.
- Express your appreciation often; send thank-you notes.

Many of these acts do not require much time or effort. An example of a simple act of caring was demonstrated by a manager who made an effort to put a small, thoughtful "gratitude" quote on her nurses' computers at the beginning of each week. Another manager would round once a day simply to "check-in" with his staff. In one of my previous positions, my manager was a former triage nurse and would plug in and manage phone calls when we were busy. Research shows that effective managers are "visible, accessible, available and responsive" (p. 23).[3]

NURSES

It is not the exclusive responsibility of managers to take care of the physical, professional, and personal needs of their nursing staff. If you are a staff nurse, you can incorporate behaviors that will increase your longevity not only in telephone triage, but in nursing. And this improved wellness will spill into your personal life, too. You must care for yourself!

Physical Care

If you have an ergonomically appropriate workstation, comply with all the recommendations and utilize all ergonomic accessories as recommended. Many times employers will provide necessary tools, but employees express being "too busy" to use them. Employees also have to prioritize personal wellness. Since telephone triage work is static, incorporate regular exercise and exercise "bursts" during your workday. You can maintain your heath by jogging in place, doing jumping jacks, and stretching in various yoga positions. Simple steps can maintain your health.

Stay home when you are ill. It may seem tempting since you do not usually have face-to-face contact with your patients, but stay home and rest. Even if you have the benefit of home access, do not "push" yourself to plug in when you do not feel well. Patients may not receive the focused care they deserve when you are ill, and you may also inhibit your own recovery.

Aim to avoid weight gain and chronic illness by eating healthy and drinking water. Since you are less active when practicing telephone triage, you need to evaluate your calorie consumption. Everyone has heard about the Freshman 15, but have you heard about the *Telephone Triage 20*? If you have switched from an active job, you may have to reduce your calorie intake. You may want to have a nutritional evaluation from a registered dietician.

It is also important for you to take your breaks. You may be tempted to work through your breaks when the call volume is high. This is not physically or mentally healthy. Taking calls continuously for 8 hours or more is exhausting and can even be risky. After you listen to series of symptoms hour after hour, fatigue may negatively impact your assessment skills, and there is the real potential for error.

Professional Care

On an ongoing basis, consider how you want to grow as a professional. If you have an annual review, be sure to not only identify your strengths, but also list areas of opportunities. Your goals should always include a list of realistic action steps.

To continue to grow professionally, you must embrace lifelong learning by seeking formalized education, obtaining specialty certification, or simply addressing your personal knowledge deficits. Growing professionally does not necessarily mean getting an advanced degree; it can be reading nursing journals, attending conferences, or engaging in professional roundtable discussions. There are volumes available to you on trusted web sites, health resource libraries, or on pages of professional publications. You can learn every day; read about new medications, search for information about unknown conditions, and study protocols that are unfamiliar. Whenever an opportunity presents, participate in *in-the-moment* learning.

Personal Care

In the Manager section, I listed a number of "Simple Acts of Caring." The manager is the "captain" of the team, but you are one of the members. A jointly caring effort can create a team that is cohesive and supportive. You will experience a sense of well-being. Review the list and adopt some of these practices.

Many years ago I decided to contribute to increasing a positive atmosphere at work as a New Year's resolution. My plan was to compliment someone at work at least one time during a shift. The compliment had to be appropriate, thoughtful, and genuine. It had to be expressed at the right time and place. For example, if the person was shy, I would avoid a public affirmation. In another example, one of the triage nurses was gifted at managing the hysterical parent calls. I let her know how much I admired her exemplary style. I will remember the smiles that resulted from my compliments. I received a "gift" in return.

Quint Studer, best-selling author, national speaker, and CEO of a health care outcomes company, summarized the importance of caring for the caregiver. "Nurses are the heart and soul of everything you do. Pay close attention to their wants and needs, and take meaningful steps to address them, and you can transform your entire organization. When nurses are happy, patients are happy — and everything else naturally falls into place."[4]

References

1. Bureau of Labor Statistics, U.S. Department of Labor, Occupational Outlook Handbook. (2012). *Registered nurses.* Retrieved from http://www.bls.gov/ooh/healthcare/registered-nurses.htm
2. Sumner, J., & Townsend-Rocchiccioli, J. (2003). Why are nurses leaving nursing? *Nursing Administration Quarterly, 27*(2), 164-171.
3. Duffield, C.M., Roche, M.A., Blay, N., & Stasa, H. (2011). Nursing unit managers, staff retention and the work environment. *Journal of Clinical Nursing, 29*(1-2), 23-33. doi: 10.1111/j.1365-2702.2010.03478.x
4. Studer, C. (2006). Beyond nurses week: How (and why) to nurture nurses. *HealthCare News.* Retrieved from http://healthcarenews.com/article.asp?id=1348

Provision of telephone triage services to special populations poses unique challenges and opportunities. Certainly college health is one of those special populations. This group represents patients of all ages, usually reasonably healthy, who are pursuing higher education or teaching/working in an academic setting. The mission of college health centers is to keep their population healthy enough to attend classes, function to their ability, and complete their course of academic study successfully. Because the college health population often comprises relatively recent high school graduates, this setting may represent their first foray into caring for themselves and making independent but informed health care decisions. In addition to helping their patients maintain optimum wellness, nurses who are providing telephone triage services to this college health population are also engaging in activities which have the potential to mold the health care attitudes and behaviors of our next generation(s). The following example from the Nurse Manager for Pat Walker Health Center at the University of Arkansas in Fayetteville, Arkansas, illustrates how telephone triage in the college health setting is represented to the students, enabling them to act as their own health care advocates.

PROMOTING NURSE TRIAGE IN A COLLEGE HEALTH CENTER SETTING

Lyn Edington, RNC-TNP

H1N1 Influenza hit our campus during the 2009 fall semester. Triage calls increased by over 50% when compared to the previous year. The clinic was not able to accommodate the demand for same-day appointments. About that time, a satisfaction survey was distributed to all patients who were seen in the clinic by a nurse or medical provider or had a telephone encounter with a triage nurse. Triage took several hits on this survey. Patients did not understand why they had to talk to a nurse in order to get an appointment. Triage seemed to be viewed as a barrier to care.

The nurse manager suspected that the negative comments on the patient satisfaction survey did not come from patients who had actually spoken to a triage nurse but rather from those who opted to hang up and seek care elsewhere. Outcome studies done in the past have always reflected very high patient satisfaction with walk-in and telephone nurse triage.

During the spring semester steps were taken to evaluate the triage process, identify problems, and promote triage as a valuable resource for students. Two outcome studies and a time study were conducted to evaluate the triage program. A nurse advice outcome study indicated satisfaction with nurse advice and 96% of patients indicated they would call and speak to a triage nurse again. The second outcome study addressed appropriateness of same-day referral. The medical providers felt that the triage nurses were making appropriate same-day referrals 89% of the time. When triage nurses err, it should be on the side of caution. Better to bring someone in that could have waited than delay care and cause harm. We can live with 89%.

The time study validated that calls were returned according to policy and the call lengths were consistent with national statistics. The wait times for a call back averaged from 8 to 25 minutes. Call lengths averaged from 9 to 11 minutes.

As suspected, patients who actually had an interaction with a triage nurse were satisfied and felt like their needs had been met. The process at intake was evaluated. When a patient called and requested a same-day appointment, the receptionist typically said, "I don't have any appointments for today. I can have a triage nurse call you back." They were just told that there were no appointments. How would talking to a nurse help? It is unknown how many simply hung up and sought care elsewhere.

The first challenge was to promote telephone triage as a valuable resource for students. The following article, "The Next Best Thing to Mom and Chicken Soup: The Triage Nurses at the Health Center," explaining the role and value of the triage nurses was posted on the health center web page. This was also included in a newsletter to the parents of new students. The article was also shared with the Student Health Advisory Board. Intake staff referred patients to the web page to get more information on the triage process.

The Best Thing Next to Mom and Chicken Soup: The Triage Nurses at the Health Center

You may not know it but you have a wonderful resource at your disposal: The triage nurses at the health center. These nurses, perhaps one of our best-kept secrets, are here to help you!

What Is a 'Triage Nurse'?

Triage means "sorting out." A telephone triage nurse is specially trained to assess problems over the phone. Telephone triage is actually a nursing specialty area. If you talk to a triage nurse you are talking to a "specialist." It requires lots of special training, clinical and life experience to be a telephone triage nurse. Only the most experienced registered nurses perform triage in the medical clinic. Two of our triage nurses are actually certified in telephone triage.

Why Talk to a Triage Nurse?

If you need a same-day appointment a triage nurse can:

- Make sure you are scheduled with the right provider.
- Make sure you are scheduled at the right time.

  An example of this is a young man who called and was given a same-day appointment for nausea and vomiting. While he was happy to have an appointment, the trouble was, his appointment was at 4:15 p.m. He had been sick for 2 days and by the time he was seen and lab work was completed, the clinic was about to close. He was referred to the emergency room for IV fluids. Had he spoken with a triage nurse, the nurse would have instructed him to come in immediately and he could have been taken care of in the clinic and avoided the trip to the emergency room.

- Prevent a bad outcome because of a delay in care.
- If possible, help you avoid treatment in the emergency department or a more costly walk-in clinic.
- If indicated, direct you to an urgent care facility and make contact with that facility prior to your arrival.
- Make sure you are *taken care of* just like mom would!

Why Should I Call at All? If I Am Sick, Can't I Just Walk in and Be Seen?

Certainly you can. But it is usually better if you call first. "Walk-in" or unscheduled patients are evaluated by one of the triage nurses. They are not seen on a first-come first-served basis. The most urgent are evaluated first. Your wait time can be very long if there are several patients ahead of you. Calling first gives you faster access to a nurse and can even save you a trip.

Why Give Advice to Someone Who Just Wants an Appointment?

Not everyone who feels bad needs to come to the clinic. You may not need an appointment but you need someone to help you. Sometimes it is in your best interest to stay at home in bed and take care of yourself. Who wants to get out of a warm bed, spend at least an hour at the clinic, only find out that there is no "magic pixie dust" to make the symptoms go away in one day? You may just need rest, fluids, and over-the-counter medications. Not antibiotics. You may also be exposing yourself (or others) to other infections by going to a busy clinic during an outbreak of flu or other viral illnesses.

A perfect example of this is a young lady who made an appointment during a flu outbreak to come in for evaluation of annoying allergy symptoms. She was evaluated and given over-the-counter medications for her allergies. Three days later she was back with flu symptoms. She may have been exposed to the flu while she was in the clinic. Her allergy symptoms probably could have been managed over the phone by a triage nurse.

What if I Don't Want to Come In?

Sometimes you just don't feel like coming in and want to stay home in bed. Sometimes you are not sure if you even need to come in. A triage nurse can help you make a decision on whether or not you should come in. If the triage nurse feels it is safe for you to manage your symptoms at home, you will be given advice for self-care. You will also be instructed on over-the-counter medications, diet, activity, and what to do about missed classes or work. Have you looked at the selection of over-the-counter cold and flu medications lately? It is not easy to select the right ones for your symptoms. A triage nurse can help. If, however, the triage nurse feels like you should be evaluated by a medical provider, you will be given a time to come in. This will greatly reduce your wait time when you feel terrible.

Again, sometimes, for your safety, we feel better if we can take a quick look at you. It is very difficult to evaluate some symptoms over the phone. Skin problems or rashes are especially challenging. The triage nurse may ask you to come in so one of them can look at you.

What if I Just Have a Question or I Am Concerned about a Friend or Roommate?

We are always happy to answer your questions or give advice. We are here for you! Just call and ask to speak to one of the triage nurses. You don't have to give a reason if you are uncomfortable talking with the receptionist.

Common Concerns or Questions

"Why are you making it so hard? Are you trying to keep me out of the clinic? My doctor at home would probably call in a Z-Pak® for my symptoms. What's up with this?"

We are not trying to keep you away. Quite the opposite! You are why we are here and we like being here to help you. We have a huge demand for our services and have a very good system in place to make sure our acutely ill or injured students who call us are seen in a timely manner. We want to provide the best possible care with the least amount of complications and disruptions to you.

Some Things You Can Do to Help Us Help You

- Talking to a triage nurse is a good thing! Don't assume that you won't get to come in if you are referred to a triage nurse. Don't just hang up and call another clinic and don't go to the emergency room with cold or flu symptoms. About 60% of the patients that the triage nurses talk to are given a same-day appointment.

- Be available to take a call when we call you back. Make sure we have your correct contact info. Currently our calls show up as an unknown number on caller ID. Please pick up. We play a lot of "phone tag." We want to talk to you, not your voice mail.

- If you haven't heard from us within an hour please call back. We try to return every call within 30 minutes but sometimes our call volume is very high or we are dealing with an emergency in the clinic. If we cannot reach you we may have the wrong number or may not be able to leave a message. If all attempts to reach you fail, we will send you an e-mail request to call us. It really worries us if we can't reach you.

- If you have talked to a triage nurse and you do not improve or get worse, please call us back. We will get you in. We assume you are doing OK if we don't hear back from you.

Take advantage of having such great access to nurses while you are here. Let them fill in when Mom can't. When you get out in the "real world of health care," you sure will miss them!

Additional Interventions

The next challenge was to change the perception that it is difficult to access same-day care.

The following script was developed along with some guidelines for the intake staff.

Intake Script

Receptionist: "Name of facility. This is __________ how can I help you?"

Patient: "I would like to make an appointment."

Receptionist: "Certainly." *Get identifying information. Verify eligibility.*

Receptionist: "When would you like to come in?" *Any time other than today. Get appropriate info and make appointment.*

Patient: "I want to come in today." (*For other than routine visit*)

Receptionist: "Certainly. Our triage nurses make our same-day appointments. I need some information and I will have one of them call you back." *Get contact info.* ***Ask*** *for their phone number (do not ask them if it is 000-000-0000). Obtain a very brief complaint.*

Patient: "Can't I just walk in?"

Receptionist: "Yes, you always of have the option to walk in. If you speak to one of the nurses and they feel that you should be seen today you will be given a time to come in. They know what is happening in the clinic and can get you to the appropriate provider at the appropriate time.

"If you choose to walk in without an appointment, you will be evaluated by a triage nurse. Walk-in patients are not seen on a first come, first-served basis so I cannot tell you how long your wait will be before the nurse can evaluate you. Based on your evaluation, if the nurse decides that you need to be seen by a medical provider, you may have to wait to be worked into the provider's schedule. You will reduce your wait time if you speak to a triage nurse on the phone. Sometimes they can help you over the phone so you don't have to come in. If you are not feeling well, you probably do not want to sit in a waiting room for hours."

Hopefully they will opt to talk to a nurse. Get contact info.
Receptionist to all callers referred to phone triage:"Our nurses try to return calls within 30 minutes. The call may read as an unknown number on your caller ID so expect a call like that. If you have not heard from a nurse in one hour please call back. They may be having difficulty reaching you. Thank you for calling."

Intake Guidelines

- During the fall and spring semesters, all requests for same-day appointments and requests to speak to a nurse should be routed to triage.
- Patients who were seen previously and are not better or are worse should go to triage, no matter which provider they saw.

- During the summer, there usually are enough appointments spots to accommodate all requests for same-day appointments but some symptoms should be evaluated as soon as possible. These things should go to triage, regardless of availability of appointments:
    - Nausea/Vomiting/Diarrhea calls
    - Abdominal pain and fever
    - Motor vehicle accident
    - Head injury
    - Patients who want to discuss their symptoms; not sure if they need to come in
    - Patients who request to talk to a nurse, have general questions, or concerns about a friend or roommate
    - Any *severe* symptom
- Remember, you can refer to the health center web page section on triage nurses.

Results

The changes at intake immediately took some pressure off the intake staff and made patients feel someone was going to help them. The next patient satisfaction survey in the fall of 2010 was much more positive and contained no complaints about triage. More patients are calling now *requesting* to talk to a triage nurse, especially the students not taking classes in the summer. When cost is an issue, they prefer self-care advice if at all possible. They are learning to be smart health care consumers and appreciate that they have access to triage nurses.

Triage Pearls from College Health Triage Veterans

- *Be nice and make a good first impression.* A triage encounter is often the first encounter at a clinic. It will lay the foundation for future visits. You may not be able to offer them a magic bullet for their cold symptoms, but you can make them feel like you care that they feel bad as you give self-care advice.

- *Any "severe" symptom needs evaluation.* Enough said.

- *Never second-guess a patient.* Wait until you get a history to form a conclusion. Remember that they called or came in because they have something going on that is important to them. It may be your 15th call about a cough today but it is their first.

- *Most 19 year-old males have problems verbalizing symptoms ("I'm just sick").* Ask any college health nurse. It is like pulling taffy to get specific symptoms from this group. But keep pulling, it will come.

- *Patients who are given self-care advice should always be instructed on the usual duration and progression of symptoms.* Be sure they know when to call back if symptoms persist or worsen.

- *Don't get too much information but make sure you have enough to make a decision.* A medical provider should be able to read a triage note and know exactly why you made your triage decision. Include all *pertinent* information. Typically, the longer the call, the more likely it will be an advice call. Unless you are talking to a 19 year-old male.

- *Beware of third-party calls.* If at all possible, talk to the patient. We have learned not to schedule appointments through a well-meaning friend, roommate, or parent. More often than not, the appointment information does not get relayed and the patient is a "no show." Instead, we assure the caller that we will contact and assist the patient.

- *Have a contingency plan if unable to contact patient.* Nothing is worse than knowing that a patient needs help and you are unable to contact him or her. Try alternate numbers, e-mail, call the resident advisor, or send the police to check on him or her if necessary.

- *Beware of the hidden agenda.* As you conclude the triage encounter, ask if there is anything else they need. You may get the real reason for the call or walk-in visit. We have had many sore throat calls or visits turn into STD concerns.

- *Alcohol consumption.* Don't forget to ask about alcohol intake history when indicated. Look at the birth date. Unfortunately, many college students celebrate their 21st birthday by consuming large amounts of alcohol. GI symptoms the day after a 21st birthday or unexplained injuries any time should raise some red flags.

- *You can't please everyone; act on valid complaints, don't take invalid ones personally.* Expectations are sometimes unrealistic, especially in the college population. Every triage encounter is an opportunity for patient education. Complaints are an opportunity to improve your system.

- *If you don't know what to do, ask someone who does.* It is perfectly acceptable to tell a patient that you are going to consult with someone and call them back. Consult with another triage nurse or medical provider.

- *Be flexible. Alter your program as patient and staffing needs change.* During a busy influenza season, you may need to suspend routine appointments and procedures to free up more acute care appointments. Shift more resources to triage.

- *Utilize outside resources when indicated.* Examples are crisis centers, poison control hot line, state and local health departments, local pharmacy, mental health facility, health educators, or even a veterinarian.

- *Not everyone* ***wants*** *to come in.* Some patients only want advice but really should be seen. You may have to convince them that they could have a bad outcome without evaluation and treatment. It's OK to say something like, "I am concerned that your abdominal pain could be due to something serious like an appendicitis or severe infection." Do whatever it takes to get their attention.

It is obvious that telephone triage requires a special commitment and understanding of the practice of nursing over the telephone. Recruitment and retention of the ideal staff are critical to program success. The following example, written by the Manager, Answer Line, St. Louis Children's Hospital and BJC HealthCare, illustrates how the FISH! philosophy has been incorporated into a medium-sized call center with the end result of significant employee satisfaction. Additionally, strategies to hire staff who have a high likelihood of success are described in the following best practice.

CALL CENTER INNOVATIONS IN REWARD, RECOGNITION, AND SELECTIVE RECRUITMENT

Suzanne Wells, MSN, RN

It is no surprise that registered nurses compose the largest group of providers in the health care industry. The profession's nursing shortages throughout the years, however, have had an impact on our ability to deliver safe, effective care. The good news, due to the country's current economic condition, is that both men and women are currently entering the profession. The not-so-good news is that not only are nurses an aging workforce, but they are also leaving the profession due to job dissatisfaction.[1] The continual simmering of these issues within our profession demands a proactive approach to the management of people on the part of the leader in order to recruit and retain qualified nurses.

Most managers believe employees care most about their pay, when in reality what employees want is to have interesting work and be "in the know." Employees also want to be valued, listened to, and appreciated for the work they do. For the nurse working in telephone triage, whether in a primary practice or call center setting, there are intrinsic issues that affect the nurse's ability to perform his or her job. Issues such as handling call after call, the isolation of working in cubicles, ergonomics, visibility of management, and the ability to stay current on department information all have an effect on the morale of the individual nurse and the team as a whole. It is the manager's responsibility to effectively address these issues in support of their staff.

To deliver safe and effective care to patients, and provide an environment where people want to come to work, it is imperative that as formal leaders, managers create a positive and responsive work environment. Incorporating open communication and fostering effective relationships are paramount in building a culture of employee engagement. Other key components to foster employee engagement and assure successful retention are respect, recognition, education, and career development.

Since 1988, St. Louis Children's Hospital Answer Line, part of BJC HealthCare and the BJC Call Center, has offered 454-KIDS, a free community service, providing pediatric health and wellness information and assessment of illness symptoms. Over the years, the staff has grown from 12 to almost 60 experienced, pediatric registered nurses. After Hours, a service that began in 1996, provides triage for over 250 community-based pediatricians in both the St. Louis metropolitan area and outstate Missouri and Illinois, when their offices are closed.

The Answer Line has implemented two innovative approaches for the purposes of talent recruitment, proactive management, and reward and recognition of employees. The FISH! Philosophy, the department's reward and recognition initiative, has enhanced the culture of the department through its promotion of staff satisfaction and retention. The Chally Group Worldwide[2] assessment, administered during the hiring process, promotes selective recruitment.

The FISH! Philosophy

The Answer Line supports staff professionalism, autonomy, accountability, and partnerships. A collaborative environment exists among the staff nurses, ancillary staff, and our community pediatricians, which enhances the nurse's ability to safely and effectively identify the caller's needs and assess the patient. Building on this culture of collaboration, the Answer Line leadership embraced the FISH! philosophy early in 2001. Our intent was to enhance the work environment in an effort to exceed both staff and customer satisfaction.

Developed by John Christensen, the FISH! philosophy is based on the experiences of the fish mongers at the Pike Place Fish Market in Seattle, Washington.[3] At the core of the FISH! philosophy are four tenets: be there, make their day, choose your attitude, and play. In the book titled *FISH!*, the reader is encouraged to "imagine a workplace where everyone chooses to bring energy, passion, and a positive attitude to the job every day. Imagine an environment in which people are truly connected to their work, to their colleagues, and to their customers."

In the fall of 2001, the FISH! philosophy was introduced as a reward and recognition program at the Answer Line. The four tenets of the FISH! philosophy help one focus every day on how he or she chooses to interact with others. Adapting the concepts of the FISH! philosophy increases personal awareness about chosen attitudes, attentiveness to co-workers and customers, and promotes the concept that it is okay to have fun, or "play," at work. To guarantee a successful launch, leadership at the Answer Line initially selected high-energy staff to develop the department's implementation of the FISH! philosophy. The implementation team, adorned in fishing gear, introduced the FISH! philosophy video at the monthly staff meeting. After viewing the video, groups of staff gathered in different areas to brainstorm what each tenet would look like when brought to life in the call center. Leadership reviewed the staff's input that came from the brainstorming activity and implemented many of their ideas swiftly.

It has not been by coincidence that the FISH! philosophy has sustained as our culture over the past 9 years. To make certain we were successful, the following areas of concern were addressed, and should also be addressed by anyone considering implementation. The support of senior leadership is paramount for success. Without high level buy-in and support there is no ability to sustain this change in culture. A department or committee should be established to be sure there is an ongoing plan. The infrastructure of the committee must initially be comprised of positive, high-energy staff in order to maintain the momentum. The FISH! philosophy should belong to the staff. They should believe and feel that they "own" it.

Therefore, the manager must transition in his or her role as formal leader of the group to that of a "sounding board," assisting them, for example, with policy and financial concerns. Learn and remember which activities were successful and repeat them. Maintain a yearly calendar of successful events to review each year. In our call center, one year during a week in February, each staff member wrote an inspirational word on a small wooden heart. All the hearts were kept in a basket (heart shaped, of course) in the call center hallway. As the employees came in for their shift they picked a word on which to focus for that particular shift. The heart words were so successful that remote nurses would ask a co-worker in the office to select their word for the shift.

Allow front-line staff to give input regarding activities and projects by establishing a vehicle for them to communicate ideas. Beware of the naysayers. They will exist. Keep moving forward and eventually they will come along. FISH! activities do not have to be expensive. FISH! can be a low-budget, no-budget initiative. At the Answer Line, the activities most enjoyed by our staff have low to no cost. Finally, consider contacting Chart House, the documentary company responsible for FISH! They are an excellent resource for just about any need, and have become good friends of our call center.

One of the most meaningful stories illustrating our FISH! culture occurred several years ago. Employees working off-shift in the call center have no access to food, as our cafeteria is closed during the evenings and weekends. At the time, management made an attempt to provide staff with the opportunity to purchase a box lunch through the cafeteria. Our hospital vice president happened to be attending the staff meeting when this process was under discussion. The conversation was about the high cost we would be charged for the meals by the cafeteria and the potential to not be able to provide box lunches. By the time I returned to my office following the meeting, my voice mail light was on. The message was from our hospital vice president telling me that he'd not only come up with a plan to make this work during his five block walk back to the hospital, but he had already put the plan in place! He had arranged for us to have lunches made daily by the cafeteria at the hospital, rather than in our building. The meals would be sent to the department daily by courier. He even paid for the 3-month pilot out of his budget. The program was eventually unsuccessful, but that is not what our staff remembers. What they do remember was the strong support our vice president demonstrated for them and for their needs.

Over the years, the FISH! philosophy has shaped our culture at the Answer Line. Applicants hear about our FISH! culture during their interview. New hires view the FISH! video during orientation. Fostering the FISH! philosophy is a goal on each and every employee's annual review. The department's FISH! committee continues to meet monthly, planning activities, games, and events throughout the year. The committee regularly provides a FISH! presentation at staff meetings, tying customer service to the four tenets of the FISH! philosophy. The Answer Line is proud to hold one of our hospital's highest employee engagement scores year after year. Over the years we have supported other hospital departments with their implementation of the FISH! philosophy. Lastly, we are valued across our hospital system and our community as best practice for reward and recognition, in large part due to the FISH! philosophy.

Selective Recruitment

More recently, St. Louis Children's Hospital Answer Line collaborated with the Chally Group Worldwide in the development of an online assessment to evaluate for four characteristics of a successful triage nurse. The entire Answer Line RN staff provided the baseline sample population for the Chally Group Worldwide assessment tool, designed to profile the best candidate for a call center position. In situations when qualifications for final candidates are equal, those final candidates being considered for a position are asked to complete the online character assessment as a last step in the interview process. The assessment is not administered in every hiring situation. The Chally Group Worldwide administers the assessment via email at the manager's request. Results are sent to the manager approximately 24 hours after the candidate completes the assessment. Answer Line leadership estimates the use of this tool as 30% of the decision to hire new nurses. Both the Chally Group Worldwide assessment and the involvement of staff in the interview process promote selective recruitment of new staff members.

In an effort to hire "the best" candidate, the Answer Line has incorporated several strategic components into the hiring process. Following review of applications, the nurse recruiter conducts a phone screening before forwarding top candidates to the manager for initial screening. The manager's initial screening allows the opportunity to verify information on the application, and also to evaluate the candidate for voice quality and tone. Once qualified applicants have been identified, the manager arranges a shadowing opportunity in the department. Shadowing allows current staff to interact with applicants and provides the manager with staff impressions. Shadowing also provides the candidate with a deeper understanding of his or her potential role as a triage nurse. Applicants are asked to contact the manager after shadowing to discuss their observations. Qualified candidates who express interest in pursuing a position move on to the first interview with the hospital's nurse recruiter. At this time a keyboarding test is administered to assess proficiency. Upon successful completion of the interview and keyboarding test, the applicant has a second interview with the department's assistant nurse managers. The final interview is with the department manager. If necessary, final qualified candidates are asked to complete the Chally Group Worldwide online assessment as a last step in the interview process.

Once a new employee joins the Answer Line, preceptors provide their unit training, which involves the use of the clinical guidelines, partnership with physicians, and an introduction to our FISH! philosophy culture. Leaders in the department are fair, consistent, accessible, and speak the golden rule, that is, "success breeds success!" By treating each staff member as a unique individual, the Answer Line values a turnover rate of less than 10%, and we often have alumni return.

Since the implementation of the FISH! philosophy and the Chally Group Worldwide assessment, both customer and physician satisfaction scores at St. Louis Children's Hospital Answer Line have improved. In addition, as previously stated, annual employee engagement scores reveal that our nurses feel very positive about their workplace and work-life balance. Our sustained employee engagement scores, high retention rates, and longevity of staff are evidence of an environment rich with innovative approaches in maintaining and improving nurse satisfaction.

AIDET

In 2011, as part of the department's Six Sigma project to establish a standard call flow process, all staff were oriented to AIDET^{sm}, a Studer Group product.[4] AIDET provided us with a measurable tool to build patient and family trust and rapport. When the training materials were evaluated by our Six Sigma team, the concept "just made good sense."

AIDET is an acronym for *acknowledge, introduce, duration, explanation,* and *thank you.* Each of these elements is incorporated into the conversation with the caller/patient, in an effort to decrease anxiety and better serve his or her needs.

Designing our own training vignettes, the call center implemented AIDET into the call flow process in March 2011. Along with the other components of call flow, AIDET is currently being measured through a new audio audit tool.

While we do not yet have measurable results from our audio audits, anecdotal feedback has been impressive. Approximately 2 weeks after implementation, an employee working for a different service in the call center who was unaware of our implementation, mentioned that she was hearing "something different." Over the cubicle walls, and only able to listen to one side of the conversation, she could strongly sense a "different" conversation with our callers, one that was calmer and more collaborative. A second anecdotal story came from the individual who works on our caller satisfaction survey, again, unaware of the AIDET initiative. During her conversations with callers she mentioned that she was receiving feedback telling her something was positively "different" about the caller's perception of the call, as well.

Any change is challenging. AIDET, because it is a relationship-building tool that "made sense," has been a relatively easy implementation for us all. We have since shared our success with Process Improvement leaders in our institution, hoping other departments will evaluate it for their patient relationship needs.

References

1. Scanlon, W.J. (2001). *Nursing workforce recruitment and retention of nurses and nurse aides is a growing concern.* United States General Accounting Office. Retrieved from http://www.gao.gov/new.items/d01750t.pdf
2. Chally Group Worldwide. (2005). *Telephone triage nurse.* Technical report. Dayton, OH: Author.
3. Lundin, S.C., Paul, H., & Christensen, J. (2000). *Fish! A remarkable way to boost morale and improve results.* New York, NY: Hyperion.
4. Studer Group. (2005). AIDET. *Five fundamentals of patient communication.* Gulf Breeze, FL: Firestarter Publishing.

Use of decision support tools as discussed throughout this book may appear to be a double-edged sword. While they provide decision support, they are often misused, disempowering (rather than empowering) the nurses who use them. Written by a Nurse Administrator at Mayo Clinic, the following best practice describes a process in which the organization utilized nurses as content and process experts to develop and refine decision support tools that capitalize on, rather than undermine, the autonomy and expertise of the nurse.

NURSE-DEVELOPED ALGORITHMS AND PROTOCOLS IN ELECTRONIC DECISION SUPPORT TOOLS FOR TELEPHONE TRIAGE PRACTICE

Debra Cox, MS, RN

The office-based call center at Mayo Clinic in Rochester, MN, provides support to pediatric, adult, and geriatric patients across six clinic locations. In 2010, annual call volumes were approximately 200,000 calls, with 58,000 calls requiring triage expertise utilizing an electronic decision support tool.

Development and Use of Triage Algorithms

The electronic decision support tool developed by a nurse-led interdisciplinary team utilizes branching logic to store and apply patient-specific information as it pertains to each individual patient. Patient information from each question asked, and a corresponding positive/negative response, populates a final note which is reviewed by the RN author and released to the electronic health record. All regulatory and professional nursing standards requiring documentation are present in the patient record.

Based on their knowledge and experience, nurses provide the foundation for the development of the clinical algorithms present in the electronic decision support tool. Information technology programming experience is not necessary to build the algorithms; nurses function within a proprietary software system which supports the algorithm "building" process. Nurses who function well in this activity are usually quite analytical and are "consecutive thinkers." Nurse "builders" are able to respond quickly to change requests from users. During the H1N1 pandemic, nurse and physician builders initiated a new algorithm and had it available for use within 24 hours. Frequent suggested adaptations from the CDC were implemented quickly, which kept contagious patients from venturing into the office setting and allowed increased clinic capacity for more acutely ill patients requiring on-site care team services. The high volume of calls was absorbed by the call center staff due to a well-constructed algorithm which provided accurate and reassuring information to callers.

Nurses participate in an annual algorithm review process with physician colleagues. This review includes an updated literature search for new evidence of treatment changes or recommendations, review of issues identified by tool users through an electronic "issue tracker," and evaluation of data analytics available from the software database. Quality assurance analysis is available regarding actual utilization of each algorithm, including the number of questions required to arrive at a disposition recommendation. Nurses reported "abdominal pain symptoms" as a highly used algorithm requiring a great deal of time and large numbers of questions to maneuver the patient through the assessment. An MD/RN team analyzed trigger questions and decreased the actual number of questions required to deliver an appropriate disposition for abdominal pain by 70%. Patient clinical outcomes were then reviewed to match patients' recommended dispositions to their actual outcomes. The nurses in builder team roles have remarkable skill and critical thinking ability in developing algorithms with the electronic decision support tool. This will continue to be another avenue for nursing practice support in the future.

Use of Protocols to Direct Delegated Medical Acts

Ambulatory care nursing practice continues to grow in complexity in response to patient's changing needs. Nursing protocols provide a tool that supports nurses' critical thinking and decision making regarding patient interventions. Protocols are a population-based tool designed to direct the triage, advice, education, and counseling process between nurses and patients.

Protocols are documents that are developed by multidisciplinary teams that result in clinical decisions being made or medications being ordered by licensed allied health professionals without direct physician intervention. Nurses are able to provide safe, efficient care to patients while maximizing their scope of practice. State Boards of Nursing determine acceptable protocol practices within each state/jurisdiction. Physicians and nurses participate in an annual review process to re-evaluate protocols for necessary changes or improvements in regard to new clinical evidence and patient outcome data.

Nursing protocols have been utilized in the ambulatory practice for greater than 10 years at our academic institution. Protocols have provided an efficient means for nurses to assess patient symptoms and provide treatment through standardized application of the protocol, including some predetermined prescriptions. The protocols are population focused and only apply to patients presenting with a specific set of symptoms. The protocol is specific to the circumstances. For example, a medication may be prescribed in a way that is informative enough to ensure that it will only be used for patients whose condition falls within predetermined parameters. Protocols are written so that nurses have a high rate of reliability in applying to patient populations. Compliance with this format delegates authority to the registered nurse who otherwise does not have prescriptive authority. The RN provides his or her signature and notes the MD author of the protocol. This practice has been of particular benefit to the office-based call center working with established patients. Patients appreciate the convenience of receiving telephone treatment for common, acute symptoms such as ear pain, conjunctivitis, etc.

Data Analysis and Revision of Decision Support Tools

Triage nurses shape their professional practice through analysis of data and trends. When nurses have access to their own practice patterns as well as the practice patterns for their clinic, they are able to set goals and evaluate their progress. Nurses are able to review their quarterly trend reports which include the following elements: categories of dispositions recommended to patients along with the percentage of time this occurred (ED, urgent visit, self-care, etc.); numbers and types of algorithms utilized; complete versus incomplete calls; and length of call. Nurses are also provided their percentage of algorithm override decisions (deviations resulting in an upgrade or downgrade). During orientation, nurses are instructed in the philosophy of professional nursing practice which supports the application of critical-thinking processes as being the primary strength when utilizing decision support tools. The software application allows the nurse to identify when either the RN or the patient disagrees with the recommended outcome and the final action. Patient-population trends seem to influence the percentages of agree/disagree. The geriatric patient may have additional co-morbidities that the nurse is considering in addition to the decision support information. The nurse may be very appropriately discerning that an alternate plan is best for the patient and decide to override the recommendation.

What is particularly valuable about these algorithms is that they are developed by nurses and are revised based on continually collected and analyzed evidence of how they are being used by the nurses with the specific population being treated by the Mayo clinic. For example, the algorithm is revised if the evidence indicates that significant numbers of nurses override at a particular branch in the algorithm. Data are collected and analyzed, which tells the team whether the revision worked (non-significant numbers of incidents of deviation from the recommended disposition).

Conclusion

As technology continues to evolve, increased sophistication of decision support will become more broadly available, and patient self-management and triage will become increasingly common. However, nurses will still provide the critical analysis and advice that has yet to be replicated by software.

The process of providing nursing care via telephone presents organizational challenges that must be addressed sequentially in order to achieve success in program design and implementation. The following example illustrates the process of problem identification through program implementation and initial problem resolution in a large metropolitan pediatric teaching institution.

TELEPHONE TRIAGE EDUCATION AND PROGRAM DEVELOPMENT IN AN URBAN TEACHING ENVIRONMENT

Wanda Mayo, BSN, RN

Curriculum development in nursing education is a creative process, intended to produce a meaningful learning experience. The ultimate purpose is to create learning opportunities that build professional knowledge and skills so that the nurse practices competently in a changing health care environment. This process is "characterized by interaction, cooperation, change, and possibly conflict; composed of overlapping, interactive, and iterative decisions; shaped by contextual realities and political timeliness; and influenced by the personal interests, styles of interaction, philosophies, judgments and values of stakeholders" (p. 6).[1] As an educator, it is important to be aware of the influences which affect the learning atmosphere within the clinical setting. To ensure that an educational endeavor is successful, all stakeholders should be brought to the table to provide input and to critique the process as it proceeds.

Assessing clinical nursing staff to determine learning needs and competency levels is a primary role of an educator. Having had extensive experience as an ambulatory care nurse, I had a clear understanding of the challenges and opportunities associated with practice within an ambulatory care setting. A unique and important function of the ambulatory care nurse is the provision of care over the telephone. Nurses talk on the telephone all the time providing advice, educating clients/families, and assessing patient status to determine the best intervention(s) necessary to meet the patient's need(s). Considering this, I asked two primary questions: Are nurses aware of the standards and guidelines associated with telehealth nursing? What educational content needs to be considered in order to assure high-quality care over the telephone?

Literature Search

Evidenced-based nursing practice is fundamental in making decisions that facilitate best practices. Performing a literature search was the starting point to obtaining factual information on the subject of telephone triage. The literature search provided valuable information related to telephone triage nursing including who can perform telephone triage assessments, standards related to this practice, Board of Nursing views on telephone triage nursing, and the potential impact of telephone triage on patient care.

Assessment of Current Situation

Upon completion of the literature search, the next step involved speaking with the nurses directly. Initially, I walked though several of the clinics and casually asked the nurses what they thought of telephone triage nursing, if they had ever received training on how to provide care over the telephone, and whether they had been provided with specific telephone triage policies. This random survey revealed that nurses had a lot to say about this practice. They were most concerned about their lack of basic telephone triage training and the paucity of policies to direct care. Based on the information obtained informally, a telephone triage survey was developed to more formally assess the nurses' level of understanding in this arena. The questions on the survey assessed the nurses' understanding of telephone triage, the amount of time the nurses spent on the telephone, the amount of telephone triage training received, and whether the nurses were interested in receiving further education in this area. The answers to the questions not only indicated there was a knowledge deficit in this area, but it also indicated that nurses were interested in gaining additional knowledge. Thus, the problem was identified (lack of education and policy guidance) and the next step was to present these findings to the ambulatory leadership team.

Identification of Content/Process Expert

Prior to approaching leadership, I decided I still needed more information and so I went back to the previously completed literature search to identify an expert who could provide additional information and guidance. With the help of a professional consultant, I became more aware of the nuances of the practice and, most notably, the potential risks associated with telephone triage.

Next Steps

The information obtained from the formal and informal nurse's surveys, the literature search, and the consultant was compiled and organized for presentation to the leadership team. This group reviewed the information and, before moving forward, they agreed to participate in a conference call with the consultant to gain further insight regarding telephone triage nursing. As a result of the information gleaned from this call and to ensure that all stakeholders' input was obtained, a Telephone Triage Task Force was formed consisting of ambulatory care directors, an ambulatory administrator, advanced practice nurses, staff nurses, and educators. Subsequently, the leadership team agreed to have the consultant perform a site visit to conduct a risk assessment in the clinics. Directors in Ambulatory Care communicated with the managers in the clinics to ensure that all were aware of the importance of this endeavor. The consultant visited the hospital facility and completed a risk assessment on 10 of the more than 50 clinics.

While on campus, the consultant presented an in-house educational conference on telephone triage to the ambulatory care nursing staff and leadership team. Leadership strongly recommended that clinic nurses attend the conference. Based on this recommendation, 90% of the nurses attended. Topics covered in the conference encompassed the description of telephone triage nursing practice, misconceptions about telephone triage, standards directing this practice, decision making and critical thinking including use of the nursing process, and clinical practice including patient assessment and risk management.

Findings and Recommendations

Following the conference, the findings of the telephone triage risk assessment were presented to the leadership team and the Telephone Triage Task Force. The risk assessment addressed scope of practice, compliance with standards, staffing, access, call flow, and an assessment of the organizational culture as it pertained to the practice of telephone triage. Based on this report, an organizational vision for telephone triage was developed by the leadership team. This vision included:

- Delivery of safe, effective patient care over the telephone in all areas.
- Telephone triage as an integrated element of patient/family-centered care.
- Standardized telephone triage care among all clinics and portals of entry.

Development of a Sustainable Telephone Triage Education Program

Following the consultant's visit, the next task was to develop an ongoing and sustainable telephone triage educational program. Nurses from various clinical areas, including clinic managers and educators, made up the telephone triage education group. The educational plan included computer-based telephone triage modules, a 1-day telephone triage conference, and uniform competency testing. All clinic nurses were required to complete the computer-based modules. The conference covered the reasons why a telephone triage education program was needed, professional communication over the phone, provision of care using the nursing process, review of telephone triage scenarios, and the legal concerns associated with telephone triage. The conference was taped and presented to all ambulatory nurses and ambulatory leadership who were unable to attend the live conference. Two months later, clinic nurses were expected to complete a comprehensive telephone triage computerized test. The amount of time the telephone triage education group invested to ensure all ambulatory nurses and leadership received the conference educational material covered a 3-month period.

Program Design

In providing support to this endeavor, leadership placed primary emphasis on standardized education regarding telephone triage for all nursing staff. Concentrated efforts were also made to assure that all calls requiring assessment were managed by RNs in both the primary care and specialty clinics. Beyond these measures, other efforts to standardize or centralize triage were tabled for the time being. Leadership believed that if RNs were specially trained to provide telephone triage services, they would be able to adapt to provide safe and effective care in any setting.

Lessons Learned

Looking back on this project, there were many ups and downs. The barriers encountered included getting past preconceived ideas about telephone triage, inconsistent utilization of nursing and support personnel, and lack of uniform physician support. The biggest challenge faced was probably the fact that as a brand new ambulatory clinical educator, I was learning my role while trying to meet the expectation that I take the lead in design and development of a telephone triage program for our institution. The size of this project was daunting, and at times there were communication breakdowns. In retrospect, the individuals chosen to be a part of a project of this magnitude should be experienced, committed, and represent multiple levels of nursing to ensure that all viewpoints are identified and addressed. Perhaps the most significant lesson learned is that support from leadership is essential to the successful implementation of a telephone triage program. There must also be a strong commitment from educators, nursing management, and clinical nursing staff. Physician support is also important.

Summary

This project took 2.5 years to complete from the time the first question was asked to the completion of the computerized test during a hospital-based skills day. What is especially notable about this project is how one question led to the recognition of need, the involvement of leadership, and the formation of a task force. The objectives of the project were to increase the nurse's knowledge and understanding related to telephone triage nursing, to ensure that nurses were competent in providing nursing care, and to assure the provision of safe nursing care over the telephone. The ultimate achievement of the project was uniform education of all professional clinic nursing staff. It was gratifying to realize that the educational team in conjunction with the Telephone Triage Task Force played a key role in ensuring that the clinic nurses were practicing safely and meeting the needs of our patients over the telephone.

Reference

1. Iwasiw, C.L., Goldenberg, D., & Andrusyszyn, M.A. (2009). *Curriculum development in nursing education.* Sudbury, MA: Jones and Bartlett Publishers.

In 2000, the U.S. Air Force undertook a demonstration project to standardize telephone triage throughout its military branch. To this end, a civilian consultant was engaged to provide guidance so that the Air Force could replicate the success enjoyed in the civilian sector. During this project, which involved three Air Force Military Treatment Facilities (MTFs), or clinics, a number of valuable lessons were learned, most of which are reflected in Chapters 14 and 15 as well as elsewhere in this book.

This process improvement project describes development and implementation of a telephone triage program at Keesler Air Force Base. Although this project took place in an Air Force facility, the principles and processes described herein would be equally applicable in both military and civilian settings. Although still a work in progress, the process followed by this Medical Group could serve as a blueprint for program design for other military and civilian settings.

The view(s) expressed herein are those of the authors and do not necessarily represent the official policy or position the U.S. Department of the Air Force, the 81st Medical Group, Department of Defense, or the U.S. Government.

PROCESS IMPROVEMENT FOR TELEPHONE TRIAGE AND SAME-DAY APPOINTMENT MANAGEMENT IN AN AIR FORCE FAMILY HEALTH CLINIC

Holli McDonald, MHL, BSN, RN
Allison Plunk, RN, USAF NC Col (Ret)
Maureen Koch, RN, USAF NC Lt Col (Ret)

The Family Health Clinic (FHC) in the 81st Medical Group (81 MDG) at Keesler Air Force Base (AFB) in Biloxi, Mississippi, serves approximately 14,000 enrolled beneficiaries. The FHC providers serve patients across the adult lifespan and as young as 5 years of age. The clinic had recently implemented the Patient Centered Medical Home (PCMH) model for the provision of primary care services. Under this model, providers were divided into teams, with each team consisting of a doctor and a mid-level provider, such as a physician assistant (PA) or nurse practitioner (NP). Under this new model, patients see their assigned patient care manager (PCM, otherwise known as patient care provider, or PCP, in the civilian sector), or their mid-level provider for all of their health care needs. The staffing guidelines associated with implementation of PCMH changed the nurse-to-provider ratio from 1:1 to 1:2, essentially doubling each nurses' workload.

Appointments were scheduled by the appointment center, which began taking calls at 5 a.m. for active duty personnel and 6 a.m. for military dependents and retirees seeking care on base. The appointment center was staffed by Appointment Services, a group of contracted receptionists with no medical training, who used a "red flag" list to identify patients who should be referred directly to an emergency department (ED), thereby bypassing the nurses in the clinics. Patients who did not meet "red flag" criteria were scheduled appointments on a first-come, first-served basis. In a setting with only about 40 acute appointments per day, there were many patients who were unable to obtain a same-day appointment in the FHC. When a same-day appointment was unavailable, the appointment clerks created a computerized message known as a telephone consultation (T-Con) which was then routed to the nursing staff in the clinic via AHLTA, the Department of Defense (DoD) electronic health record (EHR). These T-Cons were reviewed by the appropriate team nurse, who was to contact the patient within 2 hours of their initial call. The nurse would triage the patient, after which the patient might then be referred to other clinics that had space available, or referred off-base to a local urgent care clinic (UCC).

DESCRIPTION OF THE PROBLEM

The system described resulted in first-level triage being done by appointment clerks rather than RNs. Because the receptionists were not qualified to make clinical decisions, appointments were scheduled based upon the patients' perception of when they would like to be seen. This occasionally resulted in patients receiving a same-day appointment when it was not medically indicated or when the patient would have been better served in a different location, such as an ED. Patients were only permitted access to RNs if no acute appointments were available, and this process was risky because patients were occasionally misdirected. Thus, the potential existed for delay in care when the true nature of the patient's problem was inadvertently misrepresented by the appointment clerks. And when appointment requests could not be met, generation of a T-Con was cumbersome, resource intensive, inefficient, and unnecessarily time consuming for the nurses. The management of these appointment requests was further complicated by the fact that the nurses were also dealing with a variety of other patient care responsibilities such as requests for prescription refills, test results, and various other clinical and non-clinical duties.

The clinic nurses were often overwhelmed by T-Cons, and the workload became unmanageable, with the clinic nurses spending much of their day juggling T-Cons and playing phone tag with patients. Unfortunately, because each nurse was multitasked and usually overwhelmed by T-Cons, being able to return a call within 2 hours was often difficult or impossible. Occasionally, it even took days to successfully reach a patient who had requested a same-day appointment. Once a patient was contacted by an RN, if an appointment was indicated, the nurse could schedule the patient in another clinic, or refer the patient to an off-base UCC or ED. For patients referred off-base, the nurse was required to complete necessary paperwork, and the patient had to contact the Referral Management Center to ensure authorization before proceeding to the civilian UCC for evaluation and treatment.

The FHC nurses estimated that they spent at least half of each workday trying to triage and assist patients with same-day appointment requests. Subsequently, their many other clinic duties often had to take a back seat to issues related to access to care. This also created a potential delay in care for the patient and was certainly not customer friendly. There was also significant concern for liability because the nurses were not able to meet patients' needs within the organization's established time frames. All in all, the process for assisting patients when no acute appointment was available was risky, inefficient, time consuming, and otherwise problematic, often delaying patient care. Additionally, both the excessive workload and the multitasked nature of the nurse's job created the potential for suboptimal care. There was a clear need for improvements in same-day appointment management and the amount of time nurses were spending on the telephone. It was hypothesized that the implementation of telephone triage services would improve the ability of the nurse to meet the needs of the patients and significantly decrease the number of inappropriate T-Cons for the nurses, thus freeing them to perform other clinical duties.

FIRST STEPS

To facilitate change, a civilian telephone triage consultant was engaged. She made a site visit, first providing a 2-day educational session for the nurses and leadership and then performed an assessment of the current situation with emphasis on risk management including options to address risk, improve efficiency, and assure quality. After review by the consultant, her recommendations included a workload analysis, designation of dedicated staffing, improved access, and call routing by electronic menu. Additional recommendations included development of a Telephone Triage Steering Committee, a presentation to the providers, revision of the organizational policy or operating instructions (OI), selection of decision support tools, and development of a user-friendly documentation template. A planning session was attended by the members of the nursing leadership team/telephone triage work group, including the chief nurse executive, several mid-level leaders, and staff nurses who were currently managing patient calls. The group practice manager (GPM), known as a practice administrator in the civilian sector, was invited to join the group to assist with logistic concerns such as template management.

The topics addressed by this work group included articulation of a vision, development of goals and objectives, identification and sequencing of tasks which would be necessary to accomplish the goals, and development of a task force structure to address various program elements necessary for implementation. An initial plan was developed which included reviewing existing technology and implementing the new electronic menu. Problems needing immediate remedy were addressed as necessary and a workload analysis tool was developed to serve as a basis to address staffing, access, and call flow.

Vision, Goals, and Objectives

The group's vision was of a centralized telephone triage function staffed with dedicated RNs. Several objectives were identified that would need to be met in order to support change design and implementation. It was decided to phase the project, implementing lasting solutions rather than employing "quick fixes" that would need to be addressed again in the future. The FHC was selected to pilot changes with the intention of later incorporating additional clinics and services, building on previous successes and supported by ongoing data collection.

Organizational necessities to be addressed included staffing, access to care, call flow, and clinical practice including use of decision support tools and documentation. To optimize the role of the RN, an alternate solution for management of requests for prescription refills and test results would be sought. Additionally, the clerks needed to be relieved of the responsibility of performing initial triage with a red flag list and charged only with the responsibility of scheduling routine appointments. Access strategies were discussed and would be explored further with the medical staff and GPM. Call flow was discussed at length, with the objective of having RNs take the calls live or as promptly as possible in order to reduce the inefficiencies and risk related to potential delay in care associated with returning patient's calls.

Task forces were created with task force leaders being named and membership suggested. It was deemed important to do this now so that the momentum created by the consultation wouldn't be lost. Task forces included workload analysis, documentation, prescription refills/test results, quality assurance, "quick fixes," electronic menu, education, external marketing, and internal marketing.

Data Collection

Data were collected for every FHC patient who called the front desk, left a message for the provider or the nurse through the appointment line, or called a clinic nurse directly. Data collection was manual, utilizing a telephone call log that documented each call on a separate line to facilitate more complete data analysis. Data were collected daily for 2 weeks. Data sources included time-stamped T-Cons documented in AHLTA, the administrative and medical technicians, and the clinic nurses. After collection, all data were compiled and analyzed, and the results were shared with the FHC Flight Commander, chief nurse, and all clinic staff.

Data Analysis

During the 2-week data collection period, the clinic nurses received a total of 921 incoming T-Cons and phone calls. This did not include T-Cons generated by the providers, walk-in patients, or additional callbacks to patients for various other reasons. The top four call reasons accounted for nearly 80% of the call volume and included medication issues/refills (34%), appointment requests (17%), test results (14%), and referrals (14%). The referral category included any patient request for a specialty provider consult (both new and continued consults), as well as requests for durable medical equipment (DME).

The majority of appointment requests were for same-day appointments at 71%, with 77% of those being received between 6 a.m. and 11 a.m. The remainder of appointment requests was for routine and follow-up appointments, at 13% each, and well appointments at 3%. Additionally, when evaluating the time it took to return calls, 72% of patients received a call back within 2 hours from the time of their initial call. Eight percent of the patients waited more than 2 hours for a callback from the nurse and there was no time recorded for the callbacks on 19% of the patients. However, it is important to note that a callback noted within the 2-hour time frame means only that an attempt to contact the patient was made during that time, not necessarily that the patient was contacted or that the issue was resolved. So, although most patients received callbacks within the prescribed 2-hour time frame, patients often had to wait several hours to obtain an appointment, and because access was frequently not available, patients needing to be seen that day were often referred off-base to a civilian UCC for treatment. To further complicate matters, clinic nurses spent a good deal of time playing "phone tag" with patients, sometimes significantly extending the amount of time it took to close the encounter.

Based on this information, clinic leadership decided to implement a telephone triage program staffed by experienced clinic nurses who were dedicated to the telephones during high call volume times in order to facilitate same-day appointment access. These nurses would take calls live, creating the potential for one-call resolution.

IMPLEMENTATION PLAN

Leadership Approval

The first step in program implementation was to gain leadership approval. The FHC Flight Commander and acting nurse manager met with the chief nurse and the deputy chief nurse to present the research and recommendations. Due to previously described staffing adjustments associated with PCMH, the clinic had three unassigned FTEs. It was acknowledged that this would be meaningful use for these unassigned nurses, and the chief nurse granted permission to move forward with the project. Necessary operational changes were discussed including the need for revisions to the appointment line telephone tree and booking protocols, phone requirements, decision support tools and references to be used, and how to obtain approval for all of these items. A kickoff date was established for telephone triage services. Other implementation steps are outlined below, but it is important to note that many of these steps occurred concurrently as process changes were implemented.

Telephone Triage Staffing

The clinic nurses and flight commander met to discuss which individuals would fill the role of FHC telephone triage nurse. Options included accepting internal applicants, assignment by leadership, or rotation of all nursing staff. Assignment by leadership might have inadvertently resulted in selection of nurses who didn't value telephone triage and rotation would have broken continuity in the clinics by pulling the primary nurse away from the team. Ultimately, three experienced contract nurses who had attended the training session were selected for the new roles as telephone triage nurses.

Call System/Telephony

Clinic leadership discussed expectations and capabilities of the telephone system with the facilities telephone systems manager. Emphasis was placed on how calls were to be routed through Avia, the computerized phone system that requires a log in by each triage nurse. Same-day appointment requests and symptom-based calls were to be automatically sent to an available nurse as they came in via an automated call distribution system (ACD), and other calls were routed as described below. The system was also designed so that if none of the triage nurses was logged in, the calls would automatically route to the appointment line.

Call Routing

As recommended, a new telephone tree was created and recorded by internal staff and implemented by the Communications Squadron. All same-day appointment requests for the FHC, and anyone wanting to discuss his or her symptoms, were routed directly to one of the three triage nurses. Requests for lab orders, lab results, prescription refills, and all other questions or concerns were routed to the appointment line clerks to create T-Cons for the providers and nurses.

Revision of the call intake process and the creation of nurse-run telephone triage potentially duplicated the contract services to be provided by the appointment line. Because the contract agency which staffs the appointment line is remunerated for every appointment booked and T-Con created by their personnel, the development of nurse triage would negatively impact their revenue stream. Furthermore, the appointment line staff report to a different squadron than the nurses and thus approval for modifications to the telephone tree and the associated booking convention had to be approved by their director. To gain this approval, the chief nurse presented the proposal to the TRICARE Operations and Patient Administration (TOPA) director who agreed with the recommended changes. However, it was intended by the TOPA director that the nurse triage line would be held to the same stringent guidelines as the appointment line in terms of patient wait times, length of calls, etc. Efforts to help the TOPA director understand that this was a different type of service, and thus it could not be held to the same time parameters, were unsuccessful.

Centralized Location

As recommended, the three triage nurses were moved to a centrally located office within the FHC. To coordinate this move, several other clinic members, including clinic leadership, were relocated. The centralization was deemed necessary to prevent the triage nurses from being pulled in different directions and once again multitasked.

Decision Support Tools and Documentation

Several different decision support tools were presently in use at the 81 MDG, and it was deemed advisable to standardize resources across the medical group. Several sets of decision support tools were reviewed and ultimately, *Telephone Triage Decision Support Tools for Nurses: Guidelines for Ambulatory Care (7th edition)* by Dale Woodke, was chosen based on its comprehensiveness, its use of the nursing process, and its perceived ability to integrate with AHLTA. This reference material was then placed on the Executive Committee of the Medical Staff (ECOMS) agenda for approval. The selected decision support tool manuals were ordered directly from the publishing company. Access to the company's online web site was also obtained for each triage nurse. Unfortunately, the online templates were not fully compatible with AHLTA and thus had to be manually recreated one by one. With over 100 topics, this was extremely time consuming and labor intensive. The templates were modified to include much of the required, but repetitive, documentation items (e.g., verifying name, date of birth, allergies, references utilized) to shorten the amount of time it would take the nurses to document their patient encounters. The triage nurses trialed several options for documentation (e.g., electronically in real time, scanning hard copies, etc.), but because the assessments were lengthy and calls were to be taken live while other callers held in queue, time was of the essence. As such, real-time documentation on hard copies of the templates with subsequent transcription to the electronic record was chosen. About 20 copies of each protocol were printed and filed in alphabetical order in two large filing cabinets in the nurse triage office. This enabled the triage nurses to quickly and easily access the hard copy templates for assessment and documentation during live patient calls. Additional hard copies were made as needed.

Booking Protocols

The appointment line clerks booked non-acute FHC appointments based on established clinic-specific booking guidelines. Upon creation of nurse triage, the booking protocols for routine appointments were updated as appropriate and necessary and sent to the appointment line clerks for implementation. As discussed previously, prior to implementation of the dedicated nurse triage program, the appointment clerks had utilized a red flag list to identify high-risk patients who needed to be seen immediately. Patients calling the appointment line with these "red-flag" symptoms had been directed by the appointment clerks to go to the closest ED for further evaluation. However, upon closer consideration, it became clear that by using this reference list, the appointment line personnel had been technically triaging patient complaints, an activity which should be performed by RNs. Subsequently, it was decided that only the triage nurses were authorized to book same-day appointments between the hours of 5 a.m. to 11:30 a.m., which were the peak call volume times for acute appointment requests. After 11:30 a.m. or if the triage nurses were offline for an unexpected reason, the appointment clerks were authorized to schedule same-day appointment requests. However, use of the "red flag" list by the appointment clerks was discontinued to enhance patient safety and improve compliance with standards. These new booking guidelines were scheduled to be effective to coincide with the triage kickoff date.

Staff Education and Training

The three triage nurses, all of whom had attended the recent telephone triage educational session, were also trained on use of the appointment system, Avia, by systems personnel. The PCMH nurses were also trained by a fellow clinic nurse on documentation guidelines and utilization of the newly developed templates in conjunction with AHLTA and the hard copy decision support tools.

The providers were informed by the FHC Medical Director of the need to be flexible and cooperative with the triage nurses when they had a need to schedule or work in a patient. Providers were also informed of the requirement to sign triage notes within 24 duty hours to ensure agreement with and knowledge of the plan of care.

Control Plan

Tracking tool. To monitor the new process, a telephone triage outcome tracking tool was developed. The triage nurses documented the time of each call and their patient dispositions or outcomes (i.e., the plan of care for the patient) on a specially created Excel spreadsheet. Outcome options included home care, acute/same-day appointment, routine appointment (within 7 days), follow-up appointment (within 30 days), UCC network referral, and ED. Data were compiled monthly to determine the effect telephone triage was having on patient appointments. This information was reported to the FHC Flight Commander, Medical Director, Group Practice Manager, Chief Nurse, Squadron Commander, and the TOPA Director.

Service-level data. The appointment line supervisor monitors four specific indicators and their associated control limits for Appointment Services. Since triage is an option within the main appointment telephone tree and utilizes the same call answering system, TOPA also chose to monitor these same indicators for telephone triage. These indicators include the percentage of calls answered within 45 seconds of the patient's call (>90%), the percentage of abandoned calls (<18%), the average speed of answer (≤45 seconds), and the average call talk time. At this point, average call length is tracked electronically, but there is no distinction among different call types. Because very short non-clinical calls are tracked along with full triage calls, the average call length data are meaningless relative to telephone triage and thus not discussed here.

While these recommendations and control limits are the productivity parameters imposed on the Appointment Services line, in the absence of any clear guidelines for telephone triage, the TOPA Director opted to continue monitoring these indicators for the triage line. Due to recognition by the nurses of the very different nature of telephone triage, the triage nurses were not preoccupied with trying to meet these standards. Leadership is more concerned with the nurses taking care of the patient rather than how long it takes to do so. Based on recognition that each patient call is unique, the triage nurses are given an unlimited amount of time to fully assess the patient and provide care as appropriate. These statistics have improved over the last several months as the triage nurses have become more comfortable in their new roles but continue to need improvement according to TOPA's standards (see Table 1). Although TOPA currently elects to monitor these time-based indicators, nurse triage monitors the patient outcomes, thereby providing data that demonstrate the importance of implementing nurse triage DoD wide. And when the TOPA Director presents his productivity data to executive leadership, he also presents the triage outcomes data tracked by the triage RNs which demonstrates the positive effect triage is having on patient care (see Figure 1 for the RN data).

Table 1.
Telephone Triage Call System Indicators

Month	Calls Within Service Level	Calls Outside of Service Level	Abandoned Calls	Total Calls	Percent of Abandoned Calls	Service Level*	Average Speed of Answer (min:sec)
March	755	441	402	1,598	25.16%	47.25%	3:29
April	592	319	332	1,243	26.71%	47.63%	3:53
May	667	277	199	1,143	17.41%	58.35%	2:17
June	763	202	134	1,099	12.19%	69.43%	1:23
Clerical goals					<18%	>90%	< 45 sec

* Service level is the percentage equivalent of the total number of calls that are answered within 45 seconds of the patient's call being routed to the triage RNs. It is computed by dividing the number of calls within the service level by the total number of calls.

Data application. Based on these data, the triage program has made several changes to improve the service being offered to patients. These changes have included staggering triage shift start times, ensuring all triage nurses are working during peak call times, limiting the number of triage nurses scheduled off at any given time to one, developing templates for streamlined documentation of electronic charting, and allowing the appointment line to book acute appointments in times of unexpected minimal staffing (i.e., fewer than two triage nurses).

Peer Review

As a quality control measure, monthly peer reviews are also conducted on 5% of the triage calls performed in the prior month. The peer nurse who audits each nurse changes on a rotating basis. The records being audited are chosen by the auditing nurse utilizing each nurse's handwritten log of patient calls. The peer review is conducted for compliance with 22 indicators classified under five main categories: (a) demographics, (b) assessment, (c) planning, (d) intervention, and (e) evaluation. Examples of such indicators include using appropriate patient identifiers (i.e., name and date of birth), using the correct protocol based on assessment data provided, assessing a

Figure 1.
Nurse-Facilitated Care Outcomes (March-July 2011)

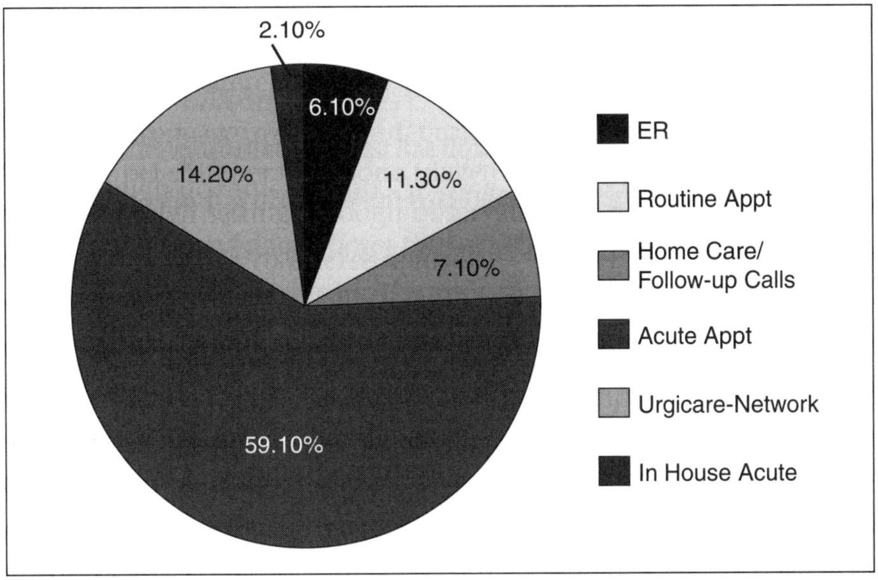

pain level, and providing a disposition consistent with the patient assessment.

Policy Manual/Medical Group Instructions (MDGI)

The medical group telephone triage instructions, MDGI 46-104, contain the roles, responsibilities, and procedures for the nursing practice of telephone triage at the 81 MDG. This MDGI includes many components of the control plan including peer review, triage nurse requirements, and telephone triage training criteria. The MDGI also contains a requirement for mandatory 24-hour provider review and sign off on all triage encounters to ensure the appropriateness of the disposition.[1]

POST IMPLEMENTATION

Call Statistics

The implementation of dedicated nurse-run telephone triage has been successful in improving the appropriateness of dispositions.

Specifically, each month on average, approximately one-fourth of the requests for same-day appointments are referred to a higher or lower level of care. Alternate dispositions included patients referred to the ED (6.1%), those scheduled for routine appointments (11.3%), and those who required only home care (7.1%). Figure 1 shows the nurse-facilitated care outcomes for the total number of requests for same-day appointments that were triaged during the first 4 months of the program. Of note is the fact that when appointments were no longer available, patients were either referred to another clinic on base (in-house acutes, 2.1%) or 14.2% were referred to UCC, each representing same-day appointment overflow. In comparison, prior to the implementation of dedicated nurse-run telephone triage, instead of referring patients to the appropriate level of care, all requests for same-day appointments were scheduled in the clinic as same-day acute appointments when available. When the supply of same-day appointments ran out, patients were given referrals for care at a local UCC in the civilian sector. This was not only very costly for the MTF, but it was also problematic in that some patients were occasionally not receiving the appropriate level of care. Unfortunately, after implementation of the triage program, when access was lacking, the UCC was still used for same-day appointment overflow. Because these patients represented 14.2% of the total dispositions, they presented an opportunity to recapture patients who were seen in the community rather than at the MTF. In summary, the data collected on triage dispositions suggested better use of same-day appointments, more appropriate dispositions for patients with acute problems, and a decrease in the number of patients who were unnecessarily referred to the community for urgent care (see Figure 1).

Satisfaction

Satisfaction measures reported directly to the chief nurse indicate that the clinic nurses are happy with the service and that it definitely frees them up to perform their other clinical duties. However, they expressed the wish for telephone triage to continue through the close of business each day because they continue to receive same-day appointment requests in the afternoon as well. To this end, a fourth nurse was reallocated to triage.

According to the clinic medical director, the majority of the clinic providers are happy with the service. They noted seeing patients with legitimately acute health care needs rather than patients who managed to secure a same-day appointment for non-acute issues. Making better use of these appointments ultimately decreases the number of work-in patients the providers must see. One physician complaint was regarding the triage nurses having control over who is worked-in to see the providers. However, of the 12 clinic providers, only two complained about this issue. In accordance with policy, each provider was asked to supply two set work-in times that are utilized at the triage nurses' discretion, based on their assessment of the patient's condition. Overall, the number of work-in patients that each provider sees is minimal as a result of these thorough nurse triage assessments, with an average of less than two work-ins per month per provider.

Many patients have expressed satisfaction with the new triage service. They enjoy being able to reach a nurse directly and not having to wait hours or days for a call back. Many patients have also noted that they are able to see their provider more often and are being referred to UCCs in the community less frequently. Early in implementation, there were some complaints about the length of time it took to reach a nurse, but Table 1 shows that the wait time is improving significantly. According to the customer service representative, there have been only a handful of complaints to date.

LESSONS LEARNED

Best Practice

Air Force Medical Operations Agency (AFMOA) conducted scheduled site visits following implementation of PCMH. The new triage service and its results were showcased to AFMOA leadership during these visits. An important outcome of these visits was that the telephone triage service was ultimately named an Air Force "Best Practice." To sustain this service, the chief nurse subsequently requested and is expected to receive three permanent government service clinical nurse positions for telephone triage as a new service line.

Process Improvements

There are several things that might have been done differently in this process improvement. Although general objectives were identified at the beginning of this process, they should have been developed in measurable terms to determine the effectiveness of the process improvement. As an example, revisions to the original generalized goals to reflect objective criteria might have looked something like this:

1. Reduce the overall number of T-Cons that FHC nurses must manage by 20% over the next 8 months.
2. Facilitate same-day appointments as requested, reducing those delayed beyond same day to 0 within 4 months.
3. Increase access for acute care by 15% within 6 months.
4. Increase percentage of T-Cons called back by close of business by 20% over the next 8 months.

In terms of data collection, in order to more fully grasp the number and type of patient calls, Appointment Services should have also been included in the data collection process by logging all calls that resulted in a scheduled appointment. These efforts would have improved the quality and reliability of the information obtained, but unfortunately Appointment Services was not given permission by their chain of command to participate in the initial data collection process.

Additionally, as part of the implementation plan, the patient population should have been educated prior to triage kickoff on the upcoming changes regarding how they would procure same-day appointments. More specifically, patients should have been educated on the purpose of triage, the changes in the process for scheduling a same-day appointment, and that changes were being made to the menu options for the appointment line. It would be particularly important to dispel the myth that triage is meant to keep patients out of the clinic and to help the patients understand that the actual goal of triage is to get patients to the right level of care within the right time frame. As an added benefit, the triage nurse attempts to improve same-day appointment access with the patient's primary care team, thereby reducing the need for referring patients off base for acute care. Due to the misconceptions about telephone triage, the program was later named Nurse-Facilitated Care to eliminate any negative connotations about triage and to refocus both staff and patients on the goal of assigning appropriate dispositions and delivering quality care.

Throughout the process, there was no actual measure of patient satisfaction. This would have been extremely important in order to appropriately monitor and listen to the voice of the customer. During the initial data collection process, the level of patient satisfaction with same-day appointment access and wait time for scheduling a same-day appointment should have been assessed as a baseline. Ideally, post implementation, these indicators could then have been reassessed and included in the control plan for consistent monitoring.

Changes for the Future

There are several recommendations for improving dedicated nurse triage. First, the TOPA service line requirements must be amended to reflect the differences between booking appointments and performing actual clinical triage services. Triage takes longer to perform and is much more in-depth than simply booking an appointment, yet both services are held to the same standards, at least on paper. As an example, TOPA requires that patients not wait more than 45 seconds before speaking with a representative. This is neither realistic nor achievable for triage services. Because of the unique nature of triage, it should be identified as a separate service line and as such, have separate service guidelines in place for control monitoring. Specifically, it is inappropriate and would possibly lead to patient safety concerns, if RNs were not afforded sufficient time to perform an adequate triage assessment.

The addition of a fourth nurse was anticipated to significantly improve performance of triage services. With three nurses, there are occasional scheduling difficulties, particularly during the summer and around holidays. Only one nurse can be off at any given time so that patient wait times do not become extensive. Furthermore, through the use of staggered start times, a fourth triage nurse would allow triage services to be available all day, thereby further freeing up clinic nurses to concentrate on their other clinical responsibilities. Improvements in the service levels would also be an expected benefit of an additional triage nurse.

To make the new provider-to-nurse ratio of 2:1 successful under the Air Force's implementation of PCMH, there must be development of creative workflow strategies to take some of the burden off of the clinic nurses. However, it is not sufficient to merely recommend processes for improvement as has been done in the past. MTFs must be given sufficient resources and guidelines for implementation to make these strategies, and ultimately PCMH, successful. As such, it is strongly recommended that the triage service be included in the Air Force's PCMH model as a new and necessary service line and that it be authorized its own manning separate from the FHC.

A recommended long-term goal, particularly if dedicated nurse triage becomes a part of the Air Force's implementation of PCMH, is that there be uniform training and development of better documentation templates that are compatible with AHLTA. Real-time documentation would be ideal in order to reduce the amount of time currently devoted to documentation and to ensure that the note is available to the provider prior to any appointments. To be successful, this may entail partnership with a decision support tool publisher. Through standardization, dedicated nurse triage could become an Air Force "best practice."

CONCLUSION

The creation of telephone triage has led to first call resolution for most patients requesting same-day appointments. This has dramatically decreased patient wait times for scheduling such appointments, ensuring that patients are directed to the right level of care within the right time frame, thereby improving patient safety and decreasing the facility's potential for liability. As added benefits, access to acute care and clinic morale have both improved significantly. With dedicated telephone triage now named as an Air Force "best practice," the Air Force model of PCMH should be modified to include additional or reallocation of staffing for a telephone triage service line to improve overall quality of care and efficiency of nursing in the Air Force.

Reference

1. Department of the Air Force. (2011). *Medical group instruction 46-104: Telehealth nursing/nursing telephone triage.* Keesler Air Force Base, MS: Author.

The following exemplar is from Langley Air Force Base and is important because it illustrates that dedication and vision, problem solving, and identification and use of existing resources (including experienced others) can and does pay off. This project was managed by a junior officer (Captain) who took the ball, and with a lot of support from her leaders and her peers, ran with it!

The view(s) expressed herein are those of the authors and do not necessarily represent the official policy or position the U.S. Department of the Air Force, Langley Air Force Base, Department of Defense, or the U.S. Government.

ONE MILITARY TREATMENT FACILITY'S JOURNEY IN SETTING UP NURSE-LED TELEPHONE TRIAGE

Capt Elizabeth Anne Hoettels, NC, USAF

Part of the joy of being a nurse in the military is that you are never "just a nurse." Jobs rotate and by virtue of stepping into new positions, you are provided often unexpected opportunities to expand your skills and professional expertise. Often you truly do not realize the increasing scope of responsibility that accompanies these duties. Such was the case with telephone triage. The only "additional duty" for a small group of three was to review the current Medical Group Instruction (MGI; i.e., policy) on Telephone Triage. The challenge during the review was to assess current practices and update the Instruction with materials to reflect the most current practice; in other words, to see if we were following our own policy. Little did we know all that would transpire by stepping into the realm of nurse-led telephone triage.

After informally interviewing nurses from various patient care areas such as the Family Health Clinic, Internal Medicine, Pediatrics, the Women's Health Clinic, and Labor and Delivery – all who have the potential to actively perform triage telephonically – the group realized some areas were not practicing consistently. Guidance, at the time of the review, left the determination to participate in telephone triage to the chief nurse executive. Our chief nurse executive believed that standardized and evidence-based telephone triage protocols provide patient-centered care while offering effective risk management. The question for the group then became: How do we implement effective nurse-led telephone triage?

Like any other clinical undertaking, our small group set out on an information-gathering expedition. In reviewing the current literature, we found telephone triage has become an increasingly accepted avenue for providing patient care, with "steady increase in telephone triage and advice services over the past decade demonstrat[ing] public demand" (p. 483).[1] It provides access to education, information, and advice while empowering patients to manage their own health care.[2] In addition, telephone triage helps manage the increasing demands for same-day appointments and ensures more efficient use of health care resources, including decreasing unnecessary patient visits to the hospital emergency room, and decreasing the costs associated with sending beneficiaries to outside urgent care centers.[1,3]

The MGI stated that we used a variety of resources to support the practice of telephone triage. Our group obtained and reviewed all the resources referenced as well as several different sets of protocols and decision support software. While there were many adult-focused sets, protocols written by Barton Schmitt and distributed by the American Academy of Pediatrics seemed to be the gold standard for pediatrics. Our group reviewed the American Academy of Ambulatory Care Nursing *Telehealth Nursing Practice Administration and Practice Standards*[4] to ensure that we were using the most up-to-date nursing practice information and to identify current practice references, requirements, and guidelines. We also researched other Air Force hospital facilities doing nurse-led telephone triage to see how they were ensuring standards. Compiling the research and updating the MGI took approximately 1 month to accomplish. The next task was to create an implementation plan.

The Answer to Everything in Life – Training

Our first step with program implementation was education. An informal poll of clinic nurses revealed very few actually had any formal telephone triage training. Most just had on-the-job training. The literature review revealed that nurses must "have specialized training and good judgment" to ensure the nurses provide safe, effective, and appropriate assessment; patient and/or parent education; and crisis intervention while using standardized protocols.[5] During the research period, one team member recalled a nationally recognized telephone triage consultant who previously provided training at another Air Force military facility. We contacted the consultant and received information on a potential training package that would be tailored to the needs of the facility – 2 days of training and education, and 1 day of a risk assessment in conjunction with a strategic planning session – a package type provided for similar military facilities.

The predominant numbers of nurses in the facility – active duty, government service, and contract – had not received official training in telephone triage. Sending all the nurses to conferences outside the state would be cost prohibitive. Additionally, the time frame to get all of our nurses trained would extend implementation because we could not send them all on business trips simultaneously, nor could we fund contract nurses for this training. Bringing the consultant to the facility enabled nurses across the Military Treatment Facility (MTF) spectrum to receive training and give them a common reference point — an advantage to new program implementation. After a cost/benefit analysis, the group concluded that having the consultant provide local on-site training would prove more beneficial overall.

Like many things in a small hospital, word spread about the upcoming training. Nurses started mentioning this training, stating it was exactly what they needed. They wanted to use the nursing knowledge they worked so hard to obtain, rather than just making appointments and refilling medications. Other nurses said they were frustrated when the medical technicians or appointment clerks answered symptom-based phone calls and referred the patients outside the MTF.

Day 1 of training arrived and almost 60 nurses with a wide variety of backgrounds showed up with manuals in hand, some a bit hesitant about this whole concept, while others were quite energized to learn more. The instructor spoke to the importance of nurses performing triage; telephone triage allows nurses to use their expertise to practice autonomously while promoting collaboration with the health care team. The speaker highlighted that the foundation of establishing effective telephone triage was to evaluate the system to determine how to best make it more efficient. The legal aspects associated with telephone triage were also addressed. Finally, Health Insurance Portability and Accountability Act (HIPAA) compliant symptom-based telephone calls were played to demonstrate the telephone triage process. Attendees reported that this was an effective training experience. One very important aspect was that the chief nurse executive and other Medical Group nursing leadership attended training right next to the more novice nurses, demonstrating not only their commitment to learn and understand what our nurses were doing, but also that this program was supported at the executive level. At the conclusion of two 8-hour days, the nurses were energized to return to their respective units and implement the process improvements.

The training was the easy part; the challenge ahead was keeping that momentum and using it to help with forward progress. The nurses left the conference empowered with knowledge and determination to ensure nurses were doing just that — practicing professional nursing. Understanding the need to keep the enthusiasm, rapid implementation was vital.

Implementation: 'The Best Laid Plans…'

To assist the chief nurse executive with a comprehensive yet tailored strategy for telephone triage at USAF Langley Hospital, the consultant spent her 3rd day conducting a risk assessment of the current telephone triage process. With a systematic approach, the consultant started from point of origin in the telephone room, following the patient's call request back to the clinic provider. With information gathered, the consultant assisted the nurse leaders with mapping a course for implementation. Part of this included identifying a "driver" (chief nurse executive) and a "worker" (someone to do the labor of gathering, coordinating, and implementing the telephone triage process), as well as key leaders and nurse volunteers who were interested in contributing to the entire process. From redesigning the flow of the telephone tree to creating templates that would be user-friendly for nurses to document, lists with details for every requirement were created, tasks assigned, buy-in achieved, and the green light given.

The team was off and running on their trek, or at least so they believed. Something as seemingly simple as revising a telephone tree would require 30 days implementation due to the contract that was in place with the current telephone intake system. Space was at a premium in the facility; obtaining a dedicated room to meet the requirements for telephone triage from the Facilities Utilization Board was extremely challenging. Finally, with staffing always a concern, we were unsure where we would find dedicated phone triage staff. Statements of work would have to be created and submitted in the hopes of obtaining contracting money to hire nurses; in the meantime, active duty nurses would need to be reallocated to different roles. While simple in concept, a few of the tasks were somewhat more complicated than they originally appeared; however, the group was not deterred. They were determined to "adapt and overcome."

Realizing this was not the first attempt for a military facility to implement centralized telephone triage, we sought other facilities that had embarked on the journey. Fortunately, the team was able to tap into the knowledge of a similar-sized Air Force hospital that began implementation just months prior. Their team graciously shared processes, staffing ratios, implementation products such as the electronic health record (EHR) templates, and even some growing pains they experienced along the way. The new group practice manager (GPM) at Langley had experience with phone tree development and shared her great ideas on how to revise the phone tree. The EHR template manager networked to find templates that could be adapted to meet requirements for documentation. Additionally, one of the flight commanders had extensive experience in nurse-led telephone triage and offered her insight to ensure success of our program. The input from these resources made transition and implementation easier for the Langley team.

Just Do It

Pieces and parts of the program had been coming together, but it seemed as if the team could not find a way to get all the stars aligned; there was always just one piece that made the team hesitate to start. Armed with encouragement from the Executive Staff, the team decided to "just do it."

The team opted for a "soft approach," easing their way into telephone triage, starting low and going slow. The plan was to start with a trial of the new process for 7 days beginning on a Tuesday, a traditionally slower day for phone volume. Three experienced active duty nurses initiated the process. Their new home for telephone triage would be in the MTF main telephone room, along with the clerks who answered the hospital phone lines. The three telephone triage nurses consisted of nurses from Family Health, Internal Medicine, and Pediatrics. The choice of nurses was planned so that they could assist each other in their respective areas of expertise. They were assigned to telephone triage duties during the traditionally identified heaviest volume hours: Monday through Friday, 0730-0930. The goals were to reclaim all of the active duty population with a symptom-based call; and then support the beneficiary population to the best of our capabilities to get the patient to the right level of care at the right time. While we did not have a personalized template as of yet, the EHR manager obtained a standardized AFMS nurse triage form for the nurses to use for documentation purposes. The nurses had acquired the basics to commence with the program; with the knowledge that this would be a starting point and the awareness of our culture of continuous improvement, we began telephone triage at our MTF.

The Road Less Traveled Is Sometimes a Little Rough: Just Wear Trail Shoes

On day 1 of this part of the journey, the nurses determined their first challenge was access. The goal of nurse-led telephone triage is to get the patient to the right level of care at the right time; it is hard to assist with getting patients to one of the "right" places – in this case the clinic – when there are limited available appointments. Understand, however, that unlike our civilian counterparts, an Air Force hospital serves as a deployment platform, meaning that on any given day our providers might be tasked to provide ramp-up medical assistance to large groups of people who are deploying or even to serve overseas thenselves. While they are meeting the greater Air Force mission, it does impact access at a local level, hampering the ability to get the triaged patients to the right place.

Not to be deterred, the team tapped into an often underutilized resource as a solution: the Independent Duty Medical Technician (IDMT). The IDMT, with oversight from a physician, has the capability and training to provide acute care to active duty members who require medical care. Working with the GPMs, appointments were created to support eight additional active duty slots for patients to be seen every day. An evaluation was conducted at the 5-week mark and confirmed that this number of same-day appointments was sufficient.

The next issue was obtaining the best mix of nursing staff for the telephone triage phone room. A request was submitted for contract nurses that would be solely dedicated to the nurse triage service. Funding for these positions was not available, meaning that the nurses would come from current active duty staff. If one of the nurses was unavailable to support the pilot program due to mission requirements, all attempts were made to ensure that another nurse from that clinic would cover the telephone triage phone lines. After a 1-month trial, the team created a rotating schedule utilizing only nurses who received telephone triage training.

The final challenge was provider and nurse buy-in. When the telephone triage nurse identified a patient needing to be seen that day by his or her provider, but no appointments were available, the triage nurse would often ask the provider or provider's nurse if it were possible to work the patient in. While some of the health care teams were amenable to assist, others questioned the nurse's judgment regarding whether the patient should be seen or not, despite triaging based upon nursing expertise and the use of an approved protocol set. Others reported being unaware of the pilot program. This was not the largest hurdle by any means, but the team solution was to continue to educate the providers, nurses, and technicians on nurse-led telephone triage.

Five Weeks and Counting

To get through the hardest journey we need take only one step at a time, but we must keep on stepping. ~ Chinese Proverb

The nurse-led telephone triage program at USAF Langley Hospital is still in its infancy. The team has only started at the tip of the iceberg, but for every challenge placed in their way, the solution is to attack and resolve each issue, one at a time. The key has been coordination with leadership and networking with counterparts who have experience with nurse-led telephone triage to collaborate and identify solutions.

To date, our triage efforts have resulted in recouping a significant number of patients for in-house care by their own providers, thereby improving patient satisfaction and saving reimbursement dollars that would otherwise have been spent on network care in the private sector. More importantly, our nurses triaged three very critical patients who had life-threatening situations. The utilization of the nursing process (assess, diagnose, plan, implement, and evaluate), superb telephone communication skills, and excellent training and experience allowed the triage nurses to get to the root of the patients' concerns quickly and assist with immediate lifesaving interventions. Those three calls made the many activities and ensuing challenging moments necessary to start a nurse-led telephone triage program entirely worth it and reassured us that we were on the right path to providing the best care for our patients.

References

1. Purc-Stephenson, R.J., & Thrasher C. (2010). Nurses' experiences with telephone triage and advice: A meta-ethnography. *Journal of Advanced Nursing, 66*(3), 482-494.
2. Penfold, J. (2011) Better telephone triage. *Primary Health Care, 21*(4), 7-8.
3. Barber, J.W., King, W.D., Monroe, K.W., & Nichols, M.H. (2000). Evaluation of emergency department referrals by telephone triage. *Pediatrics, 105*(4), 819-821.
4. American Academy of Ambulatory Care Nursing. (2007). *Telehealth nursing practice administration and practice standards* (4th ed.). Pitman, NJ: Author.
5. Hellinghausen, M. (2000). *Dialed in: Nurses prepare for the future of telephone triage.* Retrieved from http://www.nurseweek.com/features/00-05/triage.html

The work-at-home or telecommuting environment (also known as remote or virtual call centers) has grown by leaps and bounds over the past several years. The following best practice describes, in rather modest terms, an extremely successful work-at-home model implemented by a major player in the industry. Due to a variety of financial, societal, and workforce issues, it is likely that the movement toward remote telephone triage will continue to grow exponentially.

CONSIDERATIONS FOR DEVELOPMENT AND MANAGEMENT OF A WORK-AT-HOME TELEHEALTH PROGRAM

Kathryn Scheidt, MSN, MS, RN

I was employed by a very large *Fortune 500* company where the work-at-home model was successfully implemented over a period of several months. After starting with a small pilot group, the work-at-home team grew to over 800 staff in 4 years. Most of the staff were registered nurses who provided over-the-phone triage and disease management services to health plan members.

It would seem a dream come true for a RN to be able to practice nursing from a remote setting, in the comfort of his or her own home. Making the decision to work from home is not a simple one for either the employer or the employee. If you are considering this for your organization or for yourself as an employee, there is much to consider before you can successfully enter a total virtual work environment. The set of tools that make a nurse successful in a traditional hospital or clinic setting are not the same tools needed for the work-at-home setting. There are specific skill-set tools as well as office tools that are mandatory for the remote employee to be successful in this new work environment. This author experienced the transition of a staff of several hundred from a pure call center setting to a complete work-at-home setting. In this section, best practices learned from implementing our work-at-home environment are discussed from the perspectives of both the employee and the employer, as well as strategies for success in joining or launching a virtual work environment.

Nurse Characteristics Needed for Success

For nurses to consider if a work-at-home environment is right for them, they should be aware of the characteristics of the successful work-at-home employee. These characteristics are unlike those needed in most nurse employment environments and telework is not for everyone. Many people are very social and need considerable interaction with co-workers to remain satisfied with their work. Telework is not ideal for those who thrive on social interaction on a daily basis. Telework also does not work well for those who are known as loners. An isolated telework situation could be detrimental to a person who already has a self-imposed lack of contact with co-workers by exacerbating pre-existing social problems. Telework is best for those who like working alone, but do not avoid contact with others.

Teleworkers also need to be self-starters. They must have a strong work ethic, and not be the kind of person who needs close supervision in order to get work done. Working from home doesn't mean a break from action or a chance to fool around — stressed teleworkers understand that. The entire telework system will fail without self-starters in these positions.

A teleworker must have technological competence. Working from home requires proficiency with the tools used for the job and for communication, including the product-specific software programs, instant messaging, desktop faxing, Microsoft Outlook email and appointment functions, intranet or company-specific resource access, tele or web conferencing processes, and any other application that the employee may need to use. The successful teleworker is not afraid of technology; if something goes wrong with the computer system or the software, he or she will need to troubleshoot problems and either fix the problem themselves or be able to communicate the problem to a company IT employee for assistance.

Benefits for the Employer and Employee

There are benefits of a work-at-home environment that are distinctly different for the employer and the employee. When deciding to implement a work-at-home program, each must weigh the benefits. We found the following benefits to be helpful in selling the idea of going to a work-at-home environment to both the company leadership and to our current employees who would be affected by the move to working at home.

Employer Benefits of a Work-at-Home Environment

- Employee retention (annualized rate in the low teens for a Nurse Advice Line product)
- Reduced attrition
- Decreased recruiting and training costs (all training was conducted remotely using Live Meeting and other web-based technology)
- Employees able to take the job with them when they move thereby reducing turnover due to relocation
- Ease of recruiting for work-at-home
- Larger labor pool from which to draw; not limited to commuting distance from a call center
- The ability to hire RNs from any of the Compact states, thus reducing RN state licensure costs (most State Nurse Practice Act's define the practice of nursing as occurring at the location of the patient and a teleworking RN must be licensed in the state where the patient is calling from as well as in the state that the RN performs an outbound call to reach a patient)
- Reduced exposure to call center closure; usually, weather or physical disaster is a regional incident, and having employees from a broad section of the United States minimizes work lost due to these disasters

- Reduced tardiness and absenteeism, which are critical elements in a call center's ability to meet inbound call volume demands (average speed to answer and abandonment rate metrics)

Benefits to the Employee

- Quality of life improvement
- Less stress
- Can pursue hobbies
- Can see family members while on break
- Able to exercise more (walking on breaks with team challenges for accrued distances!)
- Better able to meet personal obligations
- Can arrange breaks in order to drop children off at school
- Run errands and do chores more easily
- Reduced wardrobe costs
- As-you-like-it dress code
- Ability to work during personal challenges
- Care of sick family members (under the proper circumstances)
- Return to nursing practice sooner after surgeries, births, or other conditions (medical clearance to work a portion of a day or with extended breaks during the workday are easier to accommodate in a work-at-home environment)
- Work during catastrophic health events
- Savings in automobile or commuting expenses (the commute is from your bedroom to your work desk!)

Requirements for Working at Home

Our employees had certain requirements in order to work at home and prospective work-from-home nurses would be well advised to consider these before deciding to apply for a telehealth nursing position. Generally the equipment to be used in the home workspace includes:

- Approved high-speed Internet (approved by the employer's IT department)
- Land line (cannot use cell phones for the patient contact portion of the work)
- Computer monitor of a specific size to accommodate the program application or if multiple applications need to be opened at the same time
- Office furniture dedicated to the workspace
- Ergonomic work area

We found that the most successful work-at-home employees had approached their working environment in a specific way. They had to develop an office frame-of-mind in order to step from being at-home to working-at-home. In our employee feedback and surveys, they shared these success tips:

- Create a quiet environment that is isolated from family traffic.
- Wake up at the same time each day; establish a good daily routine.
- Schedule early morning (or early shift) conference calls, meetings, or other events that help start the day or shift productively.
- Establish a ritual that marks the beginning of work every day such as reading email.
- Set up and follow a work schedule.

- Let unfinished personal projects wait until a break in work schedule.
- Make a "to do" list at the end of each day and use it to maintain focus on work the next day.
- Establish or follow scheduled breaks.
- Dress for work, even if that is very informally dressed.

As an employer, we provided the following programs, training, and equipment. Prospective employees should inquire as to whether these items will be provided by their prospective work-at-home employer before making an employment decision:

- Special training of supervisors for the challenges of remote team supervision
- Secure computer technology such as a Thin Client, or other secure systems to insure HIPAA compliance
- Policies and procedures specific for working in the remote environment including In Home Work Site Audits
- Programs for enhancing staff engagement such as a mentor program, a self-governance council of practicing nurses to discuss long-distance practice or communication issues, time for training, and virtual remote team meetings
- A process for insuring that the employees are compliant with state licensure laws. This process can be a combination of inbound call routing to specific agent groups determined by groups of states, policies for managing work lists limited to patients in the state in which the RN holds a license, the routing of inbound calls and management of calls and which state licenses an employee must obtain in order to speak with a patient (most State Nurse Practice Acts define the practice of nursing as occurring at the location of the patient).

Keys to Managing a Successful Work-at-Home Program

The primary focus at the start of the work-at-home initiative was insuring that staff had the technologies they needed to do their jobs remotely. The focus began to shift to management issues once teams were working in their new at-home workplaces. Learning how to effectively manage people who are not physically in the same workspace requires new tools and techniques.

Our supervisors were the key to building trust in their teams and making the team members feel connected. As senior managers, we armed our supervisors with the training and skills development required for managing a virtual team environment as there are not many individuals in the workforce coming to the job with virtual team management skills. The successful supervisor must be an expert electronic communicator. Many of today's seasoned nursing managers grew with emerging technology, being forced to use instant messaging, chat rooms, and secure email for what may have been face-to-face communication in years past. The supervisor must identify effective communicators within his or her team and reward them. Additionally, the supervisor must pay close attention to what has been written; tone will say much as you cannot see the emotion in the staff's faces. If the team is only partially virtual, all team members must be treated as virtual. We avoided having meetings where some members were physically present with the supervisor and others were remote, as this may be perceived as an advantage for those physically present.

A key initiative 2 years into the work-at-home project was the creation of a mentoring program that pairs each new staff member with a seasoned employee. The company set guidelines that suggest how often mentors should contact protégés – whether by phone, instant messaging, or email – and the call center nurses are given allowances for the time they spend making contact. The program has generated nothing but positive comments from not only newcomers but also veterans who have appreciated the opportunity to make more social contacts in the isolated work-at-home setting. The key to socializing in a remote setting is that it has to be ongoing and something you constantly work to improve and maintain.

The company managers as well as supervisors have also embraced new ways of staying in touch with employees. Without the chance to walk around each day and catch up with employees in person, managers learned virtual substitution; for example, instant messaging staff each day to ask how their weekend was, if a sick child was feeling better, etc. This was a shift in how the managers supervised people and established remote rapport. Team meetings are now held in a web camera Live Meeting environment, enabling everyone to "be in the same room."

In addition to daily efforts to keep staff connected, the company made an effort to bring staff together twice a year for regional meetings that combine work and social events. It is expensive, but it is well worth the money. Besides reducing staff turnover due to successful employee engagement and not having to pay for a physical plant since staff was working at home, the cost of the regional meetings was well worth the expense.

Opportunities for Success

Employers have the challenge of meeting business needs by selecting the candidate who demonstrates the greatest opportunity for success. Because there are few work-at-home positions for nurses, many applicants are approaching the work-at-home recruitment phase without prior work-at-home experience. Employers have utilized tools to assist them in identifying the best candidate. The Chally Group survey tool, discussed by Suzanne Wells, MSN, RN, in another portion of the Best Practices section, is one such tool that can assist the employer in selecting the "right person" for the telework position.

We learned much from our experience of moving all employees to a work at home environment. It has been a highly successful initiative and requires efforts on the part of both the employee and the employer.

Chapter 17

Frequently Asked Questions

This chapter is a compilation of frequently asked questions (FAQs) posed to the authors. Many of the questions address the standard of care and some have legal overtones. The necessary disclaimer is that these responses may or may not represent the standard of care for your particular situation. Because the authors are not attorneys, none of these responses can be construed as legal advice. The precise answer to each of these questions will depend on your policies as directed by your leadership in the context of your organization. If legal interpretation is required, please contact your local counsel.

The following FAQs are listed in alphabetical order:

- Ambulatory Care Nurse Certification Exam
- Approval of Protocols by Physicians
- Average Call Length
- Biggest Quality Problem in Telephone Triage
- Charting by Exception
- Collaborative Training/Shadowing in Telephone Triage
- Cost Effectiveness of Telephone Triage
- Doctors "Covering" Nurses
- Follow-Up Calls to Patients
- FTEs: RN per Provider
- How Can I Find a Job in Telephone Triage?
- Interstate Practice – Compact States

- Related Question re Nurses in Non-Compact States
- Location of Telephone Triage Nurses in the Office Setting
- Medical Assistants and Telephone Triage
- Minimum Preparation for Telephone Triage
- Non-Enrolled Patient
- Nursing Experience Necessary for Telephone Triage
- Peer Review
- Productivity Metrics
- Provider Co-Signing Triage Notes
- Recertification in Telephone Nursing Practice
- Refuse to Triage when Parent not with Child
- Replacing RNs with LPNs or UAP
- Returning Patient Calls – Time Standard
- Rotating Through Telephone Triage
- Semantics of Decision Support Tools (Protocol/Guideline/ Algorithm)
- Staffing Standards in Call Centers
- Standard of Care – Best Practice
- Taking Messages for the Doctor
- Triage Category "Urgent"
- Voicemail and Use of Front Office Personnel in Patient Intake
- Working From Home

AMBULATORY CARE NURSE CERTIFICATION EXAM

Question:

Is it possible to get certification in telehealth nursing?

Answer:

No, unless you already have it. The National Certification Corporation's (NCC) Telephone Nursing Practice (TNP) certification exam was discontinued and can only be renewed via CE credit for those who already hold the TNP certification. That being said, the relevant certification that is available to telehealth nurses is the American Nurses Credentialing Center's (ANCC) Board Certification exam in Ambulatory Care Nursing, which tests telehealth knowledge as a component of ambulatory care nursing. The AAACN endorses this as the preferred certification for telehealth and other ambulatory care nurses.

AAACN believes that telehealth nursing is an integral part of ambulatory care nursing. The thought is that a nurse cannot do a good job in telehealth nursing unless he or she has a broad base of knowledge in ambulatory care nursing *and* that essentially all ambulatory care nurses do telehealth nursing. "Ambulatory care nursing certification, especially with the enhanced telehealth component in the new electronic exams beginning April 2009, is the career credential for all ambulatory care nurses" (¶ 5).[1] The AAACN offers a review course, which many nurses have found to be of value before taking the ambulatory care nursing certification exam offered by the American Nurses Credentialing Center.

APPROVAL OF PROTOCOLS BY PHYSICIANS

Question:

We are trying to select protocols for our organization, but the prospect of getting all of our providers to agree on anything is overwhelming! In such cases, do you just keep the protocols very short and general? How do other practices deal with the challenge of enormous diversity in provider approach to the same concern?

Answer:

No doubt, this is a challenging problem. We recommend that you do a little presentation for the providers to help them understand that the primary purpose of the decision support tools is to guide nursing assessment, not to provide medical treatment. There shouldn't be much disagreement (if any) regarding how one should assess a patient with a vaginal discharge, abdominal pain, sinus symptoms, or a laceration, for example. However, some decision support tools include a section for interventions requiring a physician order such as diagnostic procedures and treatment, and that's where variability might be necessary and acceptable.

To approve the decision support tools, many organizations appoint a committee that has the responsibility of reviewing the decision support tools and reaching a consensus agreement. It doesn't have to be unanimous (and probably won't be), but your medical director should be able to devise a creative method to get everyone's input and then make the best decision for the group and its patients. It is important to keep in mind that the agreement and the collaboration does not stop at the selection of the protocols but that review and updates will also be needed at regular intervals, sometimes directed by your Board of Nursing.

Remember, the primary focus of *telephone triage* is to determine the nature and urgency of the patient's problem, identify the patient's associated needs, and direct him or her to the appropriate level of care. That makes the protocols and their format primarily a nursing concern, providing there is consensus among the provider staff about how to assess a patient with a common complaint.

However, if diagnostic or treatment recommendations are incorporated into your telephone triage protocols, the individual physician preference becomes relevant. For example, Dr. A may prefer to treat fever with ibuprofen and Dr. B may prefer acetaminophen. If you can't achieve agreement among the physicians, this is where you could allow for variation among the providers. While variation in the assessment section of the protocol is not appropriate, there is certainly a place for variability in the *treatment* section of the protocols. Protocols adapted to include treatment recommendation must reflect accurate community trends and practices (although the "community" for telehealth nursing is probably not restricted to your own geographic locale).

Additionally, if you allow for variation, you will need a policy giving clear direction to the nurse for situations such as when Dr. A is covering for Dr. B. Otherwise, you'll have unnecessary confusion and potential problems trying to determine the appropriate approach for your patients.

AVERAGE CALL LENGTH

Question:

I am an experienced RN who works at a hospital-based call center. I have done this type of nursing for several years. Recently, we have been placed under new management who states that we need to have all triage calls completed in 7 minutes or less, including documentation. This is creating a lot of stress for many people. What is the industry standard for average call length?

Answer:

There is no "industry standard" because of the many variables that impact call length. Although an average per organization can be calculated, it doesn't necessarily indicate the average length to provide quality care to your "average" patient population.

As your lead author travels around the country, teaching and consulting, she has found the average call length is creeping up. More often than not, average calls are lasting about 10-12 minutes in office/clinic settings. And some of the call centers that were expecting their nurses to take four calls per hour are now advocating three. Average call times reported in U.S. call centers have been 10 minutes for adult calls and 14.5 minutes for pediatric calls.[2]

However, in terms of trends, the overwhelming trend is *away* from targets for average call length. There is an ever-increasing recognition that the quality of care is far more important than call length. In fact, the duration of the phone call is positively correlated with the quality of nurse/patient interaction.[3] And, telephone triage research has focused mainly on the quality of the nurse patient interaction rather than the length of the call.[4,5] An effort to hold nurses to specific call length expectations is not only inadvisable, it can also increase the likelihood of a bad patient outcome. Often telephone triage calls take the place of an episodic visit. Thus, the notion of rushing through a patient encounter over the phone that usually takes 10-20 minutes in the face-to-face setting is not reasonable.

Many factors impact call length. The patient's characteristics, his or her ability to give a coherent and meaningful history, and the nurse's own instincts and professional approach will vary from call to call. Other variables, including documentation practices and the requirements of your electronic medical record, also impact call length.

Rather than helping you identify a target call length, we encourage you to determine how long an average call takes (naturally, without pressure to hurry up). Then multiply the average call length by the number of triage calls received, and that, based on productive minutes of a nurse's day, will yield the number of telephone triage nurses that are necessary to handle the call volume. Establishing artificial call length expectations in order to meet existing staffing standards is not prudent. The focus should instead be on the *quality* of care delivered. RNs are professionals who are responsible for the outcome of their patient interactions. In most cases an average call length of 5-6 minutes is insufficient to provide safe and effective care. While some calls can be handled quickly, there will be calls that last

15 minutes or more. This is especially true with elderly patients who may have difficulty hearing, multiple chronic illnesses and medications, and who may be slow to process information and to speak. Rushing these and other challenging patients could result in disaster.

BIGGEST QUALITY PROBLEM IN TELEPHONE TRIAGE

Question:

We are looking for a quality improvement project. What do you see as the biggest area of risk in telephone triage?

Answer:

We have worked a number of lawsuits related to telephone triage calls and the common thread in most of them is inadequate patient assessment and failure to *think*. Because you can't see the patient, taking the time to be certain that you have collected adequate information to support a good assessment of his or her problem is of great importance. The standard of practice dictates that nurses must use the nursing process on each call. Failure to do so can result in bad outcomes and may be indefensible in court. An effective telephone triage encounter usually includes, at a minimum, the following components:

- Safe practice demands that you open the call properly, take time to establish trust and rapport, and create a therapeutic environment which increases the likelihood of complete and accurate information sharing.
- A rapid assessment must be performed to identify life-threatening emergencies and direct appropriate action as indicated.
- Barring identification of a life-threatening emergency, baseline data should be collected to determine the context of the call. Is the patient a frail elderly patient, a young inexperienced mother, a brittle diabetic? Is the patient pregnant, nursing, immunosuppressed, diabetic, or asthmatic? What is her current state of health?

- An adequate assessment must be conducted to determine the nature and urgency of the patient's problem. This assessment should be done systematically, followed by reference to a decision support tool to assure that no critical information was overlooked and to help provide organizationally consistent dispositions and advice.

- The call must be closed properly, including determination that the patient (a) understands the instructions, (b) agrees with the plan of care and is willing to comply, (c) is comfortable with the plan of care, and (d) has no further questions. It is also essential for the nurse to give instructions to inform the patient of what to expect, what untoward symptoms to watch for, and what action to take should they occur. There must also be a plan to evaluate the effectiveness of the intervention, or at a minimum, to be certain the patient knows what to do if he or she doesn't get better.

CHARTING BY EXCEPTION

Question:

When using a protocol, is it OK to document the first positive and then state, "All previous protocol questions negative?" Also, when we give home care instructions, is it acceptable to just say, "Home care instructions per fever protocol?"

Answer:

The answer to this question depends on the policies of your organization. We recommend that the organization have a written policy specifying which protocols you are using. Then, when you state, "Care provided per fever protocol," the author and specific edition will be directly referenced in the policy. Keeping in mind that a medical record is first and foremost a communication tool, the documentation should be indicative of both your thought process and the advice you gave the caller.

So, in answer to the first question, it is *not* advisable to document "all previous protocol questions (or criteria) negative." First, the reader probably doesn't have the protocol memorized, and thus you are telling them very little. Second, you may not have actually *asked* each of those questions because you may have deemed some irrelevant. And third, without documenting your pertinent negatives, there is no evidence of critical thinking or the thought process you used in coming to a conclusion.

You are a professional and want your charting to reflect your clinical judgment. For example, it would be meaningful to document, "Denies nuchal rigidity and headache." However, there are times when you need to be more specific such as when it comes to documenting a baby's level of consciousness. Because of the importance and potential ambiguity of this assessment, you might want to document specific behaviors such as, "Playing normally, making good eye contact, audibly babbling in the background." On the other hand, on occasion, a brief comment should be sufficient. For example, it would be appropriate to say, "No evidence of dehydration" because the criteria used would be common knowledge among medical readers. That comment indicates that you assessed such criteria as mucous membranes, urine output, thirst, and activity level.

Regarding documentation of home care instructions, if you say, "Instructed per fever protocol," and there are seven criteria in the Home Care Instructions, even if you actually gave the mother all seven instructions, if you don't document them, the reader won't know what you told the mom and thus won't know what teaching to reinforce should mom call with a follow-up question. You don't have to teach the mother everything you know, but you do need to teach her everything she needs to know to provide individualized care for her child. Some teaching is common nursing knowledge and doesn't need to be spelled out exactly, but it does need to at least be documented in an abbreviated form. For example, in our opinion, it should generally be sufficient to say, "Mother instructed on management of fever and prevention of dehydration." However, if a medication is recommended, you should specify the medication, the preparation, the route, and the exact dose recommended. Or, if you instructed the mother to administer the medication "per package instructions," document that as well. Additionally, if the medication is recommended on the basis of a protocol or a direct order, the source should be documented.

Keep in mind the old adage, "If it's not written, it didn't happen." Whether that's actually true or not, it is almost certain that if it's not written, you can't *prove* it happened. Bottom line: Document more than just "assessed (or) advised per protocol." The general content of your interaction is important for both communication and legal purposes.

COLLABORATIVE TRAINING/SHADOWING IN TELEPHONE TRIAGE

Question:

Do you think there's any particular value in having non-telephone triage nurses observe what it's like in the telephone triage room?

Answer:

It's a great idea to have non-telephone triage nurses take a turn shadowing a triage nurse and, of course, that could work both ways, having telephone triage nurses shadow clinic nurses. Increasing intradepartmental or interdepartmental understanding (such as with your emergency department [ED] colleagues) can improve working relationships.

And, if you're in a residency program, encouraging the residents to sit with you for a few hours can be invaluable to them when they enter practice. This is an ideal collaborative and educational opportunity for both of you. Additionally, shadowing a physician will help hone your history-taking skills and will help you develop your diagnostic reasoning, especially if you ask the physician to think out loud or to explain their rationale.

COST EFFECTIVENESS OF TELEPHONE TRIAGE

Question:

We are launching a telephone triage program. Do you have information about how the program will reduce costs by avoiding unnecessary visits to physicians?

Answer:

There is a large body of research demonstrating that telephone triage is cost effective and safely reduces inappropriate utilization of resources.[6] Of course, any time we facilitate *appropriate* care we potentially save money, if not in the short run, in the long run through cost avoidance. It's similar to the insurance company that pays for the mammogram today so that they don't have to pay for the breast cancer treatment tomorrow.

DOCTORS "COVERING" NURSES

Question:

Is it necessary for the doctor to "cover" nurses when they do telephone triage?

Answer:

Applied to telephone triage, as long as an RN isn't making a medical diagnosis or prescribing beyond his or her scope of practice, the RN needs no direct clinical supervision. It is important to understand that the role of our physician colleagues relative to telephone triage is to support patient care; not to "cover" the RN. Our practice is not dependent upon direct collaboration with a physician or licensed provider unless medical intervention is necessary. In fact, in several cases, entrepreneurs have started telephone triage programs fully owned and operated by RNs. That's not to imply that nurses don't often have bosses, or that medical directors aren't necessary, but rather to make the point that telephone triage is independent nursing practice. However, the goal of telephone triage nursing is to provide excellent care that meets the needs of our patients, and a strong collaborative relationship with our medical directors and the physicians with whom we work is essential. Physicians are a tremendous source of medical information. Their involvement is crucial because, although nurses maintain accountability for their own actions, physicians maintain accountability for the overall management of their patient population. Having them review your patient encounters by the end of the day is a great way to keep them in the loop.

FOLLOW-UP CALLS TO PATIENTS

Question:

I am trying to find out if there is a standard regarding calling back patients who have been triaged. What we have done in the past was called everyone we directed to be seen within 24 hours in the ED. We called them back a day later. We tried three times to catch them, and after the 3rd day we removed them from our list. The question being posed now is should we try only once, leaving a message to call back as needed? Or is the accepted standard to call once a day for 3 days before not trying again?

Answer:

To date there is no written standard regarding callbacks of this nature. Of course, this is more appropriately a question for your legal counsel, but more often than not, organizations are making attempts to return calls two or three times (usually on different days and/or at different times of day) before they chalk it up to "no contact." Regarding calling back those who you send to ED, one or more of the software companies initiated that rule in the form of a recommendation several years ago, and it stuck. It is reasonable that if you've left a message, that would count as a "contact," providing you feel the message was reliable (it was identified as the patient's voice mail or the message wasn't taken by a child) and you document it. Of course, there are those for whom giving up isn't acceptable (such as with life-threatening problems).

Of greater importance to your question is that nurses need to realize the purpose of the policy (regardless of how you write it) is to assure patient safety and to encourage those who didn't seek care to do so if it's still deemed necessary. The bottom line is clinical judgment. Your nurses must keep in mind that they should act in the best interest of the patient. Here is a useful rule: If it's foreseeable that the patient might not carry out the plan of care (e.g., go to the ED) and the risk to the patient is significant (e.g., CVA or MI), the nurse should make efforts to ensure that the patient complies with the plan of care, calling back to follow-up and taking action up to and including dialing 911, over the patient's protest, if that's what's indicated.

FTEs: RN PER PROVIDER

Question:

Do you know of a benchmark for the number of nursing FTEs needed per provider FTE for telephone triage?

Answer:

There are no specific standards addressing the number of FTEs per provider. You can imagine why; there are so many variables. However, a useful rule of thumb is 3-4 providers per nurse. I've kept that in the back of my mind as a rule of thumb when I've worked with clients. It doesn't always work out that way, but it's helpful in coming up with an initial guesstimate to serve as a point of departure from which to then go up or down. We recommend a telephone workload analysis to see how many calls of various types are received over the course of a week. Use that data to identify which of those calls must be handled by an RN and which can be delegated (and to whom). Then, knowing your average call length, it's just a matter of arithmetic to come up with the right answer.

HOW CAN I FIND A JOB IN TELEPHONE TRIAGE?

Question:

I'm looking for a job in telephone triage. Can you tell me where to begin looking?

Answer:

Telephone triage is an exciting field, and many experienced nurses are well-suited for it. Begin looking the same way you would for any other job: network, check job sites, and visit Web sites of AAACN and other organizations. Finding a job, however, isn't always easy and often takes some "sleuthing." Telephone triage nurses work in a wide variety of clinical areas. Hospitals and insurance companies have call centers, and clinics and home health/hospice agencies hire telephone triage nurses as well. Other practice settings include College Health, Corrections, Same-Day Surgery, EDs, UCCs, and a variety of other clinical settings that might be managing patients over the telephone.

INTERSTATE PRACTICE – COMPACT STATES

Question:

I am looking to find out my liability for providing telephone triage to my doctor's patients who are calling from outside of my state for advice. Am I liable under the nurse practice act of the state they are calling from, or am I covered by my own state's nurse practice act? (Queried by nurse in Compact state)

Answer:

In most states, you are regarded as practicing in the state from which the patient is calling. This even extends in most states to "snow birds" and in over half of the states for vacationers, business travelers, and others who are in the state only temporarily (see Appendix A). Your state's board of nursing (BON) does not have jurisdiction in states other than your own.

The one caveat/exception to this rule is based on the Nurse Licensure Compact. This Compact was proposed by the National Council of State Boards of Nursing in 1997, but in order for it to apply, it must be passed by the state legislature in *both* of the involved states. Fortunately, you live in one of the first states that enacted the Compact. That means that if you're taking a call from a patient in another Compact state, the BON in that state has agreed to recognize your license as being valid in its state. However, it's important to be aware that even though the member boards have agreed to recognize your license, the rules and regulations regarding telehealth nursing vary from state to state and the rules you follow in your job in your state might not apply in another Compact state.

To find out which states have passed the Compact, go to www.ncsbn.org and click on "Nurse Licensure Compact." That will take you to a map of states that have enacted the Compact. If you click on "Boards of Nursing," from there, you can click on the appropriate state and go to its Web site where you can research the rules for that state.

RELATED QUESTION RE NURSES IN NON-COMPACT STATES

Question:

But what about nurses in non-Compact states? Does the same hold true for us?

Answer:

It's a little trickier for nurses in non-Compact states because, with few exceptions, you must have a license in every state from which you take calls. Even if you are talking to a patient in a Compact state, the fact that your state has not joined the Compact makes you exempt from the benefits enjoyed by nurses in Compact states who are providing care to patients in other Compact states. However, you are all in the same boat when it comes to providing care in states that have not joined the Compact.

Since you're in a non-Compact state, I urge you to contact your BON to see what you can do to help them introduce or support legislation to pass the Nurse Licensure Compact in your state.

LOCATION OF TELEPHONE TRIAGE NURSES IN THE OFFICE SETTING

Question:

Currently our triage area is in the middle of our busy office where the telephone RNs can be overheard by patients who are passing by. When I have to raise my voice to accommodate patients who are hard of hearing, patients as far as the waiting room can hear my conversation. The noise level from the activities in the office is such that I need to plug my other ear to adequately hear the patients. Additionally, we are subject to constant interruptions in our phone conversations and documentation, adversely impacting the quality of both the care I render and the legal record of my call. My office is in the process of redesign. What is your recommendation regarding the physical setting of telephone triage nurses when you consult?

Answer:

Your concerns are right on target. It is necessary for telephone triage nurses to be placed in a private area, far enough away to be "out of sight and out of mind." Besides the obvious privacy issue (which should be apparent to anyone), you have the added concern of not being able to hear well yourself and thus are at increased risk of making decisions on the basis of incomplete or inaccurate information. Also, you touched on the issue of interruptions, which raises the problem of multitasking which should be avoided. This is another important reason for you to be in a designated, remote location.

In addressing specific design, windows are nice and soundproofing is essential. There is plenty of information on the Web addressing cubicle/workstation design. When designing the area, give sufficient attention to adequate sound control but be sure that your telephone triage nurses are in close enough proximetry to each other to facilitate collaboration when necessary.

MEDICAL ASSISTANTS AND TELEPHONE TRIAGE

Question:

My clinic has recently come under new management. Emphasis is now on "productivity" over quality of care. It has turned a very difficult job into an impossible one. One of the proposed changes is to replace most, if not all, of the RNs with medical assistants including replacing RN triage nurses with MAs. This management group has done this in other practices and feels it is an acceptable practice. Do you know of any resources/literature I can access/reference for this fight?

Answer:

Unfortunately, there are few resources that speak directly to the fact that MAs can't or shouldn't do telephone triage (except in California where it's strictly and explicitly prohibited). A few other states have addressed telephone triage by MAs, but unfortunately, most haven't. One potential source for you would be your state medical board. Sometimes the medical boards speak to MA triage, but usually, if they do, what they have to say is based on the Captain of the Ship doctrine without apparent understanding of the complexity of telephone triage. Of note, however, if your board of nursing indicates that it is outside of the scope of practice for LPNs to do telephone triage, it is common sense that MAs shouldn't be doing it either.

The AAACN has a standard specifying that all calls involving assessment must be performed by a registered nurse. They also have a position statement on the Role of the RN in Ambulatory Care that speaks to the opinion that all ambulatory care settings require professional nursing services and the proper level of preparation to be accountable for delivering nursing care is the RN.

The Emergency Nurses Association (ENA) has a Position Statement on Telephone Advice which lays out the criteria for safe telephone triage. The criteria include specially trained, experienced RNs, and specifies that RNs not in compliance with the criteria described in their position statement should not be handling advice calls.

The American Accreditation Healthcare Commission (URAC) states that all calls must be managed by RNs or MDs. They provide voluntary accreditation for call centers, and they don't mince words about who should be doing it. They say MAs may not assess, triage, or make independent decisions about care of patients.

The problem is that people who don't understand just don't understand. The Greenberg Model for the Process of Telephone Nursing[7] is, in our opinion, the most compelling argument in favor of RN triage, in that it illustrates that interpreting is the central process in telephone triage (occurring from the moment we pick up the phone until we hang up the phone and beyond). An additional study found that in 46% of phone calls the nurse "...performs more than one function for the patient, i.e. arranges services, provides advice, and/or communicates instruction from the provider to the patient (p. 268).[8] The role of critical thinking in this practice can't be overestimated! In our experience as expert witnesses, poor patient outcomes are often related to an inadequate assessment and/or failure to employ clinical judgment and critical thinking.

We wish literature existed that effectively addressed the reason MAs can't do telephone triage. You might find a few reports helpful.[9,10,11,12,13] Unfortunately, these papers address "triage" by answering services and clerical personnel. It is likely those who believe MAs can do telephone triage will feel that their knowledge is superior to the answering service personnel. However, although that may be true, the issue is critical thinking and clinical judgment. Research is desperately needed that addresses MAs specifically (so we don't have to try to generalize from studies involving clerks and answering service personnel). The knowledge necessary to do telephone triage is extensive. Although in some specialty offices the MAs may be well trained to provide care for that particular specialty (e.g., ophthalmology), that knowledge can't be generalized to other specialties. For example, if patients present with problems that are not ophthalmologic in nature, the MA's limited knowledge of other organ systems and non-ophthalmologic clinical entities may pose problems.

MINIMUM PREPARATION FOR TELEPHONE TRIAGE

Question:

I'm writing to ask what you think is the minimum preparation for an experienced nurse to accept telephone triage duties. We currently have all nurses going through a 4-hour training.

Answer:

It is difficult to pinpoint minimum preparation, because so much of it is dependent upon the nurse's previous clinical and personal experiences and existing knowledge base. You might want to consider establishing a minimum number of years experience (certainly excluding new graduates), but be careful in establishing those minimums (see "Nursing Experience Necessary" in this chapter). Once you put it in writing, you must adhere to it. You might want to establish a mechanism to have a special "waiver" granted by a chief nurse executive for those "seasoned" individuals who return to nursing as a second career with a lot of life experience behind them. Life experience as well as clinical experience can be very helpful (meaning that a 35 or 40-year-old new graduate RN who has raised a family might catch on faster than a 20-year-old fresh out of school).

Now, back to the specific question of preparation. A minimum didactic training program is necessary and with demonstrated mastery of the content. This should be followed by some directed clinical experience with a mentor. Once minimum competencies are identified, you might develop a "learning contract" at the beginning of orientation which would be tailored to each new RN. Orientation programs in various organizations range from a few days to several weeks or months. We can't imagine a situation in which 4 hours would be sufficient.

NON-ENROLLED PATIENT

Question:

What is the duty to provide care when we receive a call from someone who is not our patient? We only provide triage service to patients of our practice. Sometimes we have families call us that are not our patients. Patients tend to share our phone number with friends because they like our service. We typically refer them to their own physician. If it is apparent there is an urgent situation, we will suggest they call 911 or go to the ED.

Answer:

We are happy to give you our opinion, but you answered your own question. Once you pick up the phone and say, "This is Carol; I'm an RN. How may I help you?" you have entered into a relationship with the patient and thus have a duty to provide him or her with the standard of care.[14] In our opinion, what this means is that you must perform a reasonable assessment, diagnose urgency, and refer him or her to the appropriate level of care.

As you said, if it's urgent, refer the caller to the ED or advise him or her to call 911. Here's the trick question: How did you know it was urgent if you didn't assess the caller? And if you don't believe it's urgent, that's an assessment as well. The key is to do enough of an assessment (meaning pretty thorough) to be sure you are accurately diagnosing urgency and providing the caller with a reasonable plan of care.

One example: One of us was consulting in a cardiology practice with the nurse manager when she heard a hubbub in the reception area. Going to investigate, she found the receptionist on the phone with a patient experiencing acute chest pain. The caller was not a regular patient but had found the cardiologist's number in a phone book. The receptionist was trying to explain to the patient that, not being a patient of the practice, the nurses couldn't talk to him. He, on the other hand, insisted he might be having a heart attack and wanted to talk to a nurse. The nurse manager took the phone, assessed the patient, and advised him to dial 911. Although this nurse didn't have a particular "duty" to talk to the patient, it was, in her opinion, the right thing to do.

Of course, this is a question best addressed by policy and guided by your organizational attorney.

NURSING EXPERIENCE NECESSARY FOR TELEPHONE TRIAGE

Question:

How much experience should a nurse have before being hired to work in telephone triage?

Answer:

This question pops up all the time and, unfortunately, there's no uniform answer. We've batted around numbers like 7 years, 5 years, and even 3 years (out of necessity because more experienced nurses weren't available), but there is no magic number. Three to five years of nursing experience has been the standard requirement in many countries.[15,16,17] A 2011 search for telephone triage jobs indicates that 5 years is listed most commonly as the minimum nursing experience, and a substantial number of other positions require at least 3 years. We believe competent telephone triage requires considerable experience, but there is no way to quantify that experience exactly, and the quality of the experience is just as important as the quantity.

Indeed, in recent years rather than stating the number of years of experience required, policies and guidelines are more likely to specify "competence, expertise and knowledge beyond that which is obtained in a basic nursing program" (p. 9).[18] We endorse this shift in emphasis because research shows that triage assessments and decision making are not only done better by experienced nurses, but also by nurses with more education and more training.[19,20,21] In addition, researchers have suggested that extensive life experience (e.g., raising kids, caring for aging parents, running a household) may also have considerable value.[22]

PEER REVIEW

Question:

I'm presently working as a triage nurse for my county health department. I was wondering if you think documentation of peer review is important and, if so, do you recommend any particular process for triage nurses?

Answer:

Excellent question. We do believe peer review is a critical element of quality assurance for a telephone triage program. Because nursing judgment (guided by protocols and other forms of evidence) is essential for the delivery of safe care, it's important to have a process to monitor nursing judgment. Because of the professional nature of our practice, nurses are ideally suited to evaluate the performance of other nurses. Further, the process of peer review not only helps assure quality, but it's also an outstanding teaching tool. We can often learn from each other. See Chapter 13 for a discussion of the content and process of peer review.

PRODUCTIVITY METRICS

Question:

Our call center provides appointment scheduling and nurse triage. I was surfing the Web trying to find information about telephone triage standards for: average talk time, average wrap up, average call handling time. Can you help or point me in the right direction?

Answer:

There are no universal "standards" addressing those metrics. Rather, what you might find are averages in certain settings. For example, the major decision support software vendors would know that information for their client call centers in aggregate.

The more relevant question is whether they are doing a good job or not. Are they doing an adequate assessment before they select the protocol? Are they using clinical judgment? Is there evidence of all steps of the nursing process? Are those steps documented? So many variables impact time, that taken alone it is a risky indicator. The standard should be focused on quality of care and process rather than time.

PROVIDER CO-SIGNING TRIAGE NOTES

Question:

Does the provider need to sign the triage notes? If yes, why?

Answer:

It must be noted that telephone triage is independent nursing practice, and so it's not necessary for our notes to be "co-signed" in order to "cover us" from a legal or a scope of practice perspective. We are accountable for our actions (and usually associated patient outcomes). Having the notes reviewed by the provider by the end of the day is not necessary from a scope of practice perspective, but it is important for two other reasons.

First, the provider might have a little different perspective on the patient and/or his or her issue (by virtue of his or her extensive clinical knowledge base and/or his or her personal knowledge of the patient). Therefore, having a second set of eyes review the call can occasionally provide new insights and thus catch potential errors or oversights. If we have made a mistake in patient management, it is important that it be recognized ASAP rather than waiting until it might be too late to reverse our actions. In other words, sometimes two heads are better than one.

Second, and of possibly greater significance, is the understanding that telephone triage does not exist to relieve the provider of his or her responsibility for the patient. We just serve as part of the team to facilitate prompt and appropriate care. The bottom line is that the provider has a right *and* a responsibility to know what is going on with his or her patient and therefore should be informed and involved as appropriate. Continuity of care will be enhanced by this collaboration.

Additionally, with the exception of a few states which allow recommendation of OTCs by RNs on the basis of their own license, nurses may not prescribe medications. When our activities move into that arena, we are performing a delegated medical act, which must have a supervising authority (a provider). If the medications are recommended on the basis of a signed, medically approved protocol, the authorizing authority is indicated in the protocol, so a physician signature isn't also required on the medical record for those interventions. In summary, as long as either:

1. The nurse is only engaging in independent nursing functions (including triage), or
2. The nurse is recommending medications on the basis of a signed, medically approved protocol, signatures *probably* aren't *legally* required. (We are not attorneys, so we can't answer this question with certainty. It would be wise to check with your state BON.)

In summary, the purpose of the provider co-signing the notes is to acknowledge and reinforce the notion that although triage nurses are an important part of the health care team, our practice shouldn't exist in a vacuum. It might be helpful to recall the lawsuits in which it is possible or likely that the outcome might have been different if the provider had reviewed the chart by the end of the day (e.g., the patient with the septic ACL repair for whom the LPN called in hydrocodone, the child with tonsillitis who the nurse told to go to urgent care if his breathing got worse, the child overdosed with the narcotic who died at home). In each of these cases, the physician was actively involved in the patient's treatment but was not informed of the calls and thus oblivious to the impending disasters until it was too late to intervene. However, we strongly suggest running all triage notes by the provider because it is the prudent thing to do.

RECERTIFICATION IN TELEPHONE NURSING PRACTICE

Question:

I'm having trouble finding CE credit that qualifies for my TNP recertification. Can you make any suggestions?

Answer:

According to the National Certification Corporation, as of 2009, all of the CE must be in the certification specialty. Luckily, telephone nursing practice covers a wide range of clinical topics. In addition to the special knowledge and skills needed to practice telephone nursing, topics also include primary care, home care, professional practice issues, pharmacology, physical assessment, physiological, diagnostic, and lab evaluations, OB/GYN, post partum, neonatal, and women's health. You can go to www.nccwebsite.org and use their search engine to locate codes for the TNP specialty. The core topics and instructions for the TNP recertification can be found in the maintenance catalog on the same Web site. Once you choose some areas of interest from the approved topics, there are educational opportunities offered through professional organizations such as conferences, webinars, and through professional nursing journals. Continuing education is also available online.

REFUSE TO TRIAGE WHEN PARENT NOT WITH CHILD

Question:

Recently, I have learned that many of our offices "refuse to triage" if mom is calling with a problem and the child of concern is still at daycare or school. Many times mom will be called at work or home by a daycare worker or school nurse to report her child's symptoms. Mom will then call the physician's office to obtain a same-day appointment or telephone advice based on the symptoms that have been reported to her. Our practice sites encounter this often. How should it be handled?

Answer:

This is an excellent question, and just another example of "conventional wisdom" that gets in the way of good common sense. While we're not aware of any standards that specifically state that you must triage in such a situation, we believe that failure to do so is dangerous, uncaring, and possibly unethical. And no, fortunately we are not (yet) aware of any litigation related to this refusal, but we imagine it's just a matter of time. If a parent is calling from work needing direction, we need to try to help him or her the best we can under the circumstances. Often the very reason the parent is calling is to determine whether he or she needs to leave work and go to the child. This question can usually be answered after a good conversation with the mom or dad. Three suggestions should help ease the minds of those who are reluctant to triage in these situations:

1. While the parent isn't physically with the child at the moment, he or she certainly knows the child's medical history and how the child looked this morning. Parents know about current meds, recent visits to the doctor, exposures, etc., so they are an excellent source of information (see #3).
2. Advise the parent that the advice you are providing is only as good as the information you are receiving. So, if there is important information the parent is omitting because he or she is not with the child and is thus unaware of important information, the advice could be faulty (see #3).
3. If in doubt, *call the school or daycare* for an accurate description of the child at this moment. And no, this isn't a HIPAA violation unless in the course of the conversation, the nurse discloses confidential information to the daycare worker.[23,24] If the parent provided you with the phone number, there is certainly implicit permission to contact the daycare center. This shouldn't be a problem because the purpose of the call is to get an accurate description of the child's condition at this time. If possible, a three-way call among you, the parent, and the daycare center would be ideal.

Again, this is a great question and addressing this directly in your organization can only improve patient care.

REPLACING RNs WITH LPNs or UAP

Question:

I believe that my office is planning on replacing me with a less-expensive alternative, most likely an LPN. Should I be concerned about the quality of care patients will receive, and also is it opening up my employer to liability risks?

I would also like information on the role of unlicensed assistive personnel in telephone screening and transmission of information to a provider so the provider can make a decision regarding care of the patient vs. telephone triage.

Answer:

Telephone triage is an extremely sophisticated practice requiring the nurse to make reasoned judgments based on an appropriate patient assessment. LPNs are not trained or licensed to do assessment or to perform the level of critical thinking necessary for a safe telephone triage encounter. The AAACN[25] standards and indeed international telephone triage standards are very clear in their requirement that assessment must be done by RNs.[26]

The AAACN has a position statement about the role of the RN in ambulatory care, which pretty much says it all. You can view the statement on their Web site, www.aaacn.org.

While it seems tempting to replace relatively expensive RNs with less-expensive but unqualified staff, as you pointed out, patient safety can suffer and organizational risk will escalate. It is appropriate to utilize LPNs and/or unlicensed personnel in the ambulatory care setting, but only under the supervision of an RN and only in performing tasks that are appropriate for the RN to delegate to them.

Specifically, telephone triage requires a specialized skill set and must be performed by qualified RNs.

Unfortunately, there are no standards that speak directly to the use of UAP in telephone triage. We noticed you were very careful with your wording: "Telephone screening and transmission of information to a provider so the provider can make a decision." If it were only that clear-cut! Unfortunately, as you probably realize, when we "take messages" from patients, we are doing some level of assessment just by determining which questions to ask, which information to record (and which to disregard as irrelevant), and how quickly to bring it to the attention of the provider. Bottom line: We are performing assessment-related activities, even if we don't directly recognize them as formal assessment (which we believe they are). (Refer to Chapter 3 regarding the discussion of assessment with a chain saw accident.)

Our advice is to have RNs manage these calls because patients often fail to articulate their concerns clearly. Someone who isn't trained to recognize the significance of subtle problems or who doesn't recognize important implicit information might miss the boat entirely. While it's tempting to use UAP in this manner, it's helpful to realize that telephone triage might be the most sophisticated form of professional nursing practice taking place in your setting. That realization makes it more obvious that telephone triage (or "screening patients") is not a task that should be taken lightly and delegated to personnel who don't have adequate training and aren't licensed to practice nursing.

RETURNING PATIENT CALLS – TIME STANDARD

Question:

I am not able to find anything on what the standard is for the time frame to respond to telephone consults whether for acute or routine. I've also asked some of my colleagues and they don't have anything solid either. Do you know of a source document that states what the recommended time frames are?

Answer:

As far as we know, there's no quantitative standard that sets any time frames for anything in telephone triage. The one exception is URAC standards, which do dictate an average speed of answer and average call return time for call centers that are URAC accredited.

This almost seems like a trick question because until you've called the patient back, you don't know whether it's an acute call or not. We don't mean to split hairs, but what's in the message may have little to do with why the patient is calling. The brief interaction the patient has with the clerk just isn't conducive (for many reasons) to the clerk always discerning the true reason for the call. Even if it's a request for a test result or Rx refill, the request might be precipitated by symptoms (e.g., the patient who ran out of his clonidine 2 days ago and is now symptomatic, requesting a refill).

That being said, some sites return calls within 30 minutes and others within 2 hours, but certainly all symptom-based calls should be returned by the end of the day. Even the "non-urgents" should also be returned by close of business unless you are *certain* it's not a symptom-based call.

You need to have a written policy and then stick to it. In writing your policy, be certain that it is both (a) safe and (b) achievable. The Telehealth Nursing Practice Essentials state: "Additionally, procedures need to be put in place so that requests are not left until the next day, especially assessment calls. This would be considered abandonment of care" (p. 80).[27]

Although some contracts have minimum standards regarding what types of calls need to be returned within 24, 48, or 72 hours, keep in mind that those are *minimum* standards based on a contractual agreement. They don't necessarily speak to safety.

Patients with symptoms who have not been assessed adequately are at high risk for an adverse event, and thus they should be assessed promptly.

We don't have an opinion on truly "routine" calls. We would just pose the question: How do you know they are routine until you've had a nurse assess them?

Our general advice is to have the person who is taking the message tell the patient the nurse will call back within (state your policy) and then ask the patient, "Can it wait that long?" While patients might not know the exact nature of their problem, they do know when they are concerned, and an offer to return a call "by the end of the day" or "tomorrow" is likely to be met with resistance if the caller is concerned. And if the caller is concerned, we should also be concerned and talk to the patient as soon as possible.

ROTATING THROUGH TELEPHONE TRIAGE

Question:

How do you feel about nurses rotating through triage?

Answer:

We encourage having a *designated* group of nurses for a variety of reasons; not everyone's cut out to do telephone triage. Not everyone likes it; not everyone does it well. There are other reasons to have a designated staff *including* the fact that the more you do it, the better you are at it. Also, the more you do it, the more you generally respect and understand the practice. The more experienced telephone triage nurses will likely take it more seriously and be more inclined to err on the side of caution.

We know that part of critical thinking is to reflect on past experiences. The more we reflect, the more we learn and the better we get. Therefore, we do think nurses who *like* it and do it routinely are more inclined to do a good job, but that's probably true with any practice.

SEMANTICS OF DECISION SUPPORT TOOLS (PROTOCOL/GUIDELINE/ALGORITHM)

Question:

I have a question re: protocols vs. guidelines when it comes to telephone triage. I have just read that protocols are rules and guidelines are more permissive. Several months ago I set up Telephone Triage Guidelines for our clinic. According to the reference I read, guidelines are just as fine to use as protocols. What is your opinion? In reviewing them, it seems this may be the better set up for our clinic, but I want to be legal as well!

Answer:

While we can't give you a legal definition of those terms, the reason many are now calling them "decision support tools" is because of this very controversy. We personally don't get all hung up on the difference between protocols and guidelines. Some boards of nursing use the word "protocol" in a very specific way, often referring to the relationship between an advanced practice nurse (APN) and his or her collaborating physician. So, when some Boards are asked directly, they might say RNs can't use "protocols." But if asked if they could use "guidelines" or "decision support tools," their answer would be "yes."

We think you're fine if you call them guidelines, but even better, call them "decision support tools," and it does away with the argument about differing definitions. Plus, it makes it clear that they exist to *support* your decision making, not to *make* your decisions for you. The one exception would be in the "treatment" or "intervention" section of your tool. If you are recommending medications which require a physician's order in your state, we would be inclined to call that section "protocols" unless that language is in conflict with policy established by your board of nursing.

STAFFING STANDARDS IN CALL CENTERS

Question:

I am interested in finding out what the staffing numbers are for call centers. If you have any information on this would you please forward it to me? Thank you so very much.

Answer:

You've asked a question we can't answer because the staffing will vary from call center to call center, based on population, software, policies, culture, and documentation practices, among other factors. However, we'll tell you how we would approach it if we were managing a call center.

Because establishing staffing standards would potentially dictate how much time a nurse could spend on a call, we suggest backing into the information. There are no national standards because average call times can vary so much, depending on your software, your method of call intake, your documentation practices, and your patient population (not to mention individual variations among nurses). We suggest you:

1. Determine your (actual) average call time.
2. Multiply that by the number of calls your center receives.
3. Divide that by the number of productive minutes each nurse has during his or her day. (Remember, they won't be productive every minute. Besides lunch and breaks, sometimes they need to use the restroom, look something up, or just chat with each other to decompress.)

This will tell you how many nurses you need to staff your call center. Of course, you'll need to track call volume during various times of the day so that peak call times are covered and down time is kept to a minimum. Chapter 14 provides in-depth information on this topic.

STANDARD OF CARE – BEST PRACTICE

Question:

Is there enough research in telephone nursing to say what is "best practice?" We have been told we have to do every call perfectly and if not we could be written up and reported to the board of nursing. However, as a nurse with 28 years experience, sometimes calls can't follow the exact process, or require more critical thinking. It seems like you could find something wrong in any call if you wanted to.

Answer:

While there are some "best practices," there is not consensus about one best practice. However, the standard of practice is that nurses must use their clinical judgment within the context of the nursing process, rather than merely following the protocol. In fact, following the protocols without using critical thinking and professional judgment is dangerous! While protocols provide valuable guidance, no two calls are the same and thus RNs must individualize care as appropriate for each call.

Follow-Up Question:

It sounds from what you are saying that nurses must use their clinical judgment and not just protocols to properly practice telephone nursing. Is that right? My purpose in asking this is that in my call center, experienced nurses are told that they are not providing safe care because they occasionally deviate from the protocol. They assure us that if we always follow the protocol, we will "be covered." We have continued threats of being "reported" for unsafe care if we don't follow the protocols precisely. I am truly concerned about this.

Answer:

Yes, best practice includes the use of protocols *and* clinical judgment. Strict adherence to a decision support tool is not best practice. In fact, following the protocols without using critical thinking and professional judgment is dangerous! While protocols provide valuable guidance, no two calls are the same and thus RNs must individualize care as appropriate for each. In addition, it is well-established that protocols do not and cannot cover every situation.[11,20,28,29]

> Nurses therefore tailor their use…to accommodate a number of human and organizational factors, including the precise nature of the patient's symptoms, whether patients have already received medical assistance (and, if so, what this involved), patients' levels of knowledge about their symptoms, patients' familial and social circumstances, patients' levels of anxiety (as expressed in the call), the nurses' own and their colleagues specialist knowledge and expertise, and the nurses' knowledge of how other local…services operate in practice (p. 826).[11]

Furthermore, there is substantial evidence that nurses regularly deviate from protocols.[30,31]

"Even with protocols in place, a nurse must still exercise her professional judgment" (p. 7).[14] Indeed, research shows that nurses often feel the protocols inhibit their work when they believe they must follow them without deviation, but they view protocols to be valuable in many ways when used as aids for practice rather than as rigid scripts.[5,28,31]

Does this clarification help? You are on the right track! We are sorry you are having to fight the good fight, but hopefully safe practice and reason will prevail in the end.

As to the idea that you're "covered" if you follow protocols precisely, we've done a fair amount of consulting on lawsuits relative to telephone triage, and our experience has been that using the decision support tools is not what "protects" the nurse. Use of sound clinical judgment will protect you.

TAKING MESSAGES FOR THE DOCTOR: TELEHEALTH NURSING vs. TELEPHONE TRIAGE

Question:

We thought we were following telehealth nursing guidelines in our primary care clinic. The RN speaks with the patient, finds out what the complaint is and then discusses it with the provider, who then determines the next level of care for the patient (except chest pain, 10/10 pain, loss of vision, and so on, go to ER per algorithm). We are now being questioned and told this is really triage. We're also told we should be following the triage practice book and documenting the page and book from which the questions are being asked. I just need to get your point of view as we want to do the correct thing.

Answer:

Yes. Both scenarios that you described are telephone triage. The distinction you are making seems more a matter of semantics than a substantive difference. The following paragraphs will explain our rationale for this response.

Fundamentally, we understand that all forms of professional nursing practice (telehealth and otherwise) must comply with the basic standards put forth by our profession. Perhaps the most clear and concise way to say this is that, as professional nurses, we are responsible for using the nursing process in our provision of care to patients. Although there are various forms of telehealth nursing, they all require the nurse do an adequate assessment, draw a conclusion, develop a plan of care, facilitate implementation of that plan, and evaluate the effectiveness of the plan.[25]

In your query, you are making a distinction between "telehealth nursing" and "telephone triage," but telephone triage is just a form of telehealth nursing. We actually believe the distinction between the terms *telehealth nursing* and *telephone triage* within the context you describe is largely semantic from a practical perspective.

Telephone Triage — An interactive process be-

> tween nurse and client that occurs over the telephone and involves identifying the nature and urgency of client health care needs and determining the appropriate disposition. Telephone triage is a component of telephone nursing practice that focuses on assessment, prioritization, and referral to the appropriate level of care (p. 43).[25]

Basically, when a nurse picks up a phone to interact with a patient about a symptom-based call, he or she is doing an assessment to determine the urgency and where the patient can best seek care. In other words, the nurse is practicing telephone triage.

It further appears that a primary distinction you're making between "telehealth nursing" and "telephone triage" is the use of protocols. In the first scenario, where the nurse takes the call, contacts the provider, and then responds to the patient, your responsibility as a professional nurse isn't diminished. The fact of the matter is that in determining which information is relevant, which questions to ask, and which responses to record, you are doing an assessment. The ultimate purpose of this interaction is to determine the urgency and direct the patient to the appropriate level of care – in other words, it is triage.

Because we are RNs, it is not possible to sidestep the responsibility for doing an adequate patient assessment and drawing a conclusion (or making a "nursing diagnosis") based on that assessment. Conferring with the provider, or sending him or her a T-Con (e-mail message), doesn't relieve the nurse of any of those responsibilities. In fact, there are many times when the nurse can and should make the decision without first consulting the provider. It is not necessary to restrict those occasions to chest pain, 10/10 pain, loss of vision, and other obvious problems. I'm sure your nurses recognize that this step creates an unnecessary delay when a T-Con is sent to a provider to make a disposition when the nurse already knows what the ultimate outcome should be. Additionally, use of your "emergency algorithms" does not relieve the nurse of the responsibility for making an adequate assessment and exercising clinical judgment.

Bottom line: Telephone triage is *nursing* practice. Having the nurse collect information, confer with the provider, and communicate his or her decision to the patient is underutilizing your professional nursing staff, probably creating a good deal of rework, and most likely not even resulting in a better decision. Who is better equipped to make a decision about appropriate disposition than the nurse who took the call? Certainly there will be occasions in which the nurse needs to confer with the provider, but ideally that shouldn't be a matter of routine. Under most circumstances, nursing autonomy in telephone triage is desirable; and the protocols, or decision support tools, support this autonomous practice.

On the subject of following the protocols and documenting the protocol used, this is generally standard practice for telephone triage calls (however, if you have an organizational policy that states which protocols are used, the author information doesn't have to be repeated in each patient record). Please keep in mind that whether the protocol guides your decision making or consultation with the provider guides your decision making, the ultimate responsibility for doing an adequate assessment and making an appropriate disposition rests with the nurse.

Further, if a nurse carries out an order (communicates a disposition to a patient) that is contraindicated (and the nurse should reasonably have been expected to know it was contraindicated), the fact that the provider was involved in the process does not relieve the nurse of his or her professional responsibility to the patient. In fact, because telephone triage is nursing practice, the nurse can almost definitely be held liable. In other words, the nurse will not be relieved of responsibility for accurate decision making. Use of protocols is an excellent way to assure procedural standardization and decreased ambiguity in decision making for nurses who are talking to a patient about a symptom-based call, but assessment and clinical judgment are key.

TRIAGE CATEGORY "URGENT"

Question:

There have been questions from the nurses regarding the triage category of "urgent." My organization interprets "urgent" as meaning the patient needs immediate assistance, period! Perhaps you could give me a little history on the current categories.

Answer:

The definitions and use of triage categories is really organization specific. The traditional triage categories of "emergent," "urgent," and "non-urgent" are generally well understood among triage professionals (ED personnel, EMTs, etc.), but we can see how those words could be a little confusing for others because of the non-medical definitions and connotations they carry. However, it's just semantics. Don't let your nurses get hung up on use of the words "emergent," "urgent," "non-urgent." It might be better if you use the categories "immediate," "24 hour," and "routine" because they are much more descriptive and less ambiguous. Or "red, yellow, green" would work also, as long as your written policy defines them and everyone has the same understanding. That's the key.

"Urgent" is generally defined as meaning *potentially life, limb, or vision threatening*. Because of the *potentially* life-threatening nature of these calls, these patients must be seen and evaluated promptly. It's up to the nurse's judgment, usually guided by decision support tools, to decide how quickly within that 24-hour period the patient must be seen and/or evaluated. "Urgent" could mean within the hour, before the end of the day, or first thing tomorrow. Just be sure if you put someone off until tomorrow that you are confident the patient is stable. You don't want to "bet their life" and then lose.

VOICE MAIL AND USE OF FRONT OFFICE PERSONNEL IN PATIENT INTAKE

Question:

I've been looking into it and have been told that triage calls should never go to voice mail. We are a 10-physician office and we staff 1-2 triage nurses per day. Many times some of our triage calls go to voice mail if we are on another call or finishing up on a call. Our goal is to call patients back within 1 hour, and many times it is sooner, sometimes later, dependent on our call volume at the time. We also have guidelines in place with our front desk staff for emergent type calls that require immediate attention. Does this sound like a reasonable use of voice mail?

Answer:

It's better in many ways for patients to hold to speak directly to a nurse who answers their calls in the order received, utilizing an electronic menu to do the routing. Our opinion on voice mail is that you can use it, but you need to be careful. We also have major concerns about asking the front office staff to decide which calls are too urgent to go into voice mail. Although you may use a "hot list" of "buzzwords," we know of examples of patients calling with chief complaints of "cold" or "sinus infection," which respectively turned out to be an MI and an intracranial bleed. Instead of having your secretary use the list (putting her in the position to do first-line triage), you should simply tell the patient the nurse will call him or her back "within ___ minutes/hours" and then have the secretary say (verbatim), "Can it wait that long?" The patient, like the front office person, is a lay person but probably knows better whether it can wait, because patients usually (not always) have a pretty good idea whether they think they have an emergency or not. In coming up with a policy, it needs to be practical but at the same time it should increase patient safety and decrease liability for you and your organization.

WORKING FROM HOME

Question:

I am an experienced telephone triage nurse interested in a job that allows me to work from home. Is there anything specific I need to know about working from home?

Answer:

This is a growing trend, and it's likely that home-based telehealth nursing will really catch on in coming years. One study found that nurses from home "were more productive, took fewer days sick leave and had a lower attrition rate" (p. 119).[32] The only real potential downside that we can think of (provided you don't have barking dogs or noisy children running around) is the isolation of being home alone. Experienced telephone triage nurses have learned to rely on the collegial relationships with their peers to collaborate on difficult patients or obscure presentations.[31,33] In fact, nurses have reported an increase in knowledge and experience based on the shared second opinions and experience of other nurses.[34] Some of the organizations that employ home-based triage have found creative ways to provide that contact, such as with instant messaging programs and the like.

Authors' Note:

Another version of this FAQ comes from nurses who are experiencing an extended illness, have a new baby at home, or an aging parent to care for. Without understanding the complexity of this practice, nurses looking for a job they can do from home often look to telephone triage. It is important that we all help educate our colleagues at all levels about the degree of sophistication necessary and the risks associated with this practice. This is not a job any nurse can do from home. Nurses who enter this realm must understand what they're pursuing and *want* to do telephone triage for the all the right reasons.

References

1. American Academy of Ambulatory Care Nursing. (2011). *Telehealth nursing certification.* Retrieved from http://www.aaacn.org/cgi-bin/WebObjects/AAACNMain.woa/1/wa/viewSection?s_id=1073743906&ss_id=536873025&wosid=qS1e12Aw56j025o5t7VlG1FE2LN
2. North, F., & Varkey, P. (2009). A retrospective study of adult telephone triage calls in a US call centre. *Journal of Telemedicine and Telecare, 15*(4), 165-170.
3. Derkx, H.P., Rethans, J.J., Maiburg, B.H., Winkens, R.A., Muijtjens, A.M., van Rooij, H., & Knottnerus, J.A. (2009). Quality of communication during telephone triage at Dutch out-of-hours centres. *Patient Education & Counseling, 74*(2), 174-178.
4. Omery, A. (2003). Advice nursing practice: On the quality of the evidence. *Journal of Nursing Administration, 33*(6), 353-360.
5. Purc-Stephenson, R., & Thrasher, C. (2010). Nurses' experiences with telephone triage and advice: A meta-ethnography. *Journal of Advanced Nursing, 66*(3), 482-494. doi:10.1111/j.1365-2648.2010.05275.x
6. Hertz, A., & Schmitt, B. (2011). *Decreasing ER utilization with nursing telephone triage and establishing a National Network of Medical Call centers.* Retrieved from http://www.stcc-triage.com/Decreasing%20ER%20Utilization%20with%20Nurse%20Telephone%20Triage%20July2011.pdf
7. Greenberg, M.E. (2009). A comprehensive model of the process of telephone nursing. *Journal of Advanced Nursing, 65*(12), 2621-2629. doi:10.1111/j.1365-2648.2009.05132.x
8. Vinson, M.H., McCallum, R., Thornlow, D.K., & Chanpagne, M.T. (2011). Design, implementation, and evaluation of population-specific telehealth nursing services. *Nursing Economic$, 29*(5), 265-272, 277.
9. Hildebrandt, D.E., Westfall, J.M., & Smith, P.C. (2003). After-hours telephone triage affects patient safety. *Journal of Family Practice, 52*(3), 222-228.
10. Hildebrandt, D.E., Westfall, J.M., Fernald, D.H., & Pace, W.D. (2006). Harm resulting from inappropriate telephone triage in primary care. *Journal of the American Board of Family Medicine, 19*(5), 437-442.
11. Greatbatch, D., Hanlon, G., Goode, J., O'Caithain, A., Strangleman, T., & Luff, D. (2005). Telephone triage, expert systems and clinical expertise. *Sociology of Health & Illness, 27*(6), 802-830.
12. Klasner, A., King, W., Crews, T., & Monroe, K. (2006). Accuracy and response time when clerks are used for telephone triage. *Clinical Pediatrics, 45*, 267-269.
13. Rupp, R., Ramsey, K., & Foley, J. (1994). Telephone triage: Results of adolescent clinic responses to a mock patient with pelvic pain. *Journal of Adolescent Health, 15*(3), 249-253.
14. Austin, S. (2008). Are you liable for telephone advice? *Med-Surg Insider*, 6-7.
15. Canadian Nurses Association. (2000). Telehealth: Great potential or risky terrain? *Nursing Now. Issues and Trends in Canadian Nursing, 9.* Ottawa, Canada: Author.
16. Valsecchi, R., Andersson, M., Smith, C., Sederblad, P., & Mueller, F. (2007, April). *Telenursing: The English and Sweden experiences.* Paper presented at the 25th Annual International Labour Process Conference AIAS Amsterdam. Retrieved from dspace.mah.se:8080/bitstream/handle/2043/5440/ILPC_2007%20Valsecchi%20et%20al_rev_.pdf;jsessionid=F36E781E8FB1C54FA464093848D7CB0B?sequence=1
17. Van Dinter, M. (2000). Telephone triage: The rules are changing. *American Journal of Maternal Child Nursing, 25*(4), 187-191.

18. College of Nurses of Ontario. (2009). *Telepractice: Practice guideline.* Toronto, Canada: Author. Retrieved from http://www.cno.org/Global/docs/prac/41041_telephone.pdf
19. Mayo, A.M., Chang, B.L., & Omery, A. (2002). Use of protocols and guidelines by telephone nurses. *Clinical Nursing Research, 11*(2), 204-219.
20. O'Cathain, A., Nicholl, J., Sampson, F., Walters, S., McDonnell, A., & Munro, J. (2004). Do different types of nurses give different triage decisions in NHS direct? A mixed methods study. *Journal of Health Services Research & Policy, 9*(4), 226-233.
21. Valanis, B., Tanner, C., Moscato, S. R., Shapiro, S., Izumi, S., David, M., ... Mayo, A. (2003). A model for examining predictors of outcomes of telephone nursing advice. *Journal of Nursing Administration, 33*(2), 91-95.
22. Ström, M., Marklund, B., & Hildingh, C. (2009). Callers' perceptions of receiving advice via a medical care help line. *Scandinavian Journal of Caring Sciences, 23*(4), 682-690. doi:10.1111/j.1471-6712.2008.00661.x
23. Levine, C. (2006). HIPAA and talking with family caregivers: What does the law really say? *American Journal of Nursing, 106*(8), 51-53.
24. U.S. Department of Health and Human Services. (2003). *Uses and disclosures for treatment, payment, and health care operations.* Retrieved from http://www.hhs.gov/ocr/privacy/hipaa/understanding/coveredentities/usesanddisclosuresfortpo.html
25. American Academy of Ambulatory Care Nursing. (2011). *Scope and standards of practice for professional telehealth nurses* (5th ed.). Pitman, NJ: Author.
26. International Council of Nurses. (2007). *International competencies for telenursing.* Geneva, Switzerland: Author.
27. Espensen, M. (Ed.). (2009). *Telehealth nursing practice essentials.* Pitman, NJ: American Academy of Ambulatory Care Nursing.
28. Ernesäter, A., Holmström, I., & Engström, M. (2009). Telenurses' experiences of working with computerized decision support: Supporting, inhibiting and quality improving. *Journal of Advanced Nursing, 65*(5), 1074-1083. doi:10.1111/j.1365-2648.2009.04966.x
29. Holmstrom, I. (2007). Decision aid software programs in telenursing: Not used as intended? Experiences of Swedish telenurses. *Nursing & Health Sciences, 9*(1), 23-28.
30. Dowding, D., Mitchell, N., Randell, R., Foster, R., Lattimer, V., & Thompson, C. (2009). Nurses' use of computerised clinical decision support systems: A case site analysis. *Journal of Clinical Nursing, 18*(8), 1159-1167. doi:10.1111/j.1365-2702.2008.02607.x
31. Hanlon, G., Strangleman, T., Goode, J., Luff, D., O'Cathian, A., & Greatbatch, D. (2005). Knowledge, technology and nursing: The case of NHS direct. *Human Relations, 58*(2), 147-171.
32. St. George, I., Baker, J., Karabatsos, G., Brinble, R., Wilson, A., & Cullen, M. (2009). How safe is telenursing from home? *Collegian, 16*, 119-123.
33. Knowles, E., O'Cathain, A., Morrell, J., Munro, J.F., & Nicholl, J.P. (2002). NHS direct and nurses – opportunity or monotony? *International Journal of Nursing Studies, 39*(8), 857-866.
34. Smith, C. (2008). Knowledge and the discourse of labour process transformation: Nurses and the case of NHS direct for england. *Work, Employment & Society, 22*(4), 581-599.

EPILOGUE: THE FUTURE IS NOW

If we are to truly make a difference in this world, we must have a vision for our profession.

"For a vision to truly be a force in people's hearts, it must...

- be legitimate
- be shared
- express people's highest aspirations for what they want to create in the world
- stretch beyond the limits of current realities
- conceivably be achievable"(¶ 3)[1]

In this book, we have endeavored to provide clarity about the practice of telephone triage as it is, and as it could and should be. However, before such progress can be made, there are two prevalent issues regarding telephone triage that must be brought into the light. These problems are within the domain and thus within the control of nursing.

THE ELEPHANTS IN THE ROOM

Telephone triage practices are plagued by two elephants in the room. Both of these have been amply considered in this book, but they are still rarely acknowledged or addressed in the real world of telephone triage. These largely ignored problems concern the autonomy and role of the professional nurse in telephone triage. Unresolved, these two pesky pachyderms will continue to interfere with progress toward optimal practice and the recognition of telephone triage as a unique and well-defined form of professional nursing.

The first issue has to do with the *use of protocols* as tools to dictate decision making and provide presumed clinical and legal protection. The second concerns confusion about the *scope of practice* as it presently exists in telephone triage nursing.

The autonomy of the telephone triage nurse is at the heart of both of these problems, so we would like to discuss them together before addressing each of them separately. Somewhat paradoxically, one of these areas of concern lessens the autonomy of the registered nurse, whereas the other expands it. We suggest that the true representation of our proper role lies somewhere in between.

FUNCTIONING UP TO BUT NOT BEYOND OUR SCOPE OF PRACTICE

On one hand, in the formal call center setting, we have nurses who are sometimes expected to function as near automatons, following the protocols as written and occasionally being expected to read the script verbatim. These nurses are given little if any authority to deviate from the protocol when their nursing judgment dictates it, thereby restricting their function to below their scope of practice. On the other end of the spectrum, in the clinic setting, when not performing tasks better delegated to a nursing assistant, nurses ironically are often performing functions beyond their scope of practice. For example, based on perceived "permission" of the physician, it is not uncommon for clinic nurses to independently renew prescriptions or prescribe new medications based on their own "diagnosis" of the patient's problem, involving the physician only after the fact, if at all.

As discussed in Chapter 1, the problem of reduced autonomy originally resulted from forces outside of nursing that were instrumental in the initial conception and design of telephone triage. Based on misconceptions and misunderstanding of the capabilities of the professional nurse, mechanisms were put in place to control the thoughts and actions of the nurse. However, research has shown that nurses are capable of more and often exercise independent thoughts and judgments beyond those prescribed by policy and protocol.[2,3,4]

The opposite problem of going beyond the RN's scope of practice often occurs in the informal setting of the doctor's office, but has been known to occur in more formal ambulatory care settings as well. This often results from nursing practice being defined by administrators or physicians who don't have a clear understanding of the capabilities and scope of practice of the nurse. Administrators are naturally focused on the bottom line, because their orientation is based on the business model. The actual scope of practice and abilities of nurses are often not on their radar. And physicians, having been taught in medical school that they are the captain of the ship, and lacking a clear understanding of nursing, often empower and encourage nurses to function beyond their legal scope of practice.

These two problems each represent extremes of practice. The first deprives the nurse of appropriate autonomy and the second pushes the nurse beyond his or her scope of practice. These practice dilemmas seem to be polar opposites of each other, but they are both symptoms of the same underlying deficiencies. These problems represent lack of understanding of the role of the professional nurse in telephone triage coupled with lack of nurse empowerment.

But how did this come to be? How could nurses have stood idly by watching others define their practice in ways inconsistent with what they know to be their professional responsibilities? We could blame this on outside forces, but the fact is that sometimes nurses are nursing's greatest enemy. Unfortunately, these deficiencies are more often than not the result of nurses failing to own and define their own practice.

The now graying generation was raised at a time when women were subordinate to men and nurses were subordinate to physicians. Thus, growth of the profession has often been hampered by a perceived position of powerlessness. Of course, as nursing has evolved, we have overcome Herculean obstacles such as role and gender biases, but vestiges of this era remain and have made us vulnerable, allowing outside forces to define the rules that guide our practice. Fortunately, however, over time, nursing as a profession has developed a larger scientific and evidentiary focus that supports and encourages the role of professional nurses as knowledge workers.[5] We must therefore be certain that both practice and policy are based upon the evidence supporting professional nursing.

MORE ON THE USE OF DECISION SUPPORT TOOLS

Policy related to decision support tools is often based on the perception that these tools are supposed to direct nurses' thinking and thus their decision making. This belief is presumably based in part on the assumption that these tools can provide clinical and legal protection, although they actually guarantee neither. If telephone triage nurses were to comply with this intent to the extent it is expected and touted as "safe practice" by many individuals and organizations, the practice of telephone triage by RNs would represent little more than following a recipe as one might when cooking. In some settings, RNs are actually required to read a script, effectively eliminating the possibility of independent thinking and individualization of care. For example, in one such call center, the nurses were obliged to ask every patient with a sore throat, regardless of age or circumstances, if they had engaged in oral sex.[6]

Because decision support tools are often linear, directive, and have little focus on humanistic factors, the nurse must adapt, adjust, interpret, and often override the decision support tools to better meet the needs of the individual patient.[6,7,8] Unfortunately, however, in many formalized settings, efforts of the nurse to think independently are met with disapproval. But even in such settings, nurses are expected to identify barriers and challenges patients face and address them with the patient and family, utilizing traditional nursing skills such as collaborative planning, patient education, patient advocacy, and provision of other forms of patient support. Thus, organizational policies must be improved to facilitate rather than interfere with sound telephone triage practice and clinical nursing judgment. One worthy goal for our profession is to be actively involved in improving the design and content of decision support tools so that they are less narrow and directive and more compatible with the principles of the nursing process. But even with such efforts, they will always be only aids to critical thinking and telephone triage, not dictators of the practice.

NURSING REGULATION AND SCOPE OF PRACTICE

Nursing scope of practice in less formal settings such as doctor's offices and clinics is also obscured at times. As discussed elsewhere in this book, at least three areas of potential confusion exist in nursing regulation as promulgated by the Boards of Nursing.

First, inconsistency exists in opinions regarding whether LPNs may engage in the practice of telephone triage or not. The variable opinions among the Boards likely represent differences in understanding of the complexity of this practice. We need uniform policies that clarify practice from state to state and assure patient safety by specifying that telephone triage may only be done by RNs.

Second, in many ambulatory care settings, RNs recommend medications and other treatments based on their own presumptive determination of the nature of the patient's problem, according to an "understanding" they have with the physician, or as guided and authorized by decision support tools. Further, in some clinical settings, nurses are given the autonomy to renew routine prescriptions and recommend/initiate new prescription drugs based on predetermined clinical criteria.

The question of recommendation of medications gets mixed reviews from the Boards. Interestingly, they are presently divided as to whether this activity represents simple pattern matching and compliance with medically approved protocols (similar to standing orders), or if it represents a somewhat covert process of formulating a presumptive medical diagnosis and prescribing treatment. These actions, of course, are widely regarded as being beyond the basic scope of practice for an RN. However, in the real world, these practices are common. Boards of nursing must clarify practice expectations regarding recommendation of OTCs and protocol-driven renewal or initiation of legend drugs. Again, we need uniform policies that clarify practice from state to state, are consistent with the cognitive abilities of the RN, and assure patient safety.

Finally, the question of interstate practice continues to loom large in the minds of informed telephone triage nurses and conscientious administrators. We join with the American Academy of Ambulatory Care Nursing[9] and other professional organizations in encouraging all of the Boards to seek uniform adoption. We also urge our colleagues and administrators in non-Compact states to contact their Board of Nursing to see how they can help promote adoption of the Nurse Licensure Compact in their state.

THE UNIQUE AND COMPLEX NATURE OF TELEPHONE TRIAGE NURSING: DIAGNOSTIC REASONING

As we have emphasized repeatedly throughout this book, we believe there is no more high risk or complex nursing practice than telephone triage. Over the telephone, patients present with unknown or unverified problems, and the telephone triage nurse must accurately identify the patient's problem before developing a plan of care. In doing so, the RN uses a critical thought process that incorporates clinical knowledge, experience, and professional judgment and involves sophisticated diagnostic reasoning in conjunction with well-designed decision support tools. In contrast, during the provision of care in the face-to-face setting, patients usually have at least a working diagnosis with relatively few unknowns, and there is a collaborative team with checks and balances that provide extra levels of safety. However, in telephone triage there is literally only the patient and the nurse.

The primary objective of the telephone triage nurse is to identify the nature and urgency of the patient's problem. This enables the nurse to recommend a disposition that is appropriate for that patient and to provide collaboration and support to assure that the caller's needs are met. However, without a differential diagnosis, or an idea of what's going on with the patient, it is often difficult, if not impossible, for the nurse to determine the best approach to management of the patient's problem(s). Nurses in telephone triage therefore use diagnostic reasoning to help rule out, identify, and verify symptoms or patterns. This helps to determine the acuity of the problem and the most suitable intervention. For example, diagnostic reasoning is utilized when a telephone triage nurse reassures a mother that her febrile child doesn't need an antibiotic for his cold. In this case, the nurse has tentatively determined that the problem is more likely viral than bacterial. Of course, the mother would be advised to call back if the child's condition didn't improve or worsened, leaving the door open for further evaluation if necessary. Likewise, the nurse who recommends an over-the-counter medication such as guaifenesin for a cough has determined that the patient is in need of an expectorant instead of a cough suppressant. Additionally, the nurse has also determined the source of the cough to be respiratory rather than cardiovascular in nature.

BRINGING POLICIES IN LINE WITH PRACTICE

The practice of telephone triage has developed so fast that it has outgrown our own nursing policies and our own basic nursing education. By our lack of ownership and leadership, we have allowed others to define nursing practice. Without sufficient input from nurses, policies have been developed by others such as physicians and administrators who lack a clear understanding of nursing practice. Consequently, many telephone triage nurses are working in environments in which the policies and guidelines either misdirect or do not support professional practice. Thus, nurses occasionally find themselves in a position of having to ignore policy in order to practice professional nursing and honor their nursing values and commitment to patient safety. Or worse, not owning their practice, nurses follow these misguided policies often to the potential detriment of the patient and the profession.

We need to have a stronger and clearer voice regarding our own practice in order to bring policy into conformity with our values and the processes we use to provide care.[5] As professionals and leaders, we must have policies that allow us to do our jobs. Thus, we must help organizations, leaders, and others to first understand the scope and capabilities of professional nurses and then to create policies that reflect actual practice, are reasonable, serve our patients, and are consistent with the standards of nursing practice.

There are leaders and nurses who "get it" and work diligently toward change implementation. However, many of the practicing telephone nurses have not critically examined their practice enough to advocate, teach, or buck the system if necessary. When we do speak out, we often buckle under a system historically molded by oppression. However, change is possible. The lead author of this book has conducted telephone triage seminars across the country, speaking to nurses, managers, administrators, and physicians from a vast range of settings. Over the years, the participants have left the seminars with an exquisite sense of awareness, understanding, ownership, and empowerment related to their practice of nursing over the telephone. We hope this book has provided you, the reader, with this same keen sense of the practice and value of telephone triage and has empowered you to teach and support others and to speak out for policy change as needed in your own setting.

A CALL TO ACTION

To rectify the practice challenges we have discussed, nursing has to take control of telephone triage and advance it beyond its current state. But to do so, the profession will have to overcome resistance from other parties (and even some from within our own ranks) who are entrenched in the status quo because of concerns with the costs of change, both financial and intangible. For example, we must ensure that all telephone triage calls are handled by RNs – a policy that may seem to be expensive at first glance but will be more than beneficial and cost effective in the long run. Thus, a prerequisite for implementing such improvements is recognition that we have to become bolder, more assertive, and empowered to take ownership of the future of this practice.

Fortunately this is the ideal time for nurses to step up to this challenge.[5] Nursing education has transitioned from diploma programs with training focused on the bedside to emphasis on a more theoretical and professional orientation with the BSN degree and beyond. More nurses are seeking advanced degrees[10] and promotion of the BSN as entry into practice has set the bar higher in nursing education.[11] Nursing theorists and researchers continue to expand our scientific knowledge base and provide us with new ideas of how to apply that knowledge to improve nursing care. Professional organizations have become more active in providing leadership and guidance to practicing nurses. Professional expectations have broadened such that leadership, autonomy, collaboration, and interdisciplinary practices are now the norm in many settings.

As nursing practice is changing, nurses entering the profession are changing as well. Individuals who are choosing to go into nursing today do not have to fight the odds that the previous generations did. No longer does nursing survive because it is just one of the few acceptable career choices for women, nor does the new generation of nurses view nursing as a profession to enter because they are unable to get into medical school. Nursing, when selected as a career choice, is a deliberate decision by men and women who realize they have many choices, but they have *chosen* nursing. Admission into BSN programs has become extremely competitive[10] and thus many who are entering nursing today have superior academic and social acumen. They could have done anything, but they chose to be a nurse! Armed with these advantages and awareness of what is possible, we believe that nurses are now in a great position to take control of the practice of telephone triage. With guidance and vision from experienced nurses, we must grow and support a new generation of professional nurses who embody leadership, proactivity, and advocacy, not just for the patient, but for nursing as well. However, we must be aware that nursing will only go where we take it. The continued professional growth of nursing is up to us, with the experienced nurses providing progressive mentoring and the newer nurses pressing forward into the future. It is time to take full ownership of the practice of telephone triage nursing.

A LOOK TO THE FUTURE: TELEPHONE TRIAGE IN BASIC EDUCATION

Let's briefly review the nature of the practice and offer some more specific suggestions for how we can take ownership and advance the nursing profession in general, and telephone triage in particular, to their proper place within the health care arena.

By this time, it should be quite clear to the reader that telephone triage is a sophisticated form of nursing that requires an understanding of the unique aspects of this practice and a specific skill set to assure the delivery of safe and effective care. It is likely that every nurse, at some time in his or her career, will be called upon to provide nursing care over the telephone. Because of the widespread use of telephone triage in contemporary nursing and its unique and high-risk nature, nursing students should routinely be taught the basic principles of telephone triage, just as they are taught the basic principles of critical care. Adding telephone triage content to basic nursing education will give the next generation of nurses critical insight into telephone triage practice, prevent them from thinking that answering the phone is "just another call," and reinforce their broader understanding of the nursing process.

In addition, organizations that employ nurses to practice telephone triage should provide more specialized training in the practice, beyond the basics that we are recommending as part of their BSN education. Currently, most of the training and education specific to telephone triage occurs in the work setting and lacks consistency.[12] Organizations that employ nurses to practice telephone triage should provide consistent, in-depth training that addresses the specialized skill set needed by the nurse to ensure safe and effective nursing care. There are also continuing education opportunities in telephone triage offered on-line, at private or public seminars, at professional conferences, and through our nursing organizations. The American Nurses Credentialing Center offers Board Certification in Ambulatory Care Nursing, which is currently the national certification that officially recognizes nurses as having specialty knowledge in the area of ambulatory care nursing and telephone triage.

IN CONCLUSION

We have come to the end of the book but not to the end of the story. During this journey, we have provided you with a wealth of knowledge and strategies you can use to improve your own clinical practice, your program, and its role within your health care organization. We have also provided you with five broad essential take home messages:

- Telephone triage is a unique and important form of professional nursing that epitomizes the nurse/patient interaction and the application of the nursing process.
- Sound telephone triage practice requires specialized training, experience, and appropriate program design.
- Every *symptom-based* call from a patient potentially involves triage and must be handled by an RN.
- Telephone triage requires a specialized skill set which includes erring on the side of caution at all times.
- Quality, not cost, is the bottom line in telephone triage.

FINAL THOUGHTS ON THE FUTURE OF NURSING

Trends in nursing employment fluctuate, but the demand for nurses is not only ever-present but is likely to increase in the coming decades, particularly in specialized settings.[5,13] Immediate information availability and reliance on expanding telecommunications technologies, coupled with cost consciousness of health care consumers and providers alike, will make telephone triage a continually growing presence in health care well into the future. However, regardless of the technological advances, at the base and heart of telephone triage is the essence of professional nursing. Nothing will ever change the responsibility we have to our patients. But we also have a responsibility to our profession. Although telephone triage has been the focus of this book, the underlying message is that we must honor nursing by helping it recognize its growth and complexity and evolve to the next level. Nursing will continue to be a collaborative but autonomous profession, dedicated to excellence in patient care, but as health care evolves, nurses will take on greater responsibility in the management of patients in ambulatory care settings.

Perhaps the individual nurse, feeling a commitment to affect change, wonders where to go next. Positive change is well within our grasp. We have the knowledge. We have the passion. It is time to put those into action. In other words, it isn't enough to simply know this information and be willing to apply it. We must act on it. It is critical we recognize that the future is now.

"When a critical number of people change how they think and believe, the culture will also, and a new era begins" (p. 3).[14]

References

1. International Council of Nurses. (2011). *Our vision.* Retrieved from http://www.icn.ch/about-icn/the-icns-vision/
2. Pettinari, C.J., & Jessopp, L. (2001). 'Your ears become your eyes': Managing the absence of visibility in NHS direct. *Journal of Advanced Nursing, 36*(5), 668-675.
3. Greatbatch, D., Hanlon, G., Goode, J., O'Cathain, A., Strangleman, T., & Luff, D. (2005). Telephone triage, expert systems and clinical expertise. *Sociology of Health & Illness, 27*(6), 802-830.
4. Holmstrom, I. (2007). Decision aid software programs in telenursing: Not used as intended? Experiences of Swedish telenurses. *Nursing & Health Sciences, 9*(1), 23-28.
5. Institute of Medicine. (2011). *The future of nursing: Leading change, advancing health.* Washington, DC: The National Academies Press.
6. Hanlon, G., Strangleman, T., Goode, J., Luff, D., O'Cathian, A., & Greatbatch, D. (2005). Knowledge, technology and nursing: The case of NHS direct. *Human Relations, 58*(2), 147-171.
7. Charles-Jones, H., May, C., Latimer, J., & Roland, M. (2003). Telephone triage by nurses in primary care: What is it for and what are the consequences likely to be? *Journal of Health Services Research & Policy, 8*(3), 154-159.
8. Collin-Jacques, C., & Smith, C. (2005). Nursing on the line: Experiences from England and Quebec (Canada). *Human Relations, 58*(1), 5-32.
9. American Academy of Ambulatory Care Nursing. (2009). *Nurse licensure compact (NLC) position statement.* Pitman, NJ: Author. Retrieved from http://www.aaacn.org/resources/positionStatements/positionStatementNLC.pdf
10. Raines, C.F., & Taglaireni, M.E. (2008). Career pathways in nursing: Entry points and academic progression. *The Online Journal of Issues in Nursing, 13*(3). Retrieved from http://www.nursingworld.org/MainMenuCategories/ANAMarketplace/ANAPeriodicals/OJIN/TableofContents/vol132008/No3Sept08/CareerEntryPoints.html
11. Benner, P., Sutphen, M., Leonard, V., & Day, L. (2010). *Educating nurses: A call for radical transformation.* Stanford, CA: Jossey-Bass.
12. Grady, J.L., & Schlachta-Fairchild, L. (2007). Report of the 2004-2005 International Telenursing Survey. *CIN: Computers, Informatics, Nursing, 25*(5), 266-272.
13. Auerbach, D.I., Buerhaus, P.I., & Staiger, D.O. (2011). Registered nurse supply grows faster than projected amid surge in new entrants ages 23-26. *Health Affairs, 30*(12), 2286-2292. doi:10.1377/hlthaff.2011.0588
14. Bolen, J.S. (1999). *The millionth circle: How to change ourselves and the world.* York Beach, ME: Conari Press.

Appendix A

Boards of Nursing Survey Regarding Nursing Regulation and Scope of Practice in Telephone Triage

As discussed in Chapter 5, nursing regulation and scope of practice related to telephone triage continues to be lacking and/or inconsistent. Surveys of the Boards of Nursing have been conducted several times over the past several years to identify issues and seek clarification. The results of the final survey are included here.

A survey was conducted via Survey Monkey™ of the Boards of Nursing (BONs) to inquire about issues related to nursing regulation and scope of practice in telephone triage.[1] An introductory email was sent to the Executive Director of each Board of Nursing (BON) in December 2011 and again in January 2012, with the assistance of the National Council of State Boards of Nursing (NCSBN). Follow-up emails and phone calls were made by the primary investigator until all survey responses were obtained. Responses were received 12/4/11 through 4/6/12. Attached to the email request for completion of the survey was a Background Document which included definitions of Telephone Triage and provided a scenario to improve consistency of responses. Also included was a short discussion of the primary regulatory issues facing telehealth nursing today, and it was noted that the focus of this study was telephone triage.

DISCLAIMER

Nursing regulation and scope of practice in telephone triage is a moving target. In fact, some BONs have reversed their opinions completely from one survey to the next. Because not all responses represent statute, it is imperative that each practicing nurse verify the information in this Appendix with the appropriate BON(s). For legal advice, please contact your personal or organizational attorney.

BACKGROUND DOCUMENT

The following is the introductory document provided to the BONs as background information prior to completion of the survey.

Current Issues in Telephone Triage

Nursing care has traditionally been practiced in the inpatient arena. With recent changes in the health care milieu, nursing care is shifting to ambulatory care settings with greater and greater frequency. With emerging utilization of telecommunications technology, nursing is now being practiced in a third venue, precipitating development of teleheath nursing as an area requiring regulatory guidance.

Limited research exists related to telehealth nursing. Much of what is currently known about telephone triage and other forms of telehealth nursing is based on anecdotal observations. I present seminars on telephone triage nationwide and thus have access to a diverse and geographically disparate group of nurses providing telehealth nursing services across the United States.

Telephone Triage Settings

The most visible and formal settings for telephone triage are medical call centers. These exist in three basic forms including hospital/community-based call centers, with a focus on community service and marketing; third-party payers, often with a focus on demand management and resource utilization; and entrepreneurial endeavors, which provide fee-based services to physician practices and organizations seeking to outsource their telephone triage services for their client/patient base.

However, telephone triage is practiced in a wide variety of settings including doctors' offices, clinics, home health and hospice agencies, urgent care centers, emergency departments, correctional facilities, student health centers, and other settings in both the private and public sectors. In fact, it is hypothesized that all ambulatory care nurses (and indeed, many inpatient nurses) practice telehealth nursing on a routine basis, but many do not recognize it as such.

Inconsistency in the Practice of Telephone Triage

Telephone triage, although defined by the American Academy of Ambulatory Care Nursing (AAACN)[2] as professional nursing practice, is also practiced by a wide variety of non RNs with diverse levels of preparation. While call centers employ primarily RNs for telephone triage positions, in doctors' offices and clinic settings, it is not unusual to find RNs, LPN/LVNs, and medical assistants functioning in very similar roles, with all three levels providing patient care over the telephone.

One area of significant concern in previous surveys has been the number of states that still regard telephone triage as being within the scope of practice of LPNs or LVNs, providing they are utilizing a decision support tool. Research[3] has shown that interpretation is an integral process in telephone triage from the beginning of the call to the end, and beyond, and thus even "data collection" over the telephone requires active assessment. Use of decision support tools does not negate the need for interpretation and professional assessment because critical thinking and clinical judgment are necessary for selection of the appropriate decision support tool and for its application in each clinical situation.

The practice of telephone triage is also performed in diverse manners. Medical call centers rely heavily on computerized software programs to provide decision support and capture patient data. However, other settings, such as doctors' offices and clinics, often practice with paper-based decision support tools or, more often, no decision support tools at all. In these settings, nurses and others often base their recommendations on clinical judgment or unwritten "organizational policy." It is not uncommon to find RNs, LVN/LPNs, and medical assistants recommending various medications based on their own judgment and personal experience and following unwritten "rules" provided to them by their medical staff. For example, based on unwritten "permission" from the physician, all levels of personnel often recommend over-the-counter (OTC) medications, renew existing prescriptions that have expired, and even prescribe legend drugs for their patient population without first seeking direct/written medical authorization. ***Boards of Nursing that have deemed recommendation of OTC medications to be outside of the scope of practice of a telephone triage RN, even with medically approved decision support tools, significantly restrict the usefulness of telephone triage in their state.*** Imagine a call center nurse who can't tell a mother with a febrile child to administer an antipyretic. This limitation significantly handicaps the autonomy of the telephone triage nurse, often necessitating a call to a pediatrician in the middle of the night.

The level of sophistication necessary to provide safe, effective telephone triage services is significant. Many settings such as call centers and the U.S. military routinely employ only RNs in these roles, and it isn't unusual to see significant experience requirements for nurses who practice telephone triage. Many leaders who are overseeing telephone triage services fail to recognize that "nursing services provided by electronic means is indeed the practice of nursing"(¶1)[4] and thus requires critical thinking, clinical judgment, and use of the nursing process.

Direction from the Boards of Nursing

In some states, the BONs have provided written documents in the form of position statements, FAQs, and policy statements to guide the licensed nurse in the practice of this new specialty. In other states, guidance from the BON is not forthcoming, and nurses must use their own judgment, supported primarily by decision-making models for scope of practice, to determine which activities are indeed within their scope of practice.

Three issues seem to provide the most confusion regarding the practice of telephone triage. These issues are related to:

- Interstate practice
- Recommendation of medications with and/or without decision support tools
- Varying roles and utilization of RNs, LPN/LVNs, and medical assistants, in provision of patient care by telephone

Focus of this Survey

This survey seeks to identify unique policies and interpretations of general policies that will provide guidance to practicing teleheath nurses in addressing those three areas of concern. Specifically, this survey seeks to answer the following questions.

1. To what extent, and under what circumstances, may RNs and/or LPN/LVNs recommend medications with and without medically approved decision support tools?

2. Is it within the scope of practice for LPNs/LVNs to practice telephone triage? If so, what are the limitations or caveats?
3. To what extent does the Nurse Licensure Compact pertain to patients who are temporary residents or visitors in other states?

Upon receipt and compilation of this information, it will be returned in composite to the BONs so that each may potentially learn from the experience of other Boards. These results are also anticipated to improve the understanding of telehealth nursing in hopes that more uniformity in the regulation of telehealth nursing may be achieved.

Definition of Telephone Triage

According to AAACN, Telephone Triage is described and defined as follows (p. 43).[2]

- Description:
    - A component of telephone nursing practice that focuses on assessment, prioritization, and referral to the appropriate level of care.
- Definition:
    - An interactive process between nurse and client that occurs over the telephone and involves identifying the nature and urgency of client health care needs and determining appropriate disposition.

Decision Support Tools: "Protocols" vs. "Standing Orders"

- The questions in this survey reference practice that is population-specific and guided by *Decision Support Tools* (traditionally referred to as protocols and guidelines).
- These questions do NOT refer to the use of *Standing Orders,* which would be assumed to be patient specific.

References

1. Rutenberg, C. (2012). [Results of the 2012 survey of the boards of nursing]. Unpublished raw data.
2. American Academy of Ambulatory Care Nursing. (2011). *Scope and standards of practice for professional telehealth nursing* (5th ed.). Pitman, NJ: Author.
3. Greenberg, M.E. (2009). A comprehensive model of the process of telephone nursing. *Journal of Advanced Nursing, 65*(12), 2621-2629.
4. National Council of State Boards of Nursing. (1997). *Telenursing: A challenge to regulation.* National Council, Position Paper. Chicago, IL: Author.

SURVEY QUESTIONS

The questions as asked on Survey Monkey™ are as follows:

1. **Please provide your contact information**

State:
Name:
Title:
Email Address:
Phone Number:
Today's Date:

2. **Regarding recommendation of medications by non advanced practice nurses** (yes, no, comment)

RNs may...

a. Recommend OTC drugs (e.g., guaifenesin) without a decision support tool
b. Recommend OTC drugs (e.g., guaifenesin) using a medically approved decision support tool
c. Renew prescriptions (e.g., birth control pills) using a medically approved decision support tool
d. Recommend legend drugs (e.g., amoxicillin) using a medically approved decision support tool

LP/VNs may...

e. Recommend OTC drugs (e.g.. guaifenesin) without a decision support tool
f. Recommend OTC drugs (e.g., guaifenesin) using a medically approved decision support tool
g. Renew prescriptions (e.g., birth control pills) using a medically approved decision support tool
h. Recommend legend drugs (e.g., amoxicillin) using a medically approved decision support tool

3. **LPNs/LVNs may perform telephone triage (collect data and make protocol-based decisions about urgency and patient management) in my state**

Independently,

a. With or without decision support tools
b. But only with decision support tools

Under supervision,

c. With or without decision support tools
d. Under supervision, but only with decision support tools
e. It exceeds their scope of practice under any circumstances

4. LPNs/LVNs may participate in other telephone nursing activities such as (select all that apply)

a. Call patients to report lab results, convey messages from the doctor, or other collaborative phone activities
b. Disease management (e.g., monitoring diabetes, Coumadin, or CHF by phone)
c. Behavioral modification (e.g., smoking cessation, weight reduction)

5. We do have a written policy, position paper, FAQ, or other document that speaks specifically to the role of the LPN/LVN in telephone triage or other telehealth nursing practice (yes, no, comment)

6. My state has a written policy, position paper, FAQ, or other document(s) that specifically addresses telephone triage or other telehealth nursing practice (yes, no, comment)

7. My state has written policies/rules that would restrict the practice of medical assistants in telephone triage (yes, no, comment)

8. Regarding interstate practice (select all that apply)

a. If the patient/caller is a permanent resident of your state, the out-of-state nurse must have a license in your state (or in a Compact state) in order to provide care to that patient.
b. If the patient/caller is a temporary resident of your state (e.g., a "snowbird"), the out-of-state nurse must have a license in your state (or in a Compact state) in order to provide care to that patient.
c. If the patient/caller is in your state only temporarily (e.g., vacationer or business traveler), the out-of-state nurse must have a license in your state (or in a Compact state) in order to provide care to that patient.
d. If a patient/caller is a permanent or temporary resident of your state but has an established relationship with a provider in an adjacent state, would you require nurses in that practice to have a license in your state (or in a Compact state) to provide care to their patient when s/he is calling them from home (in your state)? NOTE: The key point here is whether the established relationship with the provider mitigates the need for a nurse from an adjacent state to be licensed in your state in order to provide phone care to their patients.

e. The rules would be different if the nurse were in a doctor's office with an established relationship with the patient rather than in a call center.

9. **To your knowledge, has legal or disciplinary action been taken against nurses re telephone nursing practice in your state?** (yes, no, comment)

10. **If you are not a Compact State, do you anticipate your state taking action on this proposed legislation?**

a. We are a Compact State.
b. We anticipate taking action in 2012.
c. We anticipate taking action in the near future (please specify estimated date).
d. I do not anticipate our state taking action on the Compact in the foreseeable future (please specify concerns).

11. **Additional comments:**

Both quantitative and qualitative analysis are provided from the 2012 survey of the BONs.

RESPONSES

1. DEMOGRAPHIC INFORMATION

Respondents included 50 states plus Washington, DC, and CBME Northern Mariana Islands. All four LPN/LVN Boards (CA, GA, LA, and WV) responded. Four states were unable to provide any specific responses to the survey (DE, PA, SC, and WI), and IN provided limited responses. The LPN/LVN Board responses were included with the corresponding RN Boards in their states, and Northern Mariana Islands was not included in the tally of the 50 states and DC. Thus, the maximum number of responses to the questions (N) was either 46 or 47. Some questions had fewer responses because not all states answered all questions.

Comments of Four States that Didn't Respond to Specific Questions

- DE: *I have not replied because we do not have any language in statute or rules to address your survey questions.*
- PA: *This letter is in response to your request for information concerning the recommendation of medications by RNs and LPNs (as well as) whether LPNs may practice telephone triage…Nowhere do the Acts confer authority on the Board to issue advisory opinions or pre approve specific conduct….*
- SC: *The SC BON does not have an official advisory opinion or position statement on this matter.*
- WI: *…Last year the WI Board of Nursing enacted a process as it relates to agency staff or the Board members responding to inquiries that involve Scope of Practice type questions. In essence, the process dictates there will be no response to these inquiries, other than to direct the inquirer to the Department website…*

Discussion

Thirty of the 55 respondents were in the position of Executive Director or Associate Executive Director. Other responses were from Practice Consultants or Specialists, Education Directors, Program Coordinators, and other similar staff positions. It is important to note that in some cases, the responses reflected actual statute but in other situations, the responses represented Position Statements, Advisory Opinions, Declaratory Rulings, FAQs, or other written interpretive documents. Examples of verbiage used to explain the legal authority of these types of documents are provided.

- *Advisory Opinion (SD)*
  - *This opinion was rendered by the Board of Nursing upon submission of a written request. Although advisory opinions are not judicially reviewable and do not carry the force and effect of law, they do serve as a guideline to nurses who wish to engage in safe nursing practices. This advisory opinion was adopted by the South Dakota Board of Nursing, November 1994.*
- *Position Statement (VT)*
  - *This Position Statement represents the Board's current thinking. Position statements are not legally binding.*

Finally, in other cases, the responses represented only the informed interpretation of the Executive Director or his or her designee.

It is apparent from review of the responses that various boards have varying levels of knowledge and therefore differing understandings of the practice of telephone triage. It seems that not all recognize the level of assessment/critical thinking necessary in this practice, thus the high percentage of states with responses permitting LPNs/LVNs to do telephone triage with decision support tools.

2. REGARDING RECOMMENDATION OF MEDICATIONS BY NURSES

(percentages are based on yes and no responses)

RNs

a. OTCs without decision support tools: 35%
b. OTCs with decision support tools: 82%
   States not allowing RNs to recommend OTCs under any circumstances: AR, CT, FL, HI, MA, NH, WV
c. Renew existing prescriptions according to decision support tools: 51%
d. Recommend legend drugs according to decision support tools: 39%

LPN/LVNs

e. OTCs without decision support tools: 11%
f. OTCs with decision support tools: 35%
g. Renew existing prescriptions according to decision support tools: 32%
h. Recommend legend drugs according to decision support tools: 23%

Table 1.
BON Responses Regarding Recommendation of OTC and Legend (Prescription) Medications

	1999	2001	2005	2008	2012
RN					
OTC (w/o protocol)	16%	31%	30%	23%	35%
OTC (with protocol)	64%	82%	79%	77%	82%
Refill prescriptions	--	--	64%	47%	51%
Recommend legend	52%	54%	50%	30%	39%
LPN/LVN					
OTC (w/o protocol)		3%	11%	9%	11%
OTC (with protocol)	30%	36%	48%	40%	35%
Refill prescriptions			44%	30%	32%
Recommend legend	22%	25%	33%	21%	23%

Note: Percentages based on yes and no responses.

Figure 1.
Trends in BON Responses Regarding Recommendation of OTC and Legend (Prescription) Medications

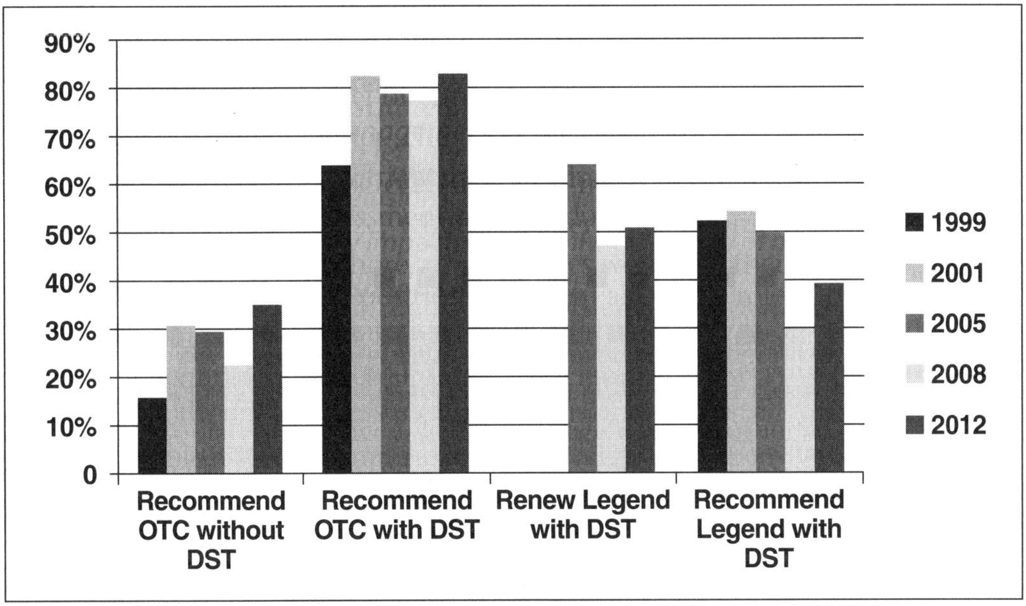

Comments by Respondents

- *Although using the term "may recommend," the context of the question seems to be about prescribing. How does one "recommend" a legend drug on the telephone without communication with the physician? Of course nurses in doctor's offices, hospitals, facilities can in fact get orders from the physician and call in prescriptions. But when you say a "medically approved decision support tool" it appears the inference is that the nurse will prescribe if the "medically approved decision support tool" allows it.*
- *(Our State) does not have an approved decision support tool at this time.*
- *(In reference to LPN renewing prescriptions) If no assessment or independent decision making is required*
- *What is meant by recommend? And by medically approved decision support tool (is that a protocol)? I would have to have the definitions of both to be able to answer this. In (Our State) neither LPNs nor RNs can prescribe although they can apply standing orders.*
- *Our statute does not address these issues specifically or the use of decision support tools.*
- *MN statute 148.171 provides that prescribing does not include recommending the use of a drug or therapeutic device which is not required by the FDA to meet the labeling requirements for prescription drugs and devices. MN Statute 148.235, Subd. 8., provides that RNs can implement a protocol that results in the prescription of a legend drug which does exclude LPNs; however Subd. 9, provides LPNs the ability to implement a protocol that results in the administration of a vaccine (a legend drug) that has been predetermined and delegated by a licensed practitioner. So, vaccines are the exception for legend drugs for LPNs in MN.*
- *We do not have any state rules related to telephone triage.*
- *There is no statutory or regulatory language that prevents a registered nurse from performing the above activities. Given the delegated role of LPNs, although there is not language about the above activities, it would be questionable whether activities including recommendation of OTC medications or renewal of prescriptions is an appropriate activity.*
- *Note: The OSBN (OR) Nurse Practice Committee is currently working on a policy for additional Board language regarding the use of Protocol/Standing Orders as they related to RN/LPN Practice which speaks to the questions above. There is currently no specific Board language addressing the above questions other than RNs and LPNs are not independent practitioners and do not have prescriptive authority.*

- *RNs and LPNs are not authorized prescribers and have no authority then to authorize the renewal or refilling of prescribed drugs in their own scope. This function would be considered delegated medical practice, a physician may choose to delegate this function as they deem appropriate with a decisioning tool, the physician is accountable for the prescription and the RN and LPN is accountable for the decision to accept the delegated task and the consequences of performing the act. No state law to my knowledge prohibits this delegation.*
- *See Texas Medical Board Rule 193.4, Scope of Standing Delegation Orders. See Texas Board of Nursing Rule 217.11 (2), Standards Specific to LVNs. See Texas NPA Sections 301.002(5) and 301.353 for directed scope of practice requirements.*
- *To renew the RN needs a detailed plan that is specific to the individual needs.*
- *What does "recommend" mean?*

3. MAY LPNs/LVNs DO TELEPHONE TRIAGE?

(percentages are based on yes and no responses although eight states didn't respond to the question)

- YES (40%)
  a. Independently with or without decision support tools: 0
  b. Independently with decision support tools: 2%
  c. Under supervision: 12%
  d. Under supervision with decision support tools: 26%
- NO (60%)
  a. It exceeds their scope of practice under any circumstances.

Comments From States Allowing Telephone Triage by LPNs/LVNs (a-d)

- *Controlled substance regulations do not allow nurses to make decisions regarding prescribing medications.*
- *Supervision does not have to be direct.*
- *They cannot deviate from the decision support tools.*
- *See Frequently Asked Question (FAQ) titled LVNs Performing Triage/Telephonic Nursing/Being On-Call for specific recommendations at http://www.bon.texas.gov/practice/faq-LVNperformingtriage.html*
- *Telephone triage may include: Symptom Assessment, Counseling, Home Treatment Advice, Referral, Information Brokering, Disease Management, Crisis Intervention. LPNs can triage in a structured setting with predictable outcomes and appropriate delegation.*

- *The Vermont Board of Nursing does not have a position on any of these nursing actions. We do have position statements on scope of practice and delegation. We have a position statement on "The Role of Licensed Practical Nurses in Triage" that states that LPNs "may collect data and ask questions that are delineated in an algorithm to assist the physician, RN, or APRN in making an assessment of a client's condition."*

Comments From States In Which Telephone Triage Exceeds LPN/LVN Scope Of Practice (e)

- *Our regulations specify the scope of assessment and practice of LPNs. Independent decision making is not in the scope of practice of LPNs. Their education does not include making this sort of decision. (AL)*
- *LPN/LVNs are not able to assess under District of Columbia Law, they are able to collect data; however, protocol-based decisions about urgency and patient management exceeds their scope of practice.*
- *The following statement specifically indicates this as a RN function. Telephonic Case Management – Advisory Opinion The South Dakota Board of Nursing affirms that out-of-state nurses who provide telephonic case management services to the citizens of South Dakota must be licensed in this state as registered nurses…*
- *No statement. Washington Administrative Code (rule) WAC 246-840-705 http://apps.leg.wa.gov/WAC/default.aspx?cite=246-840-705 (2) Licensed Practical Nurses: A routine nursing situation is one that is relatively free of complexity, and the clinical and behavioral state of the client is relatively stable, requires care based upon a comparatively fixed and limited body of knowledge. In complex nursing care situations the licensed practical nurse functions as an assistant to the registered nurse and facilitates client care by carrying out selected aspects of the designated nursing regimen to assist the registered nurse in the performance of nursing care.*

4. LPNs/LVNs MAY PARTICIPATE IN OTHER FORMS OF TELEPHONE NURSING

a. **Call patients to report lab results, convey messages from the doctor, or other collaborative phone activities: 85%**

Comments

- *As long as no independent decision making is required such as in the case of a patient asking questions.*
- *Only at the direction of the physician for the specific patient*
- *The range of participation in any listed activity is so broad that I hesitate to*

indicate that they are authorized in any area for fear that such authorization may be taken as a blanket approval of all activities within the categories. For example, an LPN can call to collaborate in following up lab work (i.e., everything was fine, no follow up necessary, or Dr. asked me to call you to make appt for follow up to discuss your lab results) vs. Dr. asked me to inform you that your Hep C results were positive and we need to make a follow up appointment. The latter communication would not be permissible.

- *When directed by Registered Nurse, physician or dentist.*
- *(Our State) Board of Nursing has not taken a position on (these actions), but, based on discussion at our Practice Committee, these patient calls do not seem to involve nursing practice, judgment, or decision-making, so would not be problematic for an LPN to do.*

b. **Disease management (e.g., monitoring diabetes, Coumadin, or CHF): 35%**

Comments

- *RN scope of practice for monitoring diseases by phone. Health education is a RN scope of practice.*
- *The LPN would need to have specific protocols for disease management and could not deviate from these protocols. If the situation falls outside of the protocols, the LPN would need to refer the situation to the RN or other higher level provider.*

c. **Behavioral modification (e.g., smoking cessation, weight reduction): 41%**

Comments

- *May do follow-up on education programs.*
- *The LPN could provide client teaching according to an established teaching plan developed by an RN and could not deviate from this plan. If the client's situation does not fit the established teaching plan, the LPN would need to refer the situation to an RN.*

General Comments

- *All of this has to be under the direction of a physician licensed to practice medicine in (Our State) or an RN licensed nurse.*
- *Data gathering is allowed; cannot report more that what physician has scripted for response.*

- *Under indirect supervision*
- *The LPN may participate in aspects of the above activities, based on their education preparation and ability to demonstrate competence with a given skill. However, the role of the RN, within a nursing context, is responsible for assessing, diagnosing, planning care, implementing and evaluating patient care outcome.*
- *Regarding behavioral modification*

5. **WE DO HAVE A WRITTEN POLICY, POSITION PAPER, FAQ, OR OTHER DOCUMENT THAT SPEAKS SPECIFICALLY TO THE ROLE OF THE LPN/LVN IN TELEPHONE TRIAGE OR OTHER TELEHEALTH NURSING PRACTICE:** (9 states)

- **AL – Administrative Code**
  - *Chapter 610-X-6, Standards of Nursing Practice www.abn.alabama.gov, click on "Laws" at the top and then Administrative Code and then Chapter 6*
- **IA – FAQ**
  - *FAQ: Can a LPN perform patient assessment? http://www.state.ia.us/nursing/faq/practice.html#l1*
  - *FAQ: Can a LPN triage? http://www.state.ia.us/nursing/faq/practice.html#l2*
- **MA – Regulations**
  - *Regulations at 244 CMR 9.02 Practice of Nursing and 9.03 (4) http://www.mass.gov/eohhs/docs/dph/regs/244cmr009.pdf*
- **MD – LPN Standards of Practice**
  - *The LPN Standards of Practice COMAR 10.27.10 effective 252011 prohibit the LPN from performing any triage activities*
- **MN – FAQ**
  - *Telephone Nursing*
- **MS – Telephonic Case Referrals & Management**
  - *94. Is telephonic case referrals and telephonic case management within the scope of practice of the LPN? Telephonic case referrals and case management (on-site and telephonic) are not within the scope of practice of the licensed practice nurse in Mississippi. They are within the scope of practice of the registered nurse.*

- NH – FAQ
  - *Telehealth Nursing: Can LPNs perform telephone triage?*
- TX – FAQ
  - *See Frequently Asked Question (FAQ) titled "LVNs Performing Triage/Telephonic Nursing/Being On-Call" for specific recommendations at http://www.bon.texas.gov/practice/faq-LVNperformingtriage.html*
- VT – Position Statement
  - *"The Role of Licensed Practical Nurses in Triage Position Statement"*

Figure 2.
Refers to Questions 5 & 6
Percent of States with Policy or Other Documents Regarding LPN/LVN Roles or Telephone Triage/Telehealth Nursing

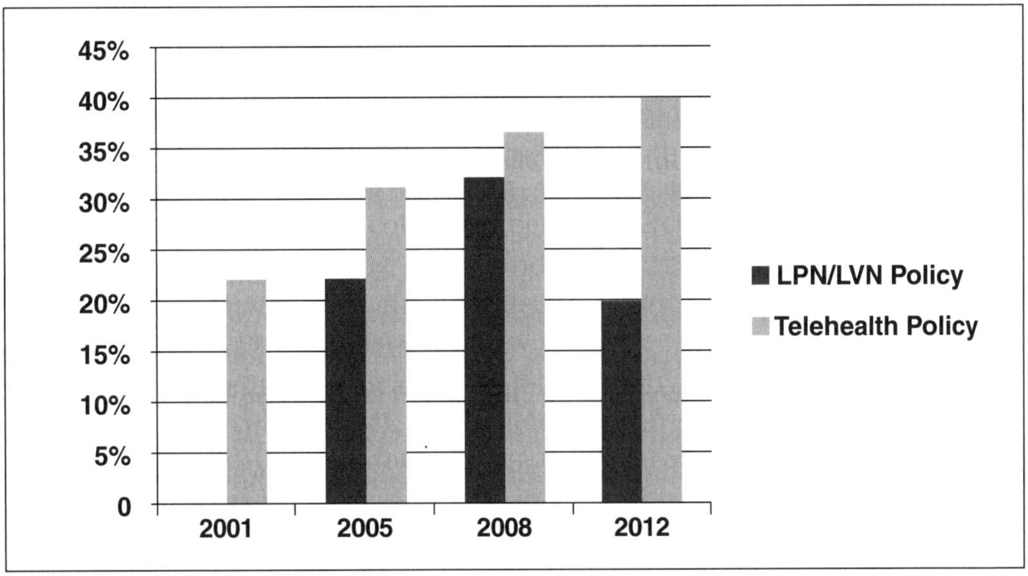

6. **MY STATE HAS A WRITTEN POLICY, POSITION PAPER, FAQ, OR OTHER DOCUMENT(S) THAT SPECIFICALLY ADDRESS TELEPHONE TRIAGE OR TELEHEALTH NURSING PRACTICE:** (18 states)

- **AL – Policy re Licensure**
  - *(4) Telephonic or electronic services used to communicate with patients and provide direction regarding nursing and medical care require an active license to practice nursing in Alabama. 610-X-4 Licensure*
- **AR – Position Statement**
  - *http://www.arsbn.arkansas.gov/lawsRules/Documents/00_2.pdf*
- **CA – Telehealth Law**
  - *California has a law, refers to what licensed individual can perform medical advice services*
  - *Statute for telephone medical advice services (statutes of 1999, Chapter 535)*
- **CO – Telenursing Policy**
  - *Nursing Board Policy POLICY NUMBER: 30-09 Title: Telenursing Date Issued: August 26, 2009 Date(s) Reviewed: References: Purpose: To define telenursing as within the scope of nursing practice in the State of Colorado POLICY: Telenursing is the practice of nursing using telecommunications technology which may cross state lines. Telenursing includes, but is not limited to, electronically receiving and sending patient's health status data; initiating and transmitting therapeutic interventions and regimens; and monitoring and recording the patient's response and nursing care outcomes. Engaging in any of the activities defined as the practice of professional or practical nursing in section 12-38-103, C.R.S., via telecommunications technology constitutes the practice of nursing in the State of Colorado. An individual engaging in such activities must be licensed to practice nursing in Colorado or be authorized to practice nursing in Colorado pursuant to the Nurse Licensure Compact, sections 24-60-3201 and -3202, C.R.S. Nursing practice occurs at the location of the recipient of nursing services. Regardless of the physical location of the individual providing the service, any one who provides any of the services listed above to a resident of the State of Colorado via telecommunications technology is engaged in the practice of nursing in Colorado. A person engaged in telenursing who is not licensed or authorized to practice nursing in the State of Colorado is subject to both administrative and criminal penalties. This policy is in accord with the positions of the American*

Nurses Association, the Association of Telehealth Service Providers, the Case Management Society of America, and the National Council of State Boards of Nursing.

- **GA – Telephonic Policy**
  - *Please visit the Board's website at www.sos.ga.gov/plb/rn, click on "Laws, Policies and Rules" and view the policy for telephonic nursing.*
- **HI – Definition**
  - *HRS §457-2 defines "Telehealth" as "the use of electronic information and telecommunication technologies to support long distance clinical health care, patient and professional health-related education, public health and health administration, to the extent that it relates to nursing."*
- **IA – Q&A re Telenursing**
  - *Provision of Nursing Services by Telecommunications/Electronic Means http://nursing.iowa.gov/nursing_practice/provision.html Nursing Practice: Nurse Licensure Compact http://www.state.ia.us/nursing/images/pdf/NLC_fact_sheet_dec_01.pdf*
- **KY (unspecified)**
- **LA – Declaratory Statement**
  - *A Declaratory Statement specific to PMHNPs in a school system was approved in Feb and will be available on our website after being published in the next issue of The Examiner in the Spring (of 2012).*
- **MA – Nursing Regulation**
  - *Regulations at 244 CMR 9.02 Practice of Nursing and 9.03 (4) http://www.mass.gov/eohhs/docs/dph/regs/244cmr009.pdf*
- **MN – FAQ**
  - *Telenursing Across State Borders*
  - *Telephone Nursing*
- **MS – Position Statement**
  - *Triage is considered a comprehensive assessment. The LPN can only perform focused assessments. Triage would be considered a patient presenting with new onset of signs and symptoms. We have just incorporated the term focused assessment into our Administrative Code and will be releasing a position statement about the role of the LPN in assessments before the end of March (or 2012). It will be available at www.msbn.state.ms.us, Position Statements*

- **NH – FAQ**
  - *FAQ Telehealth Nursing*
- **OK – FAQ re Licensure**
  - *Frequently Asked Practice Question # 5; accessible at www.ok.gov/nursing/practicefaq.pdf*
- **SD – Advisory Opinion**
  - *Telephonic Case Management*
- **TX – FAQ**
  - *See FAQ titled BON Rules and Regulations Related to Telenursing/ Telehealth at http://www.bon.texas.gov/practice/faq-telephonicnursing.html*
- **VT – Position Statement**
  - *"Licensing Requirements of Nurses Performing Telephone Triage Position Statement"*
- **WA – Interpretive Statement**

7. MY STATE HAS WRITTEN POLICIES/RULES THAT WOULD RESTRICT THE PRACTICE OF MEDICAL ASSISTANTS IN TELEPHONE TRIAGE

YES: 20% (10 states)

NO: 65%

NO RESPONSE: 15%

- **CA – Medical Board FAQ**
  - *"ARE MEDICAL ASSISTANTS ALLOWED TO PERFORM TELEPHONE TRIAGE?" "No. Medical assistants are not allowed to independently perform telephone triage as they are not legally authorized to interpret data or diagnose symptoms."*
- **CT – Delegation Rules**
- **IA – Delegation Rules**
- **KS – Statute Prohibiting Practice of Medicine/Nursing by Non-licensed Persons**
- **MS – (Unspecified)**
- **NE – Delegation Rules**

- **NH – Delegation Toolkit on Web Site**
- **ND – Rules and Regulations re Delegation**
- **SD – Statute: MA under regulation of BON and BOM**
- UT – *"In the Medical Practice Act (58-67) a medical assistant is required to practice under the direct and immediate supervision of a doctor. Telephone triage would not fit within this definition."* (2008 response, not included in 2012 data)
- **WV – Delegation Model**

8. LICENSURE REQUIREMENTS FOR INTERSTATE PRACTICE

a. For permanent residents:
   98% (44/45) Excluding NH
   Unknown DE, DC, NJ, PA, SC, WI

b. For "snowbirds"
   80% (36/45) require licensure in their state
   Excluding AL, AZ,CA, IA, NV, NH, ND, SD, WY
   Unknown DE, DC, NJ, PA, SC, WI

c. For vacationers/business travelers
   60% (27/45) require licensure in their state

d. Existing relationship in doctor's office
   71% (32/45) still require licensure in their state

e. Would the rules be different with established relationship?
   Five said "yes" (AL, CT, HI, NC, VT)

Comments

- **AZ:** *re Snowbirds and Temporary Residents: ARS 32-1631 (4) Acts and persons not affected by chapter (licensing and certification) states: The practice of nursing in this state by any legally qualified nurse of another state whose engagement requires the nurse to accompany and care for a patient temporarily residing in this state during one such engagement not to exceed six months, if the nurse does not claim to be a nurse licensed to practice in this state.* (response indicated that this might apply to telehealth nursing)
- **AR:** *If the patient is physically located in the State of AR at the time nursing care is provided, the nurse must be licensed to practice in AR. Compact licensure is considered licensed to practice in AR.*

- **CO:** *12-381 125 (d) Exclusion of resident of from another state being accompanied on a visit to CO by a nurse licensed in that same state does not apply to any of these scenarios.*
- **FL:** *Chapter 464.022 Exceptions (12), Florida Statutes, 2011: The practice of nursing by any legally qualified nurse of another state whose employment requires the nurse to accompany and care for a patient temporarily residing in the state for not more than 30 consecutive days, provided the patient is not in an inpatient setting, the board is notified prior to arrival of the patient and nurse, the nurse has the standing physician orders and current medical status of the patient available, and prearrangements with the appropriate licensed healthcare providers in this state have been made in case the patient needs placement in an inpatient setting.* (responses indicated that this does not apply to telehealth nursing)
- **GA RN & LPN:** *Please visit the Board's website at www.sos.ga.gov/plb/rn, click on "Laws, Policies and Rules" and view the policy for telephonic nursing*
- **ID:** *The nurse most hold a license or the privilege to practice in Idaho if the nursing care is occurring in Idaho.*
- **IA:** *Response is unclear regarding temporary residents. Nurses may provide care in state to transient individuals http://www.legis.iowa.gov/DOCS/ACO/IAC/LINC/12-14-2011.Rule.655.3.2.pdf 655.3.2(2b)*
- **KS:** *Kansas law does not recognize Compact licenses.*
- **LA RN:** *There are no exceptions to requirements of an RN to be licensed in LA who provides care to clients in LA regarding the issues in this question. The practice of nursing is regulated regardless of the "citizenry status" of the person receiving care from an RN. We are not a member of the Compact so do not recognize other licensures except regarding military facilities.*
- **LA LPN:** *Point of care has not been defined. These questions have not been answered by our board.*
- **MA:** *A nurse who is not licensed in MA can not practice nursing as defined at Massachusetts General Laws (MGL) Chapter 112, section 80B ("nursing practice involves clinical decision making leading to the development and implementation of a strategy of care to accomplish defined goals, the administration of medication, therapeutics and treatments prescribed"). The activities of data gathering (intake of clinical information in order to make a determination for admittance to a program where care will be delivered in another jurisdiction) and would not involve any direct clinical decision making leading to the development and implementation of a strategy of care to accomplish*

defined goals, the administration of medication, therapeutics or treatments. So the information can be gathered in MA by a nurse not licensed in MA; the nurse not licensed in MA may not practice nursing in MA. A nonresident, licensed to practice professional nursing in another jurisdiction, may attend upon a nonresident of the commonwealth that they accompany temporarily abiding here. (responses were ambiguous regarding whether this applied to telehealth nursing)

- **ME:** *The out of state nurse providing telephonic triage nursing to the temporary vacationer or business traveler would not need a license in Maine if he/she: 1. Resides and holds a Compact license in another Compact state, or 2. Meets the exception in the law that provides for a currently licensed nurse of another United States jurisdiction or foreign country to provide educational programs or consultative services within the State not to exceed 21 days per year.*
- **MI:** *Anyone who is treating a Michigan patient would be expected to hold a license in Michigan. We do have exemptions from that requirement for health professionals that live in bordering states.*
- **MN:** *A nurse must have a license in MN to speak to a patient in MN about their care. It is not based on residency but where the patient is at the time of the call. If the patient is in MN at the time, the nurse speaking to a patient in MN must have a MN license. We are not a Compact state.*
- **MT:** *If a nurse is providing nursing care to a person in our state – a license is needed. We do have an exemption for 6 months if an out-of-state nurse is providing to a person temporarily residing in the state.* (responses indicated that this does not pertain to telehealth nursing)
- **NH:** *Nurses providing advice via telephone and physically present in NH must be licensed in the state of NH or have been issued a multistate license from another Compact state. Additional information that the nurse should provide to the patient is their name, licensure status and physical location. Nurses calling NH residents from another state for purposes of telehealth must tell the NH resident their licensure status in the other state. A NH license is not required as long as the nurse has a license in the state they are calling from or hold a multi state license.*
- **NJ:** *There is no language in the statutes or regulations addressing this issue.*
- **NY:** *If a permanent resident then the nexus to the adjacent state is deemed a nullity. A relationship should be established with an instate licensed medical provider including a nurse. A temporary resident (e.g., on vacation) would be permitted to consult with the adjacent state nurse who, in fact, is the primary*

provider of medical services to the patient.

- **NC:** *The rules would be different if the nurse were in a doctor's office with an established relationship with the patient rather than in a call center.*
- **OH:** *A nurse providing nursing care to a patient located in Ohio, is engaging in nursing practice in Ohio and would require an Ohio license unless conditions meet exemption criteria contained in Section 4723.32 Ohio Revised Code.*
- **OK:** *Exceptions to application of Act in statute: 59 O.S. Section 567.11.2 The OK Nursing Practice Act shall not be construed to affect or apply to: Any nurse who has an active, unencumbered license in another state or territory who is physically present in this state on a nonroutine, nonregular basis for a period not to exceed seven (7) consecutive days in any given year.* (responses indicated that this does not apply to telehealth nursing)
- **OR:** *Our rules are such that if the patient is in Oregon and the care is provided here in Oregon the nurse needs to be licensed in Oregon to provide nursing care to that patient. We do have a policy for transport teams that cross borders and provide care in Oregon enroute to an Oregon facility but it is specific to that type of nursing care.*
- **SD:** *Telephonic Case Management – Advisory Opinion. The South Dakota Board of Nursing affirms that out-of-state nurses who provide telephonic case management services to the citizens of South Dakota must be licensed in this state as registered nurses. This opinion was rendered by the Board of Nursing upon submission of a written request. Although advisory opinions are not judicially reviewable and do not carry the force and effect of law, they do serve as a guideline to nurses who wish to engage in safe nursing practices. This advisory opinion was adopted by the South Dakota Board of Nursing, November 1994.*
- **VT:** *See the Vermont Board of Nursing position statement "Licensing Requirements of Nurses Performing Telephone Triage." Triage nurses providing care for clients living in Vermont must be licensed in Vermont except when the nurse in another state is following up on care provided in the other state. The rules would be different if the nurse were in a doctor's office with an established relationship with the patient rather than in a call center.*
- **WV RN:** *It depends on the nature of the call and the request of the patient/caller.*
- **CBME Northern Mariana Islands:** *If there is a malpractice suit due to phone triage gone wrong who provides oversight and representation? We currently have no standardized regulations in this arena.*

Figure 3.
Trends in Disciplinary Action Regarding Telephone Nursing Practice Reported by BONs

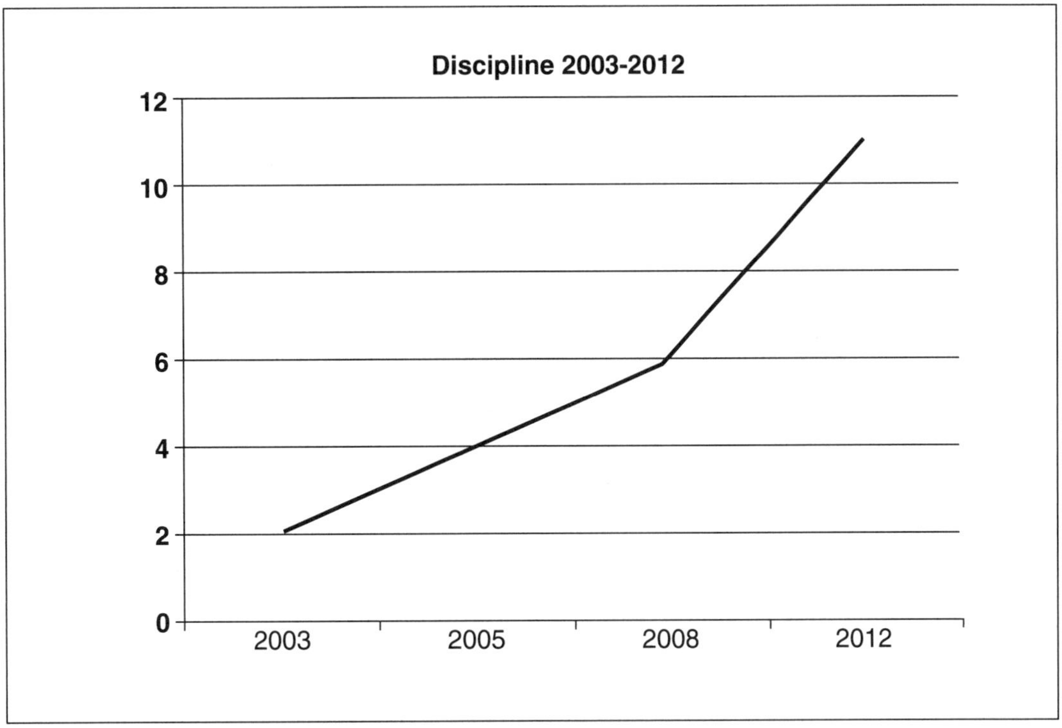

9. TO YOUR KNOWLEDGE, HAS LEGAL OR DISCIPLINARY ACTION BEEN TAKEN AGAINST NURSES RE TELEPHONE NURSING PRACTICE IN YOUR STATE? (Yes=11)

Comments

- AL: *We require self-disclosure of criminal history and substance abuse history. We've had telephone triage nurses who reported a history of substance abuse to us but not their primary state. We now require those interested in the alternative program to notify each board of nursing if they have a criminal history or substance abuse history. We've disciplined nurses for practicing in this state via telephone case management without an Alabama license.*
- CA: *The complaint had more to do with the company and the cases were referred to Telephone Medical Advice Services Bureau an agency within Department of Consumer Affairs, TMAS.*

- **CO:** *Substandard practice: I am not able to share anecdotal information.* (reported in 2008 survey)
- **GA:** *Only for unlicensed practice*
- **KS:** *...this Board has processed cases of nurses who practiced without an active license by practicing telenursing on patient's in Kansas.* (reported in 2008 survey)
- **MD:** *I do not know as Board staff may not be present for discipline cases.*
- **MN:** *Corrective actions in a few cases* (See case study below)
- **NV:** *Due to lack of Nevada licensure*

Case Study (MN): *The Board issued an Agreement for Corrective Action to the RN supervisor of a clinic for...*

- *...allowing an LPN/LVN to train, supervise, counsel, discipline, and evaluate clinic staff, including RNs, LPNs, and medical assistants (and) permitting LPN/LVNs and MAs to perform telephone triage nursing.*
  - *The LPN/LVNs and MAs triaged patient telephone calls utilizing condition-specific protocols which included independent assessments, advisements, and education to patients.*
  - *The LPN/LVN and MA triage staff did not consult with an RN regarding patient care concerns and contacted the on-call physician only if requested or if the patient condition fell outside the parameters of a protocol.*
- *The RN was unable to articulate an understanding of the scopes of practice of RN and LPN/LVN and the functions appropriately delegated to MAs. The RN also was unable to articulate an understanding a licensed health professional's legal responsibility to report unauthorized nursing practice.*
  - *The RN must differentiate between RN and LPN/LVN scopes of practice, discuss how to recognize when she and other staff are being asked to practice in an unauthorized manner, articulate her understanding of recognizing and reporting violations, and accurately define appropriate supervision of LPN/LVNs and unlicensed assistive personnel.*
- *One of the LPNs [was found to be] practicing outside the LPN scope of practice due to the telephone nursing activities she was performing. The LPN was advising and counseling patients via telephone without any documented guidelines/protocols.*

- *The Board determined the activities she was performing were RN level practice.*

- *Another LPN… was [found to be] practicing outside the LPN scope of practice while working as medical support supervisor, hiring, supervising, training, counseling, discipline, and evaluating clinic and telephone triage staff, including RNs, LPNs, and MAs.*

    - *If a nurse does not have license in Nevada, and has not applied for a license here, then the Board could issue a Citation in the amount of $500.00 for the first offense, $1000.00 for the second, and $1500.00 for each additional offense. See NRS 632.495 at http://www.leg.state.nv.us/NRS/NRS-632.html (2008)*
    - *If the nurse had applied for licensure and been found to have practiced without an active license they may be issued an administrative fine by the Board. (2008)*

- **OK:** *The OK Board of Nursing does not categorize discipline to this specific situation. Nurses have been disciplined for practicing nursing in OK without an OK nursing license.*

- **TN:** *Applies to cases when a nurse called in prescriptions for family members/friends who were not patients of the independent practitioner.*

10. IF YOU ARE NOT A COMPACT STATE, DO YOU ANTICIPATE YOUR STATE TAKING ACTIONS ON THIS PROPOSED LEGISLATION?

- **I do not anticipate our state taking action on the compact in the foreseeable future.**
    - 20 States + DC

General Comments

- *"Good topic – do get practice questions related especially to refills of medications and making those decisions without direct consultation from the prescriber – using protocols"*

- *"Very thought provoking."*

Author's note: This survey is the sixth in a series of surveys beginning in 1999. When updated information is obtained, it will be housed on our web site at www.telephone-triage.com

Appendix B

Telephone Triage Policy Manual Outline

Telephone Triage is a growing practice area in nursing and is a service that is being offered in an increasing number of clinical settings. Unfortunately, however, in spite of its complexity and the acknowledged high risk associated with this practice, many settings continue to offer care by telephone without the benefit of formal, well-developed policies to guide that practice. This appendix includes a sample Table of Contents for a policy manual for telephone triage.[1]

1. *OVERVIEW*
- 1.1. DEFINITION
- 1.2. DESCRIPTION
- 1.3. PURPOSE / OBJECTIVES
- 1.4. STANDARDS
  - 1.4.1. Professional Standards
  - 1.4.2. Accreditation Standards
  - 1.4.3. The Joint Commission
  - 1.4.4. (STATE) Department of Health
  - 1.4.5. Other

2. *STRUCTURE AND ORGANIZATION*
- 2.1. OVERSIGHT AND DIRECTION
  - 2.1.1. Telephone Triage Steering Committee:
  - 2.1.2. Administration
  - 2.1.3. Nursing
  - 2.1.4. Medical
- 2.2. ROLES AND RESPONSIBILITES
  - 2.2.1. Telephone Triage Steering Committee:
  - 2.2.2. Administration
  - 2.2.3. Medical
  - 2.2.4. Nursing
    - 2.2.4.1. Telephone Triage Nurse
      - 2.2.4.1.1. RN accountability and authority
      - 2.2.4.1.2. Role of the LPN
      - 2.2.4.1.3. Role of Unlicensed Assistive Personnel (UAP)

- 2.2.4.2. Selection/Qualifications of Telephone Triage Nurses
- 2.2.4.3. Competence and Continuing Education
- 2.2.4.4. Scope of Practice for Licensed Staff
  - 2.2.4.4.1. Recommendation of Medications
    - 2.2.4.4.1.1. Over-The-Counter Drugs
    - 2.2.4.4.1.2. Prescription / Legend Drugs
    - 2.2.4.4.1.3. Medication Refills
- 2.2.5. Chain of Command for Clinical Disputes

3. CARE DELIVERY MODEL

- 3.1. USE OF NURSING PROCESS
  - 3.1.1. Assessment
  - 3.1.2. Diagnosis
  - 3.1.3. Planning
  - 3.1.4. Intervention
    - 3.1.4.1. Continuity of Care / Referrals
  - 3.1.5. Evaluation
    - 3.1.5.1. Follow-up Calls
      - 3.1.5.1.1. By Disposition
      - 3.2.4.1.2. By Demographics
      - 3.2.4.1.3. By Clinical Concern
      - 3.2.4.1.4. By Nursing Judgment
- 3.2. DECISION SUPPORT TOOLS (PROTOCOLS / GUIDELINES)
  - 3.2.1. Selection, Approval, Routine Review
  - 3.2.2. Use
  - 3.2.3. Deviation
- 3.3. TRIAGE CATEGORIES
  - 3.3.1. Emergent / Immediate
  - 3.3.2. Urgent / 24 Hour
  - 3.3.3. Non-urgent / Routine

4. OPERATIONAL CONSIDERATIONS

- 4.1. STAFFING MODEL
  - 4.1.1. Location
  - 4.1.2. Interface with Primary Care Providers and Primary Care Nurses
- 4.2. CALL INTAKE AND FLOW (see model)
  - 4.2.1. Clerk
    - 4.2.1.1. Recognition of Obvious Emergencies
    - 4.2.1.2. Call Answering and Message Taking
      - 4.2.1.2.1 Hot Lists, High Risk Complaints
    - 4.2.1.3. Routing of Calls to Nurse
  - 4.2.2. Answering Service
  - 4.2.3. Electronic Routing
    - 4.2.3.1. Electronic Menu and Call Routing
    - 4.2.3.2. Voice Mail
    - 4.2.3.3. Management of Misrouted Calls
    - 4.2.3.4. Coverage for High Peak Call Volume

- 4.3. OUTBOUND CALLS
  - 4.3.1. Return Calls
    - 4.3.1.1. Timeframe for Call Return
    - 4.3.1.2. Inability to Reach Caller
  - 4.3.2. Follow-up Calls
- 4.4. TEMPLATE MANAGEMENT / BUSINESS RULES
  - 4.4.1. Acute:Wellness/Routine Appointment Ratio
  - 4.4.2. Hours of Operation
  - 4.4.3. Availability of Provider Staff for Today Appointments
- 4.5. SCHEDULING PATIENTS
  - 4.5.1. Nurse Authority to Schedule
  - 4.5.2. Management of Patients With No Available Appointment
  - 4.5.3. Retriaging of Patients
- 4.6. DOCUMENTATION / MEDICAL RECORD DISPOSITION
  - 4.6.1. Medical Record
    - 4.6.1.1. Medical Record Routing
    - 4.6.1.2. Medical Record Maintenance
      - 4.6.1.2.1. Maintenance of Records of Non-Enrolled Patients
    - 4.6.1.3. Review by Provider
  - 4.6.2. Log

- 4.7. SPECIAL CIRCUMSTANCES / RISK MANAGEMENT
  - 4.7.1. Patients Refusing Care
  - 4.7.2. Frequent Caller
  - 4.7.3. Patients Calling More Than Once in 8 Hours
  - 4.7.4. Difficult Callers
    - 4.7.4.1. Suspected Drug Seekers
    - 4.7.4.2. Angry / Aggressive / Abusive Callers
    - 4.7.4.3. Threats of Violence
    - 4.7.4.4. Suspected Domestic Violence
    - 4.7.4.5. Suicidal / Homicidal Patients
    - 4.7.4.6. Anonymous Callers
    - 4.7.4.7. Non Enrolled Patient Callers
  - 4.7.5. Unable to Reach Caller
  - 4.7.6. Telephone Management of Minors

5. ETHICS AND PATIENT RIGHTS

- 5.1. CUSTOMER RELATIONS
- 5.2. CONFIDENTIALITY
- 5.3. NON-PATIENT CALLERS
- 5.4. AUDITORY AND VISUAL PRIVACY
- 5.5. PROVISION OF CULTURALLY SENSITIVE CARE
- 5.6. NON-ENGLISH SPEAKING CALLERS
- 5.7. HEARING IMPAIRED CALLERS

6. ***QUALITY MANAGEMENT***
   - 6.1. DATA COLLECTION
     - 6.1.1. Call Volume
     - 6.1.2. Call Duration
     - 6.1.3. Most Common Chief Complaints
     - 6.1.4. Disposition
       - 6.1.4.1. Disposition by Original Inclination
   - 6.2. QUALITY ASSURANCE (high risk, high volume)
     - 6.2.1. Mechanism (include peer review)
     - 6.2.2. Reporting (by whom, to whom, when)
   - 6.3. QUALITY IMPROVEMENT
     - 6.3.1. Patient Satisfaction
     - 6.3.2. Staff Satisfaction
     - 6.3.3. Focus Groups
     - 6.3.4. Use of QA Findings
   - 6.4. RISK MANAGEMENT

7. ***RESOURCES***

8. ***POLICY ADDENDA***
   - 2.0.a Program Design
   - 2.0.b Organizational Chart
     - 2.2.5.a Chain of Command: Mediation of Clinical Disputes Between Triage Nurse and Provider
   - 3.1.a Telephone Triage Nurse Staffing Criteria
     - 3.2.1.a Routine Review of Decision Support Tools (Protocols)
     - 3.3.1.a Activation of EMS
       - 3.3.2.1 Management of After Hours Calls
   - 4.2.a Routing of Incoming Calls
       - 4.2.3.1.a Incoming Call Routing Menu
     - 4.5.2.a Flow Chart for Scheduling Patients When All Appointment Slots Have Been Exhausted.
     - 4.6.1.a Telephone Triage Encounter Form
     - 4.6.2.a Use of the Telephone Triage Log
     - 4.7.1.a Care of Patients Unable to Act in Their Own Best Interest
       - 4.7.4.5.a Tracing Suicide Calls
   - 6.3.a Quality Improvement Plan

9. ***COMPETENCY EVALUATION***
   - 9.1. AVOIDS COMMON ERRORS OF PRACTICE
   - 9.2. TECHNICAL SKILLS
   - 9.3. EXPERTISE & KNOWLEDGE
   - 9.4. INTERPERSONAL / COMMUNICATION SKILLS
   - 9.5. PROFESSIONAL BEHAVIORS
   - 9.6. PERSONAL CHARACTERISTICS

Reference

1. Rutenberg, C. (2009). *Customizable telephone triage policy book/how-to manual on CD*. Little Rock, AR: Telephone Triage Consulting, Inc.

INDEX

Legend
t = table
f = figure

L

M

Q

R

S

T

U

V

W

Y

The Art and Science of Telephone Triage

How to Practice Nursing Over the Phone

Carol Rutenberg, RN-BC, C-TNP, MNSc
M. Elizabeth Greenberg, RN-BC, C-TNP, PhD

A Brief Description

This book offers a comprehensive look at the growing practice of telephone triage nursing. Despite the prevalence of the practice, little education and few resources are available for nurses interested in this form of practice. The authors address the history of telephone triage, the role of telephone triage nursing in health care, theories supporting the practice, quality and risk management principles, program design, and a comprehensive look at clinical practice. Practical tips and real-life examples will illustrate and support the content.

ISBN: 978-0-9655310-4-7

Telephone Triage Consulting, Inc.
118 Clover Ridge Court
Hot Springs, AR 71913
501-767-4564; FAX 501-767-1134; E-mail: carol@telephone-triage.com; www.telephone-triage.com

Published for Telephone Triage Consulting, Inc. by
Anthony J. Jannetti, Inc., East Holly Avenue, Box 56, Pitman, NJ 08071-0056
856-256-2300; FAX 856-589-7463; www.ajj.com

DISCLAIMER

The authors and publishers of this book have made serious efforts to ensure that treatments, practices, and procedures are accurate and conform to standards accepted at the time of publication. Due to constant changes in information resulting from continuing research and clinical experience, reasonable differences in opinions among authorities, unique aspects of individual clinical situations, and the possibility of human error in preparing such a publication require that the reader exercise individual judgment when making a clinical decision, and if necessary, consult and compare information from other authorities, professionals, or sources.

Endorsed by the American Academy of Ambulatory Care Nursing

aacn American Academy of Ambulatory Care Nursing

Many settings. Multiple roles. One unifying specialty.